The GLMA Handbook on
LGBT Health

The GLMA Handbook on LGBT Health

Volume 2: Health Matters and Global Challenges

Jason S. Schneider, MD,
Vincent M. B. Silenzio, MD, MPH, and
Laura Erickson-Schroth, MD, MA, Editors

Foreword by Hector Vargas, JD

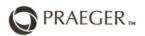

PRAEGER™

An Imprint of ABC-CLIO, LLC

Santa Barbara, California • Denver, Colorado

Library of Congress Cataloging-in-Publication Data

Names: Schneider, Jason S., editor. | Silenzio, Vincent M. B., editor. | Erickson-Schroth, Laura, editor.
Title: The GLMA handbook on LGBT health / Jason S. Schneider, Vincent M.B. Silenzio, and Laura Erickson-Schroth, editors ; foreword by Hector Vargas.
Other titles: Gay and Lesbian Medical Association handbook on LGBT health | Handbook on LGBT health
Description: Santa Barbara, California : ABC-CLIO, [2019] | Includes bibliographical references and index.
Identifiers: LCCN 2018043350 (print) | LCCN 2018044309 (ebook) | ISBN 9780313395666 (eBook) | ISBN 9780313395659 (set : alk. paper) | ISBN 9781440846847 (volume 1 : alk. paper) | ISBN 9781440846854 (volume 2 : alk. paper)
Subjects: | MESH: Sexual and Gender Minorities | Health Status | Health Services | Health Policy | United States
Classification: LCC RA564.9.H65 (ebook) | LCC RA564.9.H65 (print) | NLM WA 300 AA1 | DDC 362.1086/64—dc23
LC record available at https://lccn.loc.gov/2018043350

ISBN: 978-0-313-39565-9 (set)
        978-1-4408-4684-7 (vol. 1)
        978-1-4408-4685-4 (vol. 2)
        978-0-313-39566-6 (ebook)

23 22 21 20 19   2 3 4 5

This book is also available as an eBook.

Praeger
An Imprint of ABC-CLIO, LLC

ABC-CLIO, LLC
147 Castilian Drive
Santa Barbara, California 93117
www.abc-clio.com

This book is printed on acid-free paper ∞

Manufactured in the United States of America

Contents

Foreword

When I joined GLMA: Health Professionals Advancing LGBTQ Equality as its executive director in 2010 (then known as the Gay and Lesbian Medical Association), the nation was on the cusp of very profound changes in how it would view and treat lesbian, gay, bisexual, and transgender (LGBT) people. "LGBT American" became part of the common dialogue. Same-sex couples would soon have the freedom to marry in every state, and the White House was lit in rainbow colors. We witnessed heightened awareness and understanding about transgender individuals and the pervasive challenges they face.

This revolution cascaded into all aspects of LGBTQ life, and LGBT health was no exception. Leading health care institutions and associations—including the National Academy of Medicine, Joint Commission, American Medical Association, and American Academy of Nursing, just to name a few—studied and adopted policies addressing the health and well-being of LGBT individuals. Health professional students of all disciplines demanded their schools provide more opportunities to learn about LGBT health. The federal government implemented initiatives ensuring LGBT inclusion in health and human services programs and funding opportunities, research and data collection, and nondiscrimination policies.

As I write this foreword today, however, we live in a dramatically changed political environment. So much of the progress we have experienced in LGBT equality and health has been stymied, and we are seeing formidable attempts to erode the gains we have made, particularly in areas such as nondiscrimination in health care access and coverage and inclusion of LGBT people in national health surveys. Like other civil rights movements, we are encountering an almost inevitable deceleration after a period of significant advances.

Through its nearly 40-year history, GLMA has endured many such peaks and valleys, but our role has remained constant: to engage the scientific expertise of our LGBTQ health professional members—physicians, nurses, advanced practice nurses, physician assistants, behavioral health specialists, dentists, and many others—in education and policy initiatives to improve the health and well-being of LGBTQ people. From the organization's roots focusing nationally on services and policy for people dying of AIDS to our present-day efforts to help organize mainstream health professional associations in support of policies promoting the health of LGBTQ people, GLMA has been at the forefront of efforts to advance LGBT equality and health equity nationwide.

It is with this history and spirit that GLMA and its members are proud to offer this resource, *The GLMA Handbook on LGBT Health.* Written by LGBT health care providers who provide care for LGBT patients and clients on a daily basis, the *Handbook* is purposefully crafted for members of the general public, including LGBT people, to bring the full scope of LGBT health concerns and prevention and treatment options into two volumes in plain, easy-to-grasp language. The *Handbook* also examines related public policy, political and resource/funding issues, and their impact on the health of LGBT people.

The *Handbook* covers a broad range of topics important to the health of LGBT people. Volume One begins with an essential grounding in LGBT health by delving into the public policy landscape and public health and research considerations for the LGBT community. You will also find chapters dedicated to preventive health and sexual health as well as to specific populations, including elders, families, youth, and transgender individuals. The intersections of race and sexuality and LGBT health worldwide are also explored. Volume One also probes a topic on the minds of all LGBT people, and that is fundamental to ensuring our health and well-being—finding health care providers who are welcoming of LGBT people. Volume Two looks at specific diseases, conditions, and interventions, including mental health concerns, eating disorders, substance use, cancer, sexually transmitted infections, intimate partner violence, and cardiovascular health.

The *Handbook*'s exploration of the interrelated connection between LGBT health and policy is imperative to understanding the issues of equality and dignity that the LGBT community continues to face. One cannot fully understand the policy importance of ensuring transgender people have access to basic human services, including bathrooms consistent with their gender identity, without understanding the serious physical and mental health implications of denying such access. Learning about the advances in HIV prevention and treatment is key to the efforts to reform laws that criminalize the transmission of HIV, many of which were adopted in the early days of the AIDS epidemic when so little was known about the virus. The sobering statistics on bisexual people and suicide point to the urgent need for client-centered services for this overlooked and extremely marginalized population within the LGBT community (Pompili, et al., 2014).

Equipped with this knowledge, LGBT people can be empowered in their interactions with health care providers, and everyone can be an advocate for LGBT health and equality. The *Handbook* shows that you do not need a medical, nursing, or other specialized degree to be an agent for change—just a willingness to learn and a commitment to put knowledge into action.

I would like to take this opportunity to express my deep appreciation to the editors—GLMA past president Jason Schneider, past board member Laura Erickson-Schroth, and member and former coeditor of the *Journal of the Gay and Lesbian Medical Association* Vincent Silenzio—for their tireless efforts on this publication. And my sincerest thank-you to the many GLMA members and supporters who volunteered to share their expertise as contributors to the *Handbook*. Your passion and dedication to your work is an inspiration to me and the entire LGBT health community.

I would also like to take a moment to honor the memory of Judy Bradford, a pioneer in LGBT health, whom we lost in 2017. She was the original author of this foreword. Judy's spirit permeates the chapters in the *Handbook*, and there is not one subject covered here that does not owe some gratitude to Judy's impressive body of work. Her optimism and vision as an LGBT health leader laid the groundwork for all that we have accomplished and will accomplish in the years ahead.

Like so many GLMA members through the years, Judy dedicated her professional life to improving the health and well-being of the LGBT community. She envisioned a world where the health needs of the LGBT community are fully integrated into policy discussions, training and education of health care professionals, research efforts, and, of course, in provider interactions with LGBT patients and clients.

The GLMA Handbook on LGBT Health is firmly behind this vision, offering central building blocks of information that lead us there. The *Handbook* is geared to action, so whether you are a part of the LGBTQ community or an ally, I hope you will join GLMA members and all supporters of LGBT health equity to do your part to support education, training, and policies to ensure that LGBT people receive the clinically and culturally competent care we need and deserve. Our health depends on it.

Hector Vargas, JD, Executive Director
GLMA: Health Professionals Advancing LGBTQ Equality

REFERENCE

Pompili, M., Lester, D., Forte, A., Seretti, M. E., Erbuto, D., Lamis, D. A., . . . Girardi, P. (2014). Bisexuality and suicide: A systematic review of the current literature. *Journal of Sexual Medicine, 11*(8), 1903–1913. doi:10.1111/jsm.12581

Acknowledgments

The editors would like to particularly recognize the esteemed group of experts and scholars who gathered to complete this endeavor. Without the tireless dedication and patience of our contributors, the GLMA Handbook would not have come to fruition. Anna Artymowicz and Shea Nagle, both students at the University of Rochester School of Medicine and Dentistry, deserve special recognition for their heroic editorial assistance with several chapters. Finally, we owe significant thanks to Debbie Carvalko from ABC-CLIO for supporting this project throughout its extended timeline. Without her dedication and behind-the-scenes support, this publication would never have happened.

The chapters herein reflect the collective contributions of generations of health care professionals, scientists, public health researchers, advocates, and community members dedicated to the betterment of LGBTQ people everywhere. We stand on their shoulders.

For Judy

1

Mood and Anxiety Disorders

Brian Hurley, Justin A. Chen, and John B. Taylor

Mood and anxiety disorders occur relatively commonly among adults in the United States. The 12-month prevalence estimates for anxiety and mood disorders are 18.1 percent and 9.5 percent, respectively, in the general population (Kessler, Chiu, Demler, & Walters, 2005). Lesbian, gay, bisexual, and transgender (LGBT) populations are disproportionately affected by anxiety and mood disorders leading to significant morbidity from distress and functional impairment, and mortality from an increased risk of suicide (Cochran, Sullivan, & Mays, 2003; Haas et al., 2010; Remafedi et al., 1998). These disparities are often attributed to social stigma, individual prejudice, and discrimination faced by LGBT people (Balsam, Beadnell, & Molina, 2013; Fingerhut, Peplau, & Gable, 2010). Given the increased prevalence of mood and anxiety disorders, health care organizations serving LGBT patients are well advised to emphasize mental health screening, treatment, and/or referral protocols. Further, mental health treatment programs that include LGBT-oriented services enhance their capacity to reduce health disparities and optimize health care outcomes (Rutherford et al., 2012).

Mood and anxiety disorders are characterized by pathological disturbances in mood or anxiety states, with specific diagnostic symptoms and chronology defined by the American Psychiatric Association's *Diagnostic and Statistical Manual of Mental Disorders* (2013). More than 80 percent of patients with mood and anxiety disorders respond to some element of treatment, and there are a variety of psychotherapy, pharmacological, and somatic therapies that have been shown to be effective (Halbreich & Montgomery, 2013). Treatment can be offered in many settings, ranging from inpatient hospitals—typically used for high-acuity patients at significant risk to themselves and/or others—to outpatient clinics or partial hospital programs where the vast majority of patients obtain treatment. Patients, clinicians, and policy makers who understand the increased risk for mood and anxiety disorders in LGBT populations are better equipped to help alleviate suffering associated with these relatively common conditions.

MOOD DISORDERS

This chapter summarizes what is currently known about mood disorders in the LGBT community and describes the most common mood disorders, including major depression and bipolar disorder.

Mood disorders (also known as "affective disorders") are psychiatric illnesses whose core feature, as the name suggests, is a disturbance in mood. The term encompasses three broad categories—depression, bipolar disorder, and other mood disorders—each of which can be further classified into a number of more specific diagnoses.

Theories about social stress suggest that socially disadvantaged groups such as sexual minorities are at higher risk for mental disorders, chief among them problems with mood (Meyer, 2003). The resulting burden of illness can result in years lost to disability, overreliance on dangerous coping mechanisms such as substance abuse, and increased rates of self-injury and suicide.

Mood disorders are extremely common and associated with tremendous personal, medical, and societal costs. Each year, approximately 9.5 percent of American adults suffer from a mood disorder (U.S. Census Bureau, 2005; Kessler et al., 2003). Having a mood disorder increases one's risk of suicide 20-fold (Chehil & Kutcher, 2012). In addition, recent studies by the World Health Organization have shown that the most common of these, major depressive disorder (MDD), is the leading global cause of years lost due to disability, outpacing all other illnesses including heart disease, cancer, and HIV/AIDS, and it is the fourth-leading contributor to the global burden of disease (Murray & Lopez, 1997; World Health Organization, 2009). MDD is often functionally incapacitating, which contributes to reduced economic productivity and loss of personal identity as a contributing member of society. Bipolar disorder is associated with higher rates of suicide than depression, with frequent relapses due to treatment nonadherence.

Because mood disorders are so common, the terminology associated with them has become a part of common terminology and is frequently misused. All humans experience depressed mood at some point in their lives as a normal and appropriate response to psychological stress and life circumstances. However, the majority of people will not experience MDD, which (as discussed below) is a specific psychiatric syndrome character-ized by a combination of symptoms that must be present for a sufficient duration of time. Similarly, we have all encountered changes in mood in reaction to events that happened during the day or week—one might be sad that a hoped-for promotion fell through but become happy later that day because of a surprise birthday dinner. People with such fluctuations in mood states are sometimes incorrectly referred to as bipolar. However, these changes in mood alone are not necessarily sufficient to meet criteria for a psychiatric diagnosis of bipolar disorder.

Furthermore, because they are based on a person's moods and behav-iors, these disorders are by nature somewhat subjective, and the lines sepa-rating normal from abnormal can become blurry at times. Like most other psychiatric disorders, there are no blood tests or diagnostic imaging pro-cedures that can definitively diagnose a mood disorder. While many theo-ries have been proposed to explain what causes mood disorders, and it is clear that genetics play a role, there is still no definitive "cause" for these conditions. Therefore, similar to many neurologic, cardiac, pulmonary, and rheumatologic conditions, the diagnosis of a mood disorder must be made clinically by a medical or mental health professional based on the patient's self-reported symptoms in combination with as much objective evidence as possible, including supporting information from others who know the patient well.

Most mood disorders are generally thought to be chronic, recurrent conditions. Similar to other chronic illnesses such as diabetes or heart dis-ease, the development of a mood disorder is based on a variety of contrib-uting genetic and environmental factors. This model for developing an illness is called the "diathesis-stress" model and helps to explain why LGBT populations are at higher risk for developing mood disorders such as clinical depression.

Mood Disorders and LGBT Populations

According to the diathesis-stress model, a person's genes make him or her susceptible to an illness, but it is ultimately the interaction of a person's genetic makeup with their environment that causes the illness to develop. A common example of this is cancer; certain genes can predispose some-one to lung cancer, but their risk of actually developing the disease is greatly increased by smoking cigarettes. Similarly, mood disorders are thought to have an underlying biological or genetic basis that is then brought out by environmental triggers—the most important of which is stress.

Research in this area suggests that LGBT populations experience far greater levels of stress than their non-LGBT counterparts due to persecutory social attitudes ranging from chronic rejection to entrenched societal discrimination and stigma to outright bullying and emotional or physical assaults (Meyer, 2003). As a result, sexual minorities are estimated to be at greatly increased risk of developing a mood disorder, even though there is no evidence that LGBT people are genetically predisposed to these illnesses (Bailey, 1999). In other words, if an LGBT person grows up in a generally supportive environment, current research suggests that he or she is no more likely than a non-LGBT person to develop a mood disorder.

Sexual minorities are generally estimated to have an elevated risk of developing a mood or anxiety disorder as compared to the general population, and two to three times the risk of attempting suicide (Bolton & Sareen, 2011). However, research in this area has been limited by a number of problems related to study design, including how the subjects for the studies were identified and recruited, difficulty finding large-enough samples to draw statistically significant conclusions, and problematic definitions of sexual minority populations.

Although the sexologist Alfred Kinsey famously collapsed sexual orientation into a one-dimensional scale from 0 (exclusively heterosexual) to 6 (exclusively homosexual), later researchers have argued that sexual orientation can and should be measured along multiple different dimensions. In other words, asking people only about their sexual identity—"Do you consider yourself gay, bisexual, lesbian, or transgender?"—may inappropriately neglect large groups of individuals who experience nonheterosexual attractions or behaviors but nevertheless do not identify as LGBT. Additionally, the LGBT designation collapses sexual preference and gender identity under the same umbrella, though these are in fact different concepts. Despite these important limitations, researchers have continued to try to characterize rates of mental disorders among LGBT populations in order to highlight the needs of this community and to provide appropriate services.

In the largest and arguably best-designed study of its kind to date, researchers for the National Epidemiologic Survey on Alcohol and Related Conditions performed face-to-face interviews with almost 35,000 people over the age of 20 and asked all subjects about three dimensions of sexual orientation: identity, behavior, and attraction (Bostwick, 2010). These researchers found that for men, any sexual minority status (in any of the three dimensions above) conferred a higher lifetime prevalence of both mood and anxiety disorders.

For women, however, the story was more complicated. Lesbian, bisexual, or "not sure" sexual identities were associated with higher lifetime rates of most disorders, but women who reported exclusively same-sex sexual behavior and exclusively same-sex attraction actually had the lowest rates of most mood and anxiety disorders of any groups in the survey, lower even than heterosexual women. The authors interpreted this result to suggest that same-sex attraction or behavior among women may have protective mental health benefits. In contrast, bisexual behavior was associated with the highest odds of any mood disorder for both males and females.

Unfortunately, the prevalence of mood disorders in transgender populations has not been adequately researched to date, primarily due to small sample sizes.

In sum, while problems with methodology and recruitment of subjects has traditionally limited research in this area, the latest evidence confirms long-held beliefs that most LGBT populations are at greater risk for developing a lifetime mood or anxiety disorder, though this effect may differ for women. Mental health represents one of the areas of greatest health disparities between sexual minorities and the general population, and further well-designed research is needed to better understand specific gender differences in mental health outcomes.

Symptoms and Course of Depression

Depression is a generic term for a depressed mood state that can occur as a feature of several different psychiatric illnesses, the most common and well-known of which is MDD (also known as major depression, clinical depression, or unipolar depression). Although MDD is extremely common in the United States and around the world and responsive to treatment in over 80 percent of cases, it remains underrecognized and undertreated in the general population (National Institute of Mental Health, 2007). MDD affects about 6.7 percent of the U.S. adult population in any given year (Kessler et al., 2003). It has a median age of onset of 32 years and is the leading cause of disability among Americans aged 15 to 44 (World Health Organization, 2008; U.S. Census Bureau, 2005). It is more common in women than men (Kessler et al., 2003).

The diagnosis of MDD in the United States is most commonly established based on criteria outlined in the American Psychiatric Association's *Diagnostic and Statistical Manual of Mental Disorders* (DSM), which is currently in its fifth revision (DSM-5). Other countries around the world make use of an alternative system, the World Health Organization's International Statistical Classification of Disease and Health Problems (ICD). These two classification schemes are generally very similar, and for the purposes of this chapter, DSM criteria will be utilized (American Psychiatric Association, 2013).

The major hallmarks of MDD are a depressed or low mood and inability to experience pleasure, at least one of which must be present to qualify for a diagnosis of this disorder. MDD is often accompanied by physical symptoms, including loss of appetite, difficulty with sleep, and a lack of energy, and may also present with headaches, stomachaches, and digestive problems. Some depression subtypes involve increases in appetite and sleep. People with clinical depression often "ruminate," or repeatedly worry about the same thoughts, and may also exhibit feelings of helplessness, hopelessness, guilt, or even self-hatred.

In severe cases, clinically depressed individuals may exhibit psychotic symptoms such as delusions (fixed, false beliefs) or hallucinations (for example, hearing a voice that is not really there). If these psychotic symptoms only occur in the context of depressed mood, then they are likely related to major depression and not to another underlying psychotic disorder such as schizophrenia. Resolution of the depressive episode should also lead to resolution of the psychotic symptoms.

Among older adults, major depression may manifest as slowed movements ("psychomotor retardation") or as cognitive symptoms such as increased forgetfulness and memory loss. In fact, the term "pseudodementia" was coined to describe a syndrome in which older people appear to develop symptoms of dementia, but the cause is actually depression. Appropriate treatment of the underlying mood disturbance can successfully resolve the cognitive and memory symptoms.

A major depressive episode is defined by the presence of five of the following nine symptoms lasting most of the day, every day, for a period of at least two weeks, and with significant distress or impairment in function: depressed mood, loss of interest ("anhedonia"), impairment in energy and concentration, disruptions in sleep and appetite (either too much or too little of either), feelings of guilt or worthlessness, disruptions in movements (feeling either very restless and agitated or slowed and lethargic), and suicidal thoughts. Because of the nature of this diagnosis, clinical depression can look very different for different people, depending on which specific combination of symptoms each is experiencing.

MDD can be classified as mild, moderate, or severe, depending on the number of symptoms present and the extent of the impact on the person's functioning. If psychotic symptoms are present, the disorder is automatically classified as severe.

There are several subtypes of MDD, including:

- MDD with psychotic features (also known as psychotic depression)
- Catatonic depression, in which a person with MDD also exhibits symptoms of catatonia, including mutism (inability to speak) and

disturbances in motor behavior such as repetitive, purposeless movements, and sounds

- Postpartum depression, a specific type of clinical depression affecting 10 to 15 percent of women within three months of childbirth
- Seasonal affective disorder, which is diagnosed when a person has experienced at least two episodes of clinical depression during colder months, with none at other times over at least a two-year period
- Atypical depression, which is characterized by increased mood reactivity, increased appetite and sleep (opposite what is usually seen in "typical" depression), a feeling of heaviness in the limbs ("leaden paralysis"), and extreme hypersensitivity to perceived rejection by others, leading to social impairment

MDD may resolve after a single episode, or a person may have multiple episodes. If this is the case, the person likely has a diagnosis of "recurrent MDD." At least 50 percent of those who recover from a first episode of depression go on to have one or more additional episodes; and 80 percent of those with a history of two episodes eventually have another recurrence (American Psychiatric Association, 2013; Kupfer, Frank, & Wamhoff, 1996; Post, 1992).

Symptoms and Course of Bipolar

Bipolar disorder is characterized by episodes of elevated or agitated mood known as mania or hypomania (depending on the severity of the episode), often alternating with episodes of depression. Also known as bipolar affective disorder (BPAD), manic-depressive disorder, or manic depression, this disorder has a high rate of both under- and misdiagnosis, as its characteristic mood fluctuations may not be appropriately recognized by clinicians.

BPAD affects approximately 2.6 percent of adult Americans every year and has a median age of onset of 25 years (U.S. Census Bureau, 2005; Kessler et al., 2003). As with other types of mental disorders, there is strong evidence to suggest both genetic and environmental contributions to the development of bipolar disorder. Because the disorder is associated with high rates of suicidal thoughts ("suicidal ideation") and attempts, correct diagnosis and treatment are crucial.

Mania is the hallmark of BPAD and consists of a distinct period of elevated or irritable mood that either lasts at least one week or leads to hospitalization. Typical symptoms of mania include increased energy, decreased need for sleep, pressured speech, "racing thoughts," poor attention, and increased distractibility (sometimes associated with starting many projects but being unable to finish them), impaired judgment, uncharacteristic risky behavior such as gambling, shopping sprees, or sexual promiscuity, feelings of being special, "chosen," or "on a mission" and possessing special powers, increased religious thoughts, and increased substance use. Similar to major depressive disorder, bipolar disorder can also be associated with psychosis such as delusions or hallucinations, occasionally leading to violent behaviors.

Whereas depression is characterized by a persistently low mood, the "mood elevation" of bipolar disorder can vary substantially from person to person and can consist of anything from severe anxiety and irritability to euphoria and an inflated sense of well-being and self-esteem.

While some of these symptoms may sound appealing, the end result of mania is often significant disruption of social and occupational functioning and damage to close relationships. The risky behavior characteristic of a manic episode can lead to significant longer-term health and financial consequences. Similarly, while people with mania feel an intense motivation to engage in many activities and a heightened sense of ability and accomplishment, their impaired attention actually leads to difficulty completing tasks.

Hypomania is a milder version of mania in which similar symptoms are experienced but to a lesser degree and generally without disruption in functioning. In fact, many people with hypomania report being more productive than usual, in contrast to those with mania whose symptoms make them less effective. These symptoms most often last a few weeks to a few months, if left untreated. Hypomania is not associated with psychotic symptoms such as delusions or hallucinations.

The depression of bipolar disorder is similar to that seen in major depressive disorder, described in the previous section. However, bipolar depression is often more difficult to treat because it is less responsive to medications, and there is a risk of precipitating a manic episode with antidepressant medications.

People with bipolar disorder are also susceptible to a third mood state, called a "mixed state," in which symptoms of mania and depression are experienced simultaneously. This sensation is typically experienced as extremely unpleasant and may represent the most dangerous period of any mood disorder, with greatly elevated risks of suicide attempts and substance abuse (Goldman, 1999).

The reason for distinguishing between mania and hypomania is for purposes of diagnosis and treatment. The two main subtypes of BPAD are bipolar I disorder and bipolar II disorder. Bipolar I disorder is diagnosed when an individual has experienced one or more manic episodes. Of note, a depressive episode is often present but not required for the diagnosis of Bipolar I disorder. Bipolar II disorder, on the other hand, requires the presence of at least one hypomanic episode and at least one major depressive episode. While there is significant overlap in the medications used to treat each of these disorders, the specific combination of mood stabilizing and antidepressant medications depends on the particular features of each person's illness and their response to different treatment regimens and often must be continued chronically to prevent relapse in either manic or depressive episodes.

Unfortunately, because of the subjective nature of many of the symptoms, common misunderstandings of the terms "depression" and "mania," and the ability of certain substances to mimic the fluctuations in mood seen in affective disorders (e.g., cocaine can cause a manic-like state), an accurate diagnosis is not always obtained. Furthermore, bipolar disorder is often accompanied by poor insight into the illness and its symptoms, leading to high rates of treatment discontinuation and relapse. However, when accurately diagnosed and appropriately treated, bipolar disorder can have an excellent prognosis.

Brief Overview of Other Mood Disorders

In addition to major depressive and bipolar disorder, there are a number of other less common mood disorders. Generally, these disorders possess some but not all of the features required for a diagnosis of one of the major disorders above.

A common "subthreshold" depressive syndrome known as dysthymia is based on similar symptoms as major depressive disorder, but the symptoms are less severe and generally occur most days over the course of at least two years. Additionally, a person who experiences multiple symptoms of major depression as a result of an identifiable recent event or stressor, but does not meet full criteria for MDD, would be diagnosed with adjustment disorder with depressed mood. "Minor depressive disorder" (or "minor depression") refers to a syndrome in which at least two symptoms of MDD are present for two weeks, but the full criteria for MDD are not met.

Variants of bipolar disorder include cyclothymia, which consists of recurrent hypomanic and dysthymic (subthreshold depressive) episodes without full manic or depressive episodes. Additionally, a subcategory of bipolar disorder is "rapid cycling," defined as having at least four episodes in one year.

Finally, as described above, substance use can contribute to mood disturbances, and when these disturbances reach the threshold for a full disorder, this is referred to as a substance-induced mood disorder. Evidence suggests that problematic alcohol use can directly cause depression rather than simply being a symptom of a depressive disorder. Similarly, long-term use of benzodiazepines such as diazepam (Valium) can have a similar depression-causing effect as alcohol.

ANXIETY DISORDERS

Anxiety is a common experience faced, to varying degrees, by all people in a variety of situations throughout life (Barlow, 2004). In certain situations, it is adaptive, such as when one is under threat or experiencing something new and unexpected. Physical symptoms (nausea, headache) may be present, as well as symptoms common to a variety of psychiatric disorders (insomnia, poor concentration). Anxiety can be pathological when it extends beyond its adaptive usefulness and become chronic and pervasive; when its severity is above what might reasonably be expected for a given situation; and when its presence interferes with functioning in one or more settings. Under these circumstances, anxiety is said to be disordered (M. G. Craske et al., 2011). Anxiety disorders are a debilitating set of psychiatric illness causing much impairment and disability.

Anxiety disorders are among the most frequently occurring psychiatric disorders in the general population (Lépine, 2002). In any given year, it is estimated that almost 20 percent of people will suffer from an anxiety disorder. The likelihood that a person will develop an anxiety disorder during one's lifetime approaches 30 percent. Anxiety disorders occur more frequently in women than men.

Other disorders frequently co-occur with anxiety disorders (Grant et al., 2004; Pini et al., 1997). While each disorder has varying rates of disorder comorbidity, some generalizations can be made. When the diagnosis of an anxiety disorder is made, there is a markedly increased likelihood that comorbid diagnosis of a mood disorder (especially major depressive disorder), another anxiety disorder, or a substance use disorder is also present. It should also be noted that anxiety disorders often manifest with somatic symptoms, which can make their diagnosis difficult; for example, the symptoms of a panic attack can mimic those of a serious cardiac condition, or the symptoms of generalized anxiety disorder could be confused with symptoms of a thyroid disorder.

Since everyone experiences anxiety, delineating whether it is a naturally occurring and adaptive state, rather than a psychiatric disorder, can be challenging (Pini et al., 1997). The experience of anxiety is subjective and often difficult to characterize, manifesting as an internal sense of restlessness, difficulty concentrating to due ruminative thoughts, or constant worry. Somatic symptoms, including nausea, vomiting, headache, muscle tension, sweating, and heart palpitations can also occur. Some anxiety disorders also have more specific manifestations, such as the compulsive repetitive behaviors of obsessive-compulsive disorder or the flashbacks and nightmares of post-traumatic stress disorder. Due to the wide variety of possible symptoms and the overlap these symptoms have with other psychiatric and medical disorders, making correct diagnoses is challenging for even the most skilled practitioner (Barlow, 2004).

Understanding the Common Anxiety Disorders

A **panic attack** is characterized as a bout of extreme anxiety or fear with co-occurring physical symptoms (e.g., shortness of breath, elevated heart rate, nausea, dizziness, fear of losing control or dying, sweating, etc.). Panic attacks typically reach their peak within 10 minutes. Certain situations can trigger panic attacks in some people; in others, panic attacks occur unexpectedly and with no warning. A common trigger for panic attacks is being in public places, enclosed places, or places from which escape is difficult or not always possible, such as a large crowd or a subway train. This fear of being unable to exit public places should one have a panic attack is known as **agoraphobia**. Agoraphobia can be debilitating, leading to avoidance of public places, social isolation, and, as a result, impairment in work and relationships.

When panic attacks are recurrent, unexpected, and lead to excessive worry or anxiety about when another panic attack will occur, what the consequences of panic attack symptoms might mean, or a significant change in behavior in an effort to avoid panic attacks, this is known as panic disorder (Sunderland, Hobbs, Andrews, & Craske, 2012). People will seek out medical care for symptoms that mimic asthma or cardiac conditions unnecessarily. Avoidance of locations or people thought to trigger panic attacks is common. In some patients, agoraphobia is present along with panic disorder, leading to a debilitating condition wherein people will often become housebound in an effort to avoid panic attacks. While many people experience panic attacks, a subset experience distress that leads to the long-term modification of behavior that separates panic attacks from panic disorder.

Specific phobia is the most commonly prevalent mental disorder in women. This disorder is typified by an extreme fear that is in excess of what might be reasonable given the situation triggered by either the presence or expectancy of a specific situation or object (Becker et al., 2007). Common specific phobias include the fear of heights, spiders, snakes, germs/dirt, or medical intervention (injections or drawing blood). The response to these situations is often a panic attack. People often recognize that their response to the situation is unreasonable or over the top, but they do not feel they have control over their response. This frequently leads to avoidance of situations that will produce these symptoms. The result is often a significant impairment in the person's ability to function in their job or social life.

Social phobia (also known as social anxiety disorder) is similar to specific phobia, but with a circumscribed set of situations in which the anxiety occurs (Ruscio et al., 2008). For a person with social phobia, situations in which one needs to perform in front of a group (e.g., public speaking) or socialize with many other people (e.g., a party) with whom one is unfamiliar leads to symptoms similar to those of specific phobia. The person feels like they will be judged, embarrassed, or humiliated, whether because they will act in a particular way that will lead to judgment or because their anxiety will manifest in a way that will lead to embarrassment. As in specific phobia, the fear of embarrassment leads to avoidance of social situations or situation in which the person must perform, leading to impairment.

Of the more common anxiety disorders, **generalized anxiety disorder** is perhaps the most nebulous in terms of how it manifests, because its diagnostic criteria are so broad (Rowa & Antony, 2008). A diagnosis of generalized anxiety disorder requires excessive anxiety occurring for the majority of days over a period of six months. The anxiety can be about anything but is most often about responsibilities faced by the person—e.g., academic performance, job performance, or financial troubles. The person cannot control their anxiety, which manifests in several psychological and somatic ways (diagnosis requires three or more of the following): restlessness; becoming easily fatigued; difficulty concentration; irritability; muscle tension; or sleep disturbance, whether falling asleep, staying asleep, or both. Generalized anxiety disorder frequently co-occurs with another anxiety disorder or a depressive disorder, with estimates that over half of patients with generalized anxiety disorder have a second disorder present.

Recognizing the Less Common Anxiety Disorders

Obsessive-compulsive disorder (OCD) is a frequently debilitating disorder that is characterized by the presence of either obsessions or compulsions (Stein, 2002). **Obsessions** are defined as recurrent, persistent, intrusive thoughts, impulses, or images that are recognized as inappropriate and that cause anxiety or distress. One will attempt to ignore or suppress this intrusive thought or neutralize it with another thought or action. **Compulsions** are defined as repetitive behaviors or mental acts that the person feels driven to perform either in response to an obsessional thought or according to rigidly applied rules. In order to qualify for a diagnosis of OCD, either obsessions or compulsions must be present, but not necessarily both. The obsession or compulsions must cause marked distress and significantly interfere with the person's daily functioning. Finally, a person with OCD will recognize that the obsessions or compulsions are irrational and that their own thoughts and behaviors cause them distress; when one has feelings that conflict with one's own self-image, these are known as **ego-dystonic** thoughts, which are characteristic of the disorder.

There are other discrete disorders that have many features in common with OCD and might be best thought of as highly characterized variants of OCD. **Body dysmorphic disorder (BDD)** is a disorder wherein a person becomes preoccupied with a real or imagined physical imperfection or defect; the person will often go to extreme lengths to either hide or correct the imperfection. Disorders involving compulsive picking, such as **trichotillomania** or **excoriation (skin-picking) disorder** are grouped by DSM-5 into Obsessive-Compulsive and Related Disorders (American Psychiatric Association, 2013). In trichotillomania, one will experience great anxiety until a hair is pulled out, after which a sense of relief occurs; patches of hair loss frequently result. Considering symptoms, this is not altogether different from the compulsive hand washer who experiences skin damage. Finally, **Tourette's disorder**, a disorder characterized by physical and vocal tics that the patient will frequently attempt to resist before succumbing to, shares much with the compulsive behaviors found in OCD.

OCD has a lifetime prevalence of 1 to 2 percent (Stein, 2002), though of the anxiety disorders, it has the highest proportion of sufferers in the "severe" category rather than mild or moderate. OCD often emerges in childhood, with over half of patients experiencing an age of onset lower than 19 years. While, as with most other anxiety disorders, there is no clear precipitant for its development (the usual confluence of genetic predisposition and environmental factors are thought to be responsible), there is one variant with a clear etiology: pediatric autoimmune neuropsychiatric disorders associated with streptococcus (PANDAS) (Felling & Singer, 2011). There is an increasing literature showing a correlation between juvenile streptococcal infection and the onset of tic disorders and OCD (Swedo, Leckman, & Rose, 2012).

Post-traumatic stress disorder (PTSD) occurs, as the name implies, in response to a trauma. The DSM-5 criteria for PTSD requires that the afflicted person was exposed, either directly or indirectly, to death, threatened death, actual or threatened serious injury, or actual or threatened sexual violence (American Psychiatric Association, 2013). In addition to the trauma, the person's response must have involved fear, helplessness, or horror. *Reexperiencing* of the event must be present in some way, including nightmares or distressing dreams, recurrent intrusive distressing recollections of the trauma, acting or feeling as though the traumatic event were happening again, and distress or psychological reactivity at exposure to cues that remind one of the traumatic events. *Avoidance* and numbing must be present, which can include avoiding thoughts, feelings, conversations, people, or places that are associated with the trauma; inability to recall aspects of the trauma; feeling detached from others; diminished interest or participation in significant activities; restricted range of affect; or a sense of a foreshortened future. At least two symptoms of *hyperarousal*, including insomnia, irritability and anger, poor concentration, hypervigilance, and exaggerated startle response, must be present. Finally, in PTSD, symptoms must occur for more than one month.

Many of the symptoms listed above also occur in other disorders, e.g., major depressive disorder. The reexperiencing of an event can mimic the anxious ruminations present in a major depressive episode; diminished range of affect can occur in many disorders; diminished interest in activities, poor concentration, insomnia, and irritability can occur in numerous conditions. The primary differences that separate PTSD from other similar disorders are the presence of a traumatic event and dissociative symptoms (Gros, Tuerk, Yoder, & Acierno, 2010).

Experiencing or witnessing violence can often lead to PTSD, which explains why this disorder is so prevalent in the military population. Civilians who witness or experience violence can also develop PTSD. Other stressful situations, such as lawsuits, can also induce PTSD symptoms. In situations where long-term, repeated trauma takes place, such as a prisoner-of-war camp, repeated acts of domestic violence, or repeated acts of sexual abuse, a condition known as "complex PTSD" can develop wherein the patient not only develops symptoms of PTSD but also develops many characteristics consistent with borderline personality disorder (which, it should be noted, has several criteria which overlap with PTSD already) (Gros et al., 2010). Patients can have an unstable sense of self, chronic feelings of emptiness, chronic suicidal ideation, and recurrent self-injurious behavior.

Anxiety Disorders in LGBT Populations

Research looking at anxiety disorders as they pertain specifically to the LGBT population is lacking; this is particularly true of research on bisexual and transgender persons. A 2002 study looking at the amount of articles dedicated to LGBT medical issues found that 0.1 percent of articles not pertaining to sexually transmitted infections addressed lesbians and gay men, while bisexual persons were written about less frequently, and transgender persons least of all (Boehmer, 2002).

Studies looking at the epidemiology of anxiety disorders among the LGBT population largely indicate an increased incidence as compared to heterosexual populations, though there are conflicting data across the full range of studies (Cochran et al., 2003; Gilman et al., 2001). Homosexual men, when compared to heterosexual men, have significantly higher rates of anxiety disorders; agoraphobia, simple phobia, and obsessive-compulsive disorder had higher rates of 12-month prevalence in homosexual men (Sandfort, de Graaf, Bijl, & Schnabel, 2001). Except for generalized anxiety disorder, homosexual men have a higher lifetime prevalence of all anxiety disorders. (Sandfort et al., 2001). In females, there were no significant differences found between homosexual or heterosexual women in either the 12-month or lifetime prevalences of anxiety disorders (Sandfort et al., 2001).

One study looked at subjectively reported psychological distress and found that gay and bisexual men reported higher levels than their heterosexual counterparts. No difference in psychological distress was found between heterosexual, homosexual, and bisexual women. This study also found that gay and bisexual men are more likely to suffer from panic disorder than heterosexual men, and lesbian and bisexual women are more likely to suffer from generalized anxiety disorder than heterosexual women (Cochran, Sullivan, & Mays, 2003).

PTSD in the LGBT population has been investigated. Notably, at least 30 percent of homosexual men experience sexual assault during childhood, adolescence, and/or adulthood (Rothman, Exner, & Baughman, 2011). This rate is similar to that of heterosexual women. Unsurprisingly, an increased rate of PTSD is also found in these populations. In homosexual men, internalized homophobia was found to correlate more with severity of symptoms and treatment outcome than assault severity (Dragowski, Halkitis, Grossman, & D'Augelli, 2011).

There is speculation about why both mood and anxiety disorders might be more prevalent in the LGBT population. One hypothesis is the "minority stress" hypothesis, which supposes that psychiatric disorders are the result of discrimination and social stress that is not faced by nonheterosexuals (Fingerhut et al., 2010). Prejudice may, in fact, cause members of the LGBT community to suffer from mental illness. Another theory is that nonheterosexual men and women, who have been found to rate higher on the neuroticism personality trait than their heterosexual counterparts, might be predisposed to anxiety disorders based on personality factors found to be more prevalent in the LGBT population (Dragowski et al., 2011). As well, genetic and biological factors that influence the development of homosexuality may also increase the likelihood of the presence of psychiatric disorders.

While the amount of money devoted to LGBT research and the number of articles examining the LGBT population has increased, data looking at the mental health of transgender populations remains sparse. A small cross-sectional study examining 31 patients found that the prevalence of anxiety disorders at the time of interview was 25.8 percent, while the lifetime prevalence in this population was 22.6 percent (Hepp, Kraemer, Schnyder, Miller, & Delsignore, 2005). Another much larger study examining 579 patients in Japan found that 3.6 percent of patients met criteria for an anxiety disorder at the time of interview, though the study found markedly elevated rates of suicidal ideation and self-injurious behavior (Hoshiai et al., 2010).

TREATING MOOD AND ANXIETY DISORDERS

There are a variety of treatment options in many settings available for people suffering with mood and anxiety disorders. The first step in the treatment process for any active mood or anxiety disturbance is an assessment of the safety of the patient and their clinical situation. Patients who are in crisis, have active thoughts of hurting themselves or others, who put themselves in reckless endangerment, have severe or acute psychotic features (that is, having trouble distinguishing reality from nonreality), or who are unable to care for their fundamental needs require emergent evaluation in an emergency room setting. Patients who are in danger of losing their employment, housing, or other devastating loss, or who have nonacute psychotic features (for example, auditory hallucinations without delusional thinking), or symptoms severe enough to affect their core role functions require an urgent evaluation by a clinician specialist in mental health. The vast majority of patients do not have severe or acute features associated with a mood or anxiety episode; as such, the majority of patients are clinically appropriate for outpatient treatment programs.

LGBT people have a baseline increased risk of suicide due to minority stress (Meyer, 2003). While a safety assessment is a core first step in initiating any treatment for mood or anxiety disorders, it is particularly important for LGBT patients. Particularly vulnerable to suicide are people who are older than 48, male-identified, single, with limited social supports, access to firearms, and with active substance use (Brown, Beck, Steer, & Grisham, 2000). Prior suicide attempts also predict future suicide attempts; a thorough safety assessment will take into consideration these and other risk factors to inform the level of care required by a particular patient.

Treatment Settings

The majority of patients with mood and/or anxiety disorders are free from serious safety or severity concerns, and the usual treatment setting is outpatient treatment. Typical outpatient treatment may involve any combination of visits with a psychotherapist for psychotherapy, group psychotherapy sessions, and/or visits with a prescriber for medication management. Some patients in a combined treatment visit a psychotherapist separate from their medication prescriber. Others have a single clinician manage both psychotherapy and medications. There are a range of psychotherapies and medications that have demonstrated efficacy in treating mood and anxiety disorders, and matching the treatment to the particular patient is often a matter of both empirical trials and assiduous assessment of patient's treatment priorities and response to prior treatments.

For patients with significant mood or anxiety symptoms, or whose symptoms do not improve with treatment, some find relief from an intensification of treatment. Increased levels of care range from three-times-a-week intensive outpatient programs to five-hours-a-day-for-five-days-a-week structured partial hospital programs, to round-the-clock residential programs where patients temporarily reside on-site during a treatment course. These intensified programs almost always involve a combination of psychotherapies and consultation with a medication prescriber.

For patients who pose a safety concern—that is, are at significant risk of harming themselves or others, or who are unable to care for their fundamental needs—inpatient psychiatric care is required. Inpatient psychiatric care is 24-hours-a-day care, typically in a hospital setting, and often with locked doors. Inpatient treatment involves visits with a psychiatrist five to seven days a week, 24-hour nursing care, and usually involves a combination of psychotherapies focused on mitigating symptoms and restoring function. Many patients with high-severity symptoms impacting major life functions seek out inpatient psychiatric care to obtain rapid relief. Each state in the United States also has civil commitment laws that permit people with mental illness to be involuntary committed to inpatient psychiatric care if they pose a high safety risk to themselves or their communities because of their mental illness (Appelbaum, 1994).

Treatment Settings for LGBT Populations

There is significant variability in the breadth and depth of LGBT-specific treatment settings between various geographies throughout the United States. Further, there are no LGBT-specific treatment standards for mental health service providers working with LGBT patients (Lucksted, 2004). LGBT patients describe poorer overall satisfaction with mental health treatment than non-LGBT counterparts (Avery, Hellman, & Sudderth, 2001; Burgesset, Tran, Lee, & van Ryn, 2007; Fraser & Solovey, 2007). Despite this, there is no evidence that LGBT patients seek out services less frequently than non-LGBT populations (Grella, Greenwell, Mays, & Cochran, 2009).

The core element of any effective treatment is a functional therapeutic alliance, even if the treatment itself is not entirely voluntary (Fraser & Solovey, 2007; Happell, 2008; National Institute on Drug Abuse, 2009). Thus, LGBT patients may find it easier to access treatment for mood and anxiety disorders in LGBT-focused settings. However, there are no controlled trials demonstrating that LGBT patients have better outcomes in LGBT-specific settings than general settings. In general, the more adherent patients are with any particular mental health treatment, the better the outcome. As such, all patients (LGBT patients included) are best served in settings where they are comfortable and invested in the treatment.

While there are no LGBT-specific psychotherapies, medications, or other types of component treatments, each of these treatments can often be organized in an LGBT context. An internet search will yield a list of LGBT-focused treatment centers that advertise staff and clinicians with specific experience in working with LGBT patients or clients. There are also treatment centers that offer LGBT group psychotherapies where group members can be assumed to identify as LGBT. Individual clinicians seeking LGBT patients or clients often advertise in LGBT-specific publications or on the Gay and Lesbian Medical Association's (GLMA's) provider directory (Gay and Lesbian Medical Association, 2017). Depending on their geography and the type of insurance someone may have, provider options may range from abundant to sparse.

For LGBT patients whose identification as an LGBT person is directly connected with distressing mood or anxiety symptoms, LGBT-oriented settings may offer a therapeutically useful context to address LGBT issues within the focus of treatment. For other LGBT people, being LGBT may be entirely incidental to their mood or anxiety symptoms. In either instance, patients are best served in treatments where they are empowered to involve as much of their life experience as is relevant to their recovery (The National Alliance on Mental Illness [NAMI], 2009). While it would be optimal for all mental health providers to have equivalent skill and experience in working with LGBT populations, in reality, many patients are left to trial and error in finding a clinician or treatment program with the necessary fit.

Psychotherapies for Mood and Anxiety Disorders

Psychotherapy is a particular type of conversation between a patient and therapist, or between patients in a facilitated group, organized to relieve distress and achieve well-being. While there are a myriad types of psychotherapies, these treatments can be grouped into four main categories: psychodynamic therapy, cognitive-behavior therapy, supportive psychotherapy, and non–talk psychotherapies.

Psychodynamic psychotherapy is a technique focused on "exploring those aspects of self that are not fully known, especially as they are manifested and potentially influenced in the therapy relationship" (Shedler, 2010). In a psychodynamic psychotherapy, the therapist or group facilitator focuses on emotion and the attempts patients may make to avoid distressing emotions. Recurring themes are identified, and past experiences are reviewed. As emotions and attempts to avoid distressing emotion become manifest in the relationships between patients and the therapist, these are identified. The patient is encouraged to make sense of their experience and avoid behaviors that interfere with optimal function. In doing so, patients achieve emotional insight that leads to change and improved capacity to find greater enjoyment and meaning in life (Shedler, 2010). Psychoanalysis is a particular type of psychodynamic psychotherapy and typically involves more frequent meetings between patient and therapist than other types of psychodynamic psychotherapies.

Cognitive behavioral therapy (CBT) is an umbrella term for a variety of psychotherapies focused on patients' current thoughts, behavior patterns, and active feelings, in contrast to unconscious processes. In cognitive psychotherapy, a therapist works with the patient to identify maladaptive thoughts, self-statements, or beliefs, and frequently employs a series of exercises designed to change these thoughts and beliefs. In behavioral psychotherapy, interventions are applied to decrease maladaptive behaviors and increase adaptive ones. Cognitive-behavior therapies share a common "science and theory of behavior and cognition, and the centrality of problem-focused goals (M. Craske, 2009)." A few examples of psychotherapies within the CBT umbrella include interpersonal psychotherapy, behavioral activation therapy, acceptance and commitment therapy, dialectic behavioral therapy, problem-solving therapy, process-experiential therapy, and life-review therapy (Cuijpers et al., 2012).

Supportive psychotherapy is a less structured therapy "without specific psychological techniques other than those belonging to the basic interpersonal skills of the therapist, such as reflection, empathic listening, encouragement, and helping people to explore and express their experiences and emotions" (Werman, 2014). In psychodynamic psychotherapy, therapists offer interpretations. In cognitive behavioral psychotherapy, tasks are organized around finding solutions or teaching new skills. In supportive psychotherapy, each of these tasks are largely absent, in favor of active listening and offering support focusing on participants' problems and concerns (Areán et al., 2010). Supportive psychotherapy is also referred to as counseling or as a nonspecific talk therapy when used with individual therapists, and as a support group when used in groups (Bower & Rowland, 2006).

Psychotherapy treatments are described in a variety of formats that range from individual patient-therapist dyads to couples, family, or network therapies, or group psychotherapies (Gurman, Lebow, & Synder, 2002; Yalom & Leszcz, 1995). Depending on the diagnosis and nature of the mood and anxiety disorder features, a treatment plan that incorporates one or more of these psychotherapies might be indicated. While there is no evidence that LGBT-focused therapies are required to be effective for LGBT patients, multiple authors posit that a basic familiarity with LGBT mental health issues supports treatment effectiveness (Blumer, Green, Knowles, & Williams, 2012; Hartwell, Serovich, Grafsky, & Kerr, 2012).

While the aforementioned psychotherapies are based on spoken conversations between patients and therapists, there is a fourth category of psychotherapies focused on different types of expression. Examples of these treatments include dance-movement therapies, music therapies, and various types of expressive art therapies. For patients who find speaking about their thoughts and experiences to be challenging, using these techniques can be therapeutic (Bates, 2008; Knill, Levine, & Levine, 2005).

There is no evidence that any particular category of psychotherapy is more effective than any other for mood or anxiety disorders, or for LGBT patients versus non-LGBT patients (Luborsky, 1995; Luborsky, Singer, & Luborsky, 1975). A variety of authors suggest that nonspecific factors underlie the shared effectiveness of psychotherapies. The literature supports psychotherapy being most effective when the therapeutic alliance between patient and provider is strong, and when the practitioner is experienced with the technique being employed (Cuijpers et al., 2012; Thoma et al., 2012). As different psychotherapies have different types of time commitments (multiple times a week versus once a month or less frequently) and durations (ongoing with no predefined duration versus a fixed number of sessions), patient preference regarding financial and time commitments often influence which psychotherapies are initially pursued. As the therapeutic alliance is of paramount import to treatment success, finding the sufficient patient-therapist fit is a crucial consideration for patients initiating a psychotherapy treatment.

LGBT patients are best served in deciding how important a provider's understanding and familiarity with LGBT terminology, identities, and common issues is to them when seeking care. There are some LGBT providers that openly advertise their own LGBT identities and who might specialize in working with LGBT patients; others may not identify professionally as LGBT but possess robust clinical familiarity with LGBT issues; others may lack specific expertise but remain be open to understanding what being LGBT might mean for patients. As long as the therapeutic alliance is effective, any of these clinicians could deliver an effective treatment. For patients, knowing how important LGBT savvy might be to support a good fit with their psychotherapist can help guide how much weight to put on seeking providers with LGBT expertise.

Medications for Mood and Anxiety Disorders

There are a variety of medications that can relieve clinically significant mood and anxiety symptoms, in many classes that include antidepressants, mood stabilizers, and anxiolytics. Cells in the brain communicate to each other by releasing chemicals called neurotransmitters. Psychiatric medications work, generally, by binding to one or more specialized proteins in the brain that change neurotransmitter signaling (Schatzberg, Cole, & Debattista, 2010).

Patients considering medications for mood or anxiety symptoms usually begin by discussing medication options with their primary care provider. The first step in medication management should including a medical evaluation for underlying nonpsychiatric treatable conditions that might mimic mood or anxiety symptoms. In many cases, this includes a history, physical exam, blood tests, and an electrocardiogram. For major depressive disorder without psychotic features or uncomplicated anxiety syndrome, there are primary care providers well equipped to effectively manage first-line antidepressants and anxiolytic medications.

For patients with bipolar disorder, psychotic symptoms (that is, with signs of difficulty distinguishing reality from nonreality), debilitating symptoms that affect their job performance or other core life function, or who are at risk of harming themselves or others, usually psychiatric specialty care is indicated. As previously discussed, patients can access care emergently through emergency room services at hospitals, or in less emergent cases, meet with a psychiatric specialist who can provide expert evaluation and management.

Whether managed within a primary care setting or by a psychiatric provider, patients interested in medication options can expect to discuss one or more initial medication options with their prescriber. Some psychiatric medications work within moments after taking them; others require weeks to months of daily adherence before the full effect is achieved. There are psychiatric medications that generate tolerance and therefore lose their effect over time, and often, medications with this property have an addictive potential. It is reasonable to expect a discussion of the intended effects, risks, benefits, alternatives, expected duration of treatment, and common side effects that might be experienced with any particular medication.

During a course of psychiatric medication treatment, prescribers monitor for common adverse medication effects as well as the extent to which intended benefit is achieved. In some cases, patients may experience side effects so strongly that they cannot tolerate taking the medication at all.

More commonly, medication adverse effects may be present initially but resolve over time with taking continued doses. As such, many psychiatric medications are started at a low dose to assess that they can be tolerated before their dose is increased over time to achieve a therapeutic effect. If a medication does not yield much benefit when balanced against side effects, the prescriber may recommend switching to another medication. For most psychiatric medications that have been taken for weeks or longer, it is recommended that the dose be lowered gradually rather than abruptly stopped.

Antidepressants have been hypothesized to work through amplifying the effects of the brain chemicals serotonin, noradrenaline, and/or dopamine. The most commonly prescribed type of antidepressants block the reuptake of serotonin and are called selective serotonin reuptake inhibitors. Other medications affect both serotonin and noradrenaline; these are called serotonin and norepinephrine reuptake inhibitors. There are also other classes of medications that include tricyclic antidepressants and monamine oxidase inhibitors. Each medication has its own unique set of risks and adverse effects (for example, patients taking certain types of monamine oxidase inhibitors are recommended to follow a specialized diet to avoid serious side effects). Most medications in these classes must be taken daily for six to eight weeks before their full effect is achieved.

Nearly 70 percent of patients with a depressive disorder experience a significant relief of their depressive symptoms with one or more of these medications (Gaynes et al., 2012). For patients with ongoing depressive symptoms, psychiatric specialist prescribers sometimes add on antipsychotic or anti-parkinsonian medications (which typically affect dopamine transmission) or specific hormone medications, which have been shown to boost the effect of antidepressants. Additionally, patients with depressive symptoms resistant to medications altogether often find significant relief with electroconvulsive shock therapy, which is an approved treatment for major depressive disorder.

Patients who experience manic or hypomanic episodes have bipolar disorder, and separate classes of medications categorically referred to as mood stabilizers are indicated to treat mood episodes in individuals with bipolar disorder. There are many different types of mood stabilizers with myriad mechanisms of action. Many medications in the antipsychotic class have clinical efficacy during manic or depressive phases of bipolar disorder, and these are thought to work by blocking specific dopamine and serotonin receptors. Some mood stabilizers require regularly checking the medication levels in blood as part of monitoring against medication toxicity. Prescribers should discuss the mood stabilizer options, risks, benefits, and monitoring protocols with patients for whom these medications are indicated.

For patients with anxiety disorders, many of the above-mentioned serotonin- and norepinephrine-focused medications also reduce anxiety symptoms if taken at an adequate dose over a sufficient duration (typically weeks to months) (Ravindran & Stein, 2010). There are other types of anti-anxiety medications that have an immediate effect on anxiety symptoms, most notably the benzodiazepine and barbiturate classes. Although they work quickly, benzodiazepines and barbiturates carry the risk of both physical tolerance and have a significant addiction potential. Additionally, they can cause sedation, dizziness, and can even cause people to stop breathing if used in excessive doses or in combination with alcohol or other sedating medications.

There are other types of medications that are frequently employed to quickly lower acute anxiety symptoms when taken on an as-needed basis. These include some antihistamine medications, certain types of seizure medications, and select blood pressure medications. Only a few of the medications in these classes have been approved by the U.S. Food and Drug Administration to treat anxiety conditions, and therefore many are prescribed "off label." Nevertheless, these remain effective anxiolytic medication options for patients for whom they are clinically indicated.

Finding Treatment for Mood and Anxiety Disorders

In the United States, the majority of patients rely on health insurance to cover the costs of treatment (Schiller, Lucas, Ward, & Peregoy, 2012). Most insurance carriers offer mental health benefits, and those that do are required by federal regulations (the Mental Health Parity and Addiction Equity Act of 2008) to offer mental health benefits comparable to medical and surgical benefits. In many cases, insurance companies subcontract the management of mental health care insurance to a separate affiliated carrier. Regardless of which insurance a patient may carry, anyone planning to use these benefits is well served to consult their carrier's explanation of benefits relevant to mental health care. Despite federal law, there remain insurers not in compliance with parity (McCarty, 2013).

A 2010 executive order regarding hospital visitation rights for LGBT Americans, and 2010's Patient Protection and Affordable Care Act (PPACA) passed by the U.S. Congress, changed the landscape for health care access by LGBT people in the United States (Byne, 2014). Through expanded coverage, an increased focus on LGBT-specific data collection, an emphasis on preventive care, LGBT-inclusive nondiscrimination protections, and insurance market reforms, the law has the potential to expand health care options available to LGBT Americans (Cray & Baker, 2013). The extent of the impact of these reforms on LGBT mental health care is theoretically significant but remains to be fully realized in practice.

As previously mentioned, patients in crisis who are at significant risk of harming themselves or others, or who are unable to care for their fundamental needs, require emergent psychiatric evaluation. This is optimally arranged by expediting these patients' presentation to the closest emergency room, often involving emergency medical services (via calling 911). Once a level of care is determined as part of a psychiatric assessment, emergency departments perform a cross-reference of a patient's insurance coverage and available treatment options. The Emergency Medical Treatment & Labor Act, passed by the U.S. Congress in 1986, requires emergency rooms to facilitate transitions and/or referrals to an appropriate level of care (Lindor et al., 2014).

Outside of an emergency room setting, or situation where case managers are available to confirm insurance benefits and coordinate referrals, it is incumbent upon patients to identify which available treatment options are compatible with their insurance benefits. A common place to start is with one's primary care provider, who will often have referral recommendations based on their own clinical experience, coordination within a shared institution, and knowledge of shared participation in an insurance plan. Some insurance plans require a formal referral be made by a primary care provider for a patient to obtain coverage for mental health services. Other options include contacting one's insurance company for a list of participating mental health providers. Many people also rely on word of mouth and contact mental health providers and treatment centers directly.

For those patients without insurance and without the ability to pay for care out of pocket, many cities have one or more community hospitals or facilities offering mental health services to patients at nominal cost. The specific mental health services offered, as well as their breadth and depth, have considerable variability between geographies. Since the introduction of 2010's PPACA, there has been an expansion in health insurance options available to patients for whom health insurance coverage wasn't previously available, and patients with mental health treatment needs are generally best served by obtaining insurance coverage (Garfield & Druss, 2012).

LGBT patients living in proximity to cities with LGBT health centers may consider contacting their local LGBT center to find which, if any, services are offered. Many LGBT centers run supportive counseling groups and can offer referrals when other services or other levels of care are indicated. Some centers directly offer counseling and other psychiatric services to patients, while many refer patients out to community providers.

There is a minority of patients with the financial resources to pay for their mental health care directly without insurance. There are myriad of treatment providers and centers available at all levels of care that accept direct payment from patients without insurance. Some patents in this situation purchase an insurance product that reimburses a proportion of out-of-pocket fees after a billable service is delivered.

Many patients find navigating the range of insurance and provider options to be daunting. As mentioned, beginning with a primary care provider and contacting one's insurance company for a list of participating mental health providers or institutions often yields a useful set of options with which to begin. Mood and anxiety disorders can be effectively treated in a variety of settings, and patients are best served by initiating treatment as soon as symptoms become clinically significant.

CONCLUSION

Within the LGBT community, mood and anxiety disorders occur at rates higher than the general population. This is hypothesized to be due to exposure to chronic stress specific to this community that, at a certain threshold, develops into a disorder. In addition, the risk of suicide in the LGBT population is higher. It is therefore important to be vigilant and screen for mood and anxiety disorders. Because stigma affects both the LGBT population and psychiatric illness, it is imperative to create treatment settings that allow for the comfort to divulge sensitive information and details. Typical treatments include psychotropic medications (including antidepressants and anxiolytics), psychotherapy (including supportive therapy, cognitive behavioral therapy, and psychodynamic therapy), or a combination. Accessing psychiatric care should begin with the primary care provider, who will determine whether a specialist is needed.

REFERENCES

American Psychiatric Association. (2013). *Diagnostic and statistical manual of mental disorders* (5th ed). Washington, DC: Author.

Appelbaum, P. S. (1994). *Almost a revolution: Mental health law and the limits of change.* New York: Oxford University Press.

Areán, P. A., Alexopoulos, G. S., Raue, P. J., Kiosses, D. N., Mackin, R. S., Kanellopoulos, D., & McCulloch, C. (2010). Problem-solving therapy and supportive therapy in older adults with major depression and executive dysfunction. *American Journal of Psychiatry, 167*(11), 1391.

Avery, A. M., Hellman, R. E., & Sudderth, L. K. (2001). Satisfaction with mental health services among sexual minorities with major mental illness. *American Journal of Public Health, 91*(6), 990–991.

Bailey, M. (1999). Homosexuality and mental illness. *Archives of General Psychiatry, 56*(10), 883–884.

Balsam, K. F., Beadnell, B., & Molina, Y. (2013). The daily heterosexist experiences questionnaire measuring minority stress among lesbian, gay, bisexual, and transgender adults. *Measurement and Evaluation in Counseling and Development, 46*(1), 3–25.

Barlow, D. H. (2004). *Anxiety and its disorders: The nature and treatment of anxiety and panic.* New York: Guilford Press.

Bates, J. (2008). The hidden treasure of the self. In D. McCarthy (Ed.), *Speaking about the unspeakable: Non-verbal methods and experiences in therapy with children* (pp. 17–26). Philadelphia: Jessica Kingsley.

Becker, E. S., Rinck, M., Türke, V., Kause, P., Goodwin, R., Neumer, S., & Margraf, J. (2007). Epidemiology of specific phobia subtypes: Findings from the Dresden Mental Health Study. *European Psychiatry, 22*(2), 69–74.

Blumer, M. L. C., Green, M. S., Knowles, S. J., & Williams, A. (2012). Shedding light on thirteen years of darkness: Content analysis of articles pertaining to transgender issues in marriage/couple and family therapy journals. *Journal of Marital and Family Therapy, 38*(1), 244–256.

Boehmer, U. (2002). Twenty years of public health research: Inclusion of lesbian, gay, bisexual, and transgender populations. *American Journal of Public Health, 92*(7), 1125–1130.

Bolton, S. L., & Sareen, J. (2011). Sexual orientation and its relation to mental disorders and suicide attempts: Findings from a nationally representative sample. *Canadian Journal of Psychiatry, 56*(1), 35–43.

Bostwick, W. B., Boyd, C. J., Hughes, T. L., & McCabe, S. E. (2010). Dimensions of sexual orientation and the prevalence of mood and anxiety disorders in the United States. *American Journal of Public Health, 100*(3), 468–475.

Bower, P. J., & Rowland, N. (2006). Effectiveness and cost effectiveness of counselling in primary care. *Cochrane Database of Systematic Reviews, 3,* CD001025.

Brown, G. K., Beck, A. T., Steer, R. A., & Grisham, J. R. (2000). Risk factors for suicide in psychiatric outpatients: A 20-year prospective study. *Journal of Consulting and Clinical Psychology, 68*(3), 371–377.

Burgesset, D., Tran, A., Lee, R., & van Ryn, M. (2007). Effects of perceived discrimination on mental health and mental health services utilisation among gay, lesbian, bisexual, and transgender persons. *Journal of LGBT Health Research, 3*(4), 1–14.

Byne, W. (2014). A new era for LGBT health. *LGBT Health, 1*(1), 1–2.

Chehil, S., & Kutcher, S. (2012). *Suicide risk management: A manual for health professionals.* Chicester: John Wiley & Sons.

Cochran, S. D., Sullivan, J. G., & Mays, V. M. (2003). Prevalence of mental disorders, psychological distress, and mental health services use among lesbian, gay, and bisexual adults in the United States. *Journal of Consulting and Clinical Psychology, 71*(1), 53–61.

Craske, M. G. (2009). *Cognitive-behavioral therapy: Theories of psychotherapy.* Washington, DC: American Psychological Association.

Craske, M. G., Rauch, S. L., Ursano, R., Prenoveau, J., Pine, D. S., & Zinbarg, R. E. (2011). What is an anxiety disorder? *Journal of Lifelong Learning in Psychiatry, 9*(3), 369–388.

Cray, A., & Baker, K. (2013). How the affordable care act helps the LGBT community. Retrieved from https://www.americanprogress.org/issues/lgbt/news/2013/05/30/64609/how-the-affordable-care-act-helps-the-lgbt-community/

Cuijpers, P., Driessen, E., Hollon, S. D., van Oppen, P., Barth, J., & Andersson, G. (2012). The efficacy of non-directive supportive therapy for adult depression: A meta-analysis. *Clinical Psychology Review, 32*(4), 280–291.

Dragowski, E. A., Halkitis, P. N., Grossman, A. H., & D'Augelli, A. R. (2011). Sexual orientation victimization and posttraumatic stress symptoms among lesbian, gay, and bisexual youth. *Journal of Gay & Lesbian Social Services, 23*(2), 226–249.

Felling, R. J., & Singer, H. S. (2011). Neurobiology of Tourette syndrome: Current status and need for further investigation. *Journal of Neuroscience, 31*(35), 12387–12395.

Fingerhut, A. W., Peplau, L. A., & Gable, S. L. (2010). Identity, minority stress, and psychological well-being among gay men and lesbians. *Psychology & Sexuality, 1*(2), 101–114.

Fraser, S., & Solovey, A. D. (2007). *Second-order change in psychotherapy: The golden thread that unifies effective treatments.* Washington, DC: American Psychological Association.

Garfield, R. L., & Druss, B. G. (2012). Health reform, health insurance, and mental health care. *American Journal of Psychiatry, 169*(7), 675–677.

Gay and Lesbian Medical Association. (2017). Health professionals advancing LGBT equality. Retrieved from http://www.glma.org

Gaynes, B. N., Warden, D., Trivedi, M. H., Wisniewski, S. R., Fava, M., & Rush, A. J. (2012). What did STAR* D teach us?: Results from a large-scale, practical, clinical trial for patients with depression. *Focus Major Depressive Disorder: Maintenance of Certification Workbook, 60*, 129.

Gilman, S. E., Cochran, S. D., Mays, V. M., Hughes, M., Ostrow, D., & Kessler, K. C. (2001). Risk of psychiatric disorders among individuals reporting same-sex sexual partners in the National Comorbidity Survey. *American Journal of Public Health, 91*(6), 933.

Goldman, E. (1999). Severe anxiety, agitation are warning signals of suicide in bipolar patients. *Clinical Psychiatry News, 1*(1), 25.

Grant, B. F., Stinson, F. S., Dawson, D. A., Chou, S. P., Dufour, M. C., Compton, W., . . . Kaplan, K. (2004). Prevalence and co-occurrence of substance use disorders and independent mood and anxiety disorders: Results from the National Epidemiologic Survey on Alcohol and Related Conditions. *Archives of General Psychiatry, 61*(8), 807–816.

Grella, C. E., Greenwell, L., Mays, V. M., & Cochran, S. D. (2009). Influence of gender, sexual orientation, and need on treatment utilisation for substance use and mental disorders: Findings from the California Quality of Life Survey. *BMC Psychiatry, 9*(52), 1–10.

Gros, D. F., Tuerk, P. W., Yoder, M., & Acierno, R. (2010). Post-traumatic stress disorder. In J. C. Thomas & M. Hersen (Eds.), *Handbook of clinical psychology competencies* (pp. 785–810). New York: Springer.

Gurman, A. S., Lebow, J. L., & Synder, D. K. (2002). *Clinical handbook of couple therapy.* New York: Guilford Press.

Haas, A. P., Eliason, M., Mays, V. M., Mathy, R. M., Cochran, S. D., D'Augelli, A. R., . . . Clayton, P. J. (2010). Suicide and suicide risk in lesbian, gay, bisexual, and transgender populations: Review and recommendations. *Journal of Homosexuality, 58*(1), 10–51.

Halbreich, U., & Montgomery, S. A. (2013). *Pharmacotherapy for mood, anxiety, and cognitive disorders.* Arlington, VA: American Psychiatric.

Happell, B. (2008). Determining the effectiveness of mental health services from a consumer perspective: Part 1: Enhancing recovery. *International Journal of Mental Health Nursing, 17*(2), 116–122.

Hartwell, E. E., Serovich, J. M., Grafsky, E. L., & Kerr, Z. Y. (2012). Coming out of the dark: Content analysis of articles pertaining to gay, lesbian, and bisexual issues in couple and family therapy journals. *Journal of Marital and Family Therapy, 38*(1), 227–243.

Hepp, U., Kraemer, B., Schnyder, U., Miller, N., & Delsignore, A. (2005). Psychiatric comorbidity in gender identity disorder. *Journal of Psychosomatic Research, 58*(3), 259–261.

Hoshiai, M., Matsumoto, Y., Sato, T., Ohnishi, M., Okabe, N., Kishimoto, Y., . . . Kuroda, S. (2010). Psychiatric comorbidity among patients with gender identity disorder. *Psychiatry and Clinical Neurosciences, 64*(5), 514–519.

Kessler, R. C., Berglund, P., Demler, O., Jin, R., Koretz, D., Merikangas, K. R., . . . National Comorbidity Survey Replication. (2003). The epidemiology of major depressive disorder: Results from the National Comorbidity Survey Replication (NCS-R). *Journal of the American Medical Association, 89*(23), 3095–3105.

Kessler, R. C., Chiu, W. T., Demler, O., & Walters, E. E. (2005). Prevalence, severity, and comorbidity of twelve-month DSM-IV disorders in the National Comorbidity Survey Replication (NCS-R). *Archives of General Psychiatry, 62*(6), 617–627.

Knill, P. J., Levine, E. G., & Levine, S. K. (2005). *Principles and practice of expressive arts therapy: Towards a therapeutic aesthetics.* Philadelphia: Jessica Kingsley.

Kupfer, D. J., Frank, E., & Wamhoff, J. (1996). Mood disorders: Update on prevention of recurrence. In C. Mundt, M. J. Goldstein, K. Hahlweg, & P. Fiedler (Eds.), *Interpersonal factors in the origin and course of affective disorders* (pp. 289–302). London: Royal College of Psychiatrists.

Lépine, J. P. (2002). The epidemiology of anxiety disorders: Prevalence and societal costs. *Journal of Clinical Psychiatry, 63*(14), 4–8.

Lindor, R. A., Campbell, R. L., Pines, J. M., Melin, G. J., Schipper, A. M., Goyal, D. G., & Sadosty, A. T. (2014). EMTALA and patients with psychiatric emergencies: A review of relevant case law. *Annals of Emergency Medicine, 64*(5), 439–444.

Luborsky, L. (1995). Are common factors across different psychotherapies the main explanation for the dodo bird verdict that 'Everyone has won so all shall have prizes.' *Clinical Psychology: Science and Practice, 2*(1), 106–109.

Luborsky, L., Singer, B., & Luborsky, L. (1975). Comparative studies of psychotherapies: Is it true that 'everyone has won and all must have prizes'?
Archives of General Psychiatry, 32(8), 995.

Lucksted, A. (2004). Lesbian, gay, bisexual, and transgender people receiving services in the public mental health system: Raising issues. *Journal of Gay &
Lesbian Psychotherapy, 8*(3–4), 25–42.

McCarty, D. (2013). Parity: An ongoing challenge and research opportunity.
American Journal of Psychiatry, 170(2), 140–142.

Meyer, I. H. (2003). Prejudice, social stress, and mental health in lesbian, gay, and
bisexual populations: conceptual issues and research evidence. *Psychological Bulletin, 129*(5), 674.

Murray, C. J., & Lopez, A. D. (1997). Global mortality, disability, and the contribution of risk factors: Global Burden of Disease Study. *Lancet, 349*(9063),
1436–1442.

The National Alliance on Mental Illness (NAMI). (2009). GLBTQI mental
health: Recommendations for policies and services. Retrieved from
http://tucollaborative.org/wp-content/uploads/2017/03/GLBTQI-MH
-Recommendations-for-Policies-and-Services.pdf

National Institute of Mental Health. (2007). Depression basics. Retrieved from
https://www.nimh.nih.gov/health/publications/depression/index.shtml

National Institute on Drug Abuse. (2009). *Principles of drug addiction treatment:
A research-based guide*. Bethesda, MA: Author.

Pini, S., Cassano, G. B., Simonini, E., Savino, M., Russo, A., & Montgomery, S. A.
(1997). Prevalence of anxiety disorders comorbidity in bipolar depression,
unipolar depression and dysthymia. *Journal of Affective Disorders, 42*(2),
145–153.

Post, R. M. (1992). Transduction of psychosocial stress into the neurobiology of
recurrent affective disorder. *American Journal of Psychiatry, 149*(8),
999–1010.

Ravindran, L. N., & Stein, M. B. (2010). The pharmacologic treatment of anxiety disorders: A review of progress. *Journal of Clinical Psychiatry, 70*(7), 839–854.

Remafedi, G., French, S., Story, M., Resnick, M. D., & Blum, R. (1998). The Relationship between suicide risk and sexual orientation: Results of a
population-based study. *American Journal of Public Health, 88*(1), 57–60.

Rothman, E. F., Exner, D., & Baughman, A. L. (2011). The prevalence of sexual
assault against people who identify as gay, lesbian, or bisexual in the United
States: A systematic review. *Trauma, Violence, & Abuse, 12*(2), 55–66.

Rowa, K., & Antony, M. M. (2008). Generalized anxiety disorder. In W. E. Craighead, L. W. Craighead, & D. J. Miklowitz (Eds.), *Psychopathology: History,
diagnosis, and empirical foundations* (pp. 78–114). Hoboken, NJ: Wiley.

Ruscio, A. M., Brown, T. A., Chiu, W. T., Sareen, J., Stein, M. B., & Kessler, R. C.
(2008). Social fears and social phobia in the USA: Results from the National
Comorbidity Survey Replication. *Psychological Medicine, 38*(1), 15.

Rutherford, K., McIntyre, J., Daley, A., & Ross, L. E. (2012). Development of expertise in mental health service provision for lesbian, gay, bisexual, and transgender communities. *Medical Education, 46*(9), 903–913.

Sandfort, T. G. M., de Graaf, R., Bijl, R. V., & Schnabel, P. (2001). Same-sex sexual behavior and psychiatric disorders: Findings from the Netherlands Mental Health Survey and Incidence Study (NEMESIS). *Archives of General Psychiatry, 58*(1), 85–91.

Schatzberg, A. F., Cole, J. O., & Debattista, C. (2010). *Manual of clinical psychopharmacology* (7th ed.). Arlington, VA: American Psychiatric Publishing.

Schiller, J. S., Lucas, J. W., Ward, B. W., & Peregoy, J. A. (2012). Summary health statistics for U.S. adults: National Health Interview Survey, 2010. *Vital and Health Statistics, 10*(252), 1–207.

Shedler, J. (2010). The efficacy of psychodynamic psychotherapy. *American Psychology, 65*(2), 98–109.

Stein, D. J. (2002). Obsessive-compulsive disorder. *Lancet, 360*(9330), 397–405.

Sunderland, M., Hobbs, M., Andrews, G., & Craske, M. G. (2012). Assessing DSM-IV symptoms of panic attack in the general population: An item response analysis. *Journal of Affective Disorders, 143*(1), 187–195.

Swedo, S. E., Leckman, J. F., & Rose, N. R. (2012). From research subgroup to clinical syndrome: modifying the PANDAS criteria to pescribe PANS (pediatric acute-onset neuropsychiatric syndrome). *Pediatrics & Therapeutics, 2*(2), 1–8.

Thoma, N. C., McKay, D., Gerber, A. J., Milrod, B. L., Edwards, A. R., & Kocsis, J. H. (2012). A quality-based review of randomized controlled trials of cognitive-behavioral therapy for depression: An assessment and metaregression. *American Journal of Psychiatry, 169*(1), 22–30.

U.S. Census Bureau. (2005). Table 2: Annual estimates of the population by selected age groups and sex for the United States: April 1, 2000 to July 1, 2004 (NC-EST2004-02). Retrieved from http://www.census.gov/popest /national/asrh/NC-EST2004/NC- EST2004-02.xls

Werman, D. S. (2014). *Practice of supportive psychotherapy.* Abingdon, United Kingdom: Routledge

World Health Organization. (2008). *The global burden of disease: 2004 update.* Geneva, Switzerland: Author.

World Health Organization. (2009). Global health risks: Mortality and burden of disease attributable to selected major risks. Retrieved from http://www .who.int/entity/healthinfo/global_burden_disease/GlobalHealthRisks _report_full.pdf

Yalom, I. D., & Leszcz, M. (1995). *The theory and practice of group psychotherapy.* Cambridge, MA: Basic Books.

2

Eating Disorders

Lazaro Zayas, Louis Ostrowsky, and Brian Hurley

Eating disorders cause serious physical and mental health consequences, especially in children, adolescents, and young adults (Goldstein, Dechant, & Beresin, 2011). Many recent studies reveal that over the last 30 to 40 years, the incidence of eating disorders in the United States has been steadily rising. It has been quoted that at any given time, 10 percent or more of late adolescent and adult women report symptoms of eating disorders (Academy for Eating Disorders, 2011). Often thought of as "cognitive disorders" with adverse medical complications, eating disorders are all believed to have some relationship to avoid obesity (Williamson, Martin, & Stewart, 2004a). More specifically, the core psychological feature of all eating disorders is the overevaluation of shape and weight and their control (Fairburn, 2008). Other features that are shared among eating disorders are body image distortions, fears of weight gain, and a drive for thinness (Williamson et al., 2002). The *Diagnostic and Statistical Manual of Mental Disorders*, 5th Edition (DSM-5), includes the feeding and eating disorders of pica, rumination disorder, avoidant/restrictive food intake disorder, anorexia nervosa (AN), bulimia nervosa (BN), binge-eating disorder, as well as other specified feeding or eating disorders, and unspecified feeding or eating disorders. Under the previous edition of the *Diagnostic and Statistical Manual of Mental Disorders* (DSM-IV), the two specified eating disorders were anorexia nervosa (AN) and bulimia nervosa (BN); as well as eating disorder not otherwise specified (EDNOS) (Smink, van Hoeken, & Hoek, 2012). In this prior DSM-IV classification system, EDNOS was the most common eating disorder encountered in clinical practice across clinical and community samples, which highlights the challenge of accurately diagnosing and distinguishing one syndrome from another (Fairburn & Cooper, 2007). The DSM-5 disorders of anorexia nervosa (AN), bulimia nervosa (BN), and binge-eating disorder are the most well characterized with greatest clinical relevance to lesbian, gay, bisexual, and transgender (LGBT) populations and thus will be the dominant focus in this chapter.

Because eating disorders share the core psychological feature of over-evaluation of shape and weight and their control, the judging of self-worth of afflicted individuals is largely impacted by their perceived ability or inability to control their shape and weight. Their perceived need to control their body shape and weight leads to many of the core clinical symptoms and behaviors often observed in these disorders, including rigid and extreme dietary restraint. Table 2.1 includes a list of behaviors typically seen in patients with eating disorders.

Eating disorders often cause significant medical problems, especially if one's undereating leads to significant weight loss. In fact, anorexia nervosa has the highest death rate of any mental health disorder (Williamson et al., 2004a). Medical complications of eating disorders can be life-threatening and often include abnormalities in electrolytes, cardiovascular effects, gastrointestinal effects, endocrine imbalances, and nutritional deficiencies (Patrick, 2002).

In addition to medical complications, eating disorders can also have detrimental effects on an individual's psychosocial functioning. In children and adolescents, eating disorders disrupt their developmental trajectory, thereby placing them under an increased amount of stress (Goldstein et al., 2011). For example, the eating disorder itself might render an individual unable to engage in extracurricular and social activities given the time taken up by the behaviors mentioned. Because of underlying concerns regarding their appearance, socializing might be avoided altogether. Furthermore, academic or professional performance may worsen, given frequent disruptions due to time spent attending treatment appointments or undergoing inpatient hospitalizations.

Given the myriad medical and psychosocial complications that can ensue because of an underlying eating disorder, it is prudent that one identifies and treats these individuals expediently (The Massachusetts General Hospital, 2010). In addition to the aforementioned challenge of categorizing patients under a DSM-IV diagnosis, there are other challenges

Table 2.1   Behaviors Commonly Observed in Eating Disorders

Anorexia: Loss of appetite.

Binge Eating: A "binge" is an episode of eating during which an objectively large amount of food is eaten, given the circumstances, and there is a sense of loss of control at the time.

> *Subjective binge eating*: A "binge" in which the amount eaten is not unusually large, given the circumstances.

> *Objective binge eating*: A true "binge" as defined above.

Calorie counting: The continuous monitoring of calorie intake and the calculation of a running total. Generally, the person is trying to keep under a daily calorie limit, but often, the calorie counting is inaccurate. Underweight patients tend to overestimate their intake, whereas the opposite is more typical of overweight patients.

Debting: The creation of an energy deficit or "debt" (typically through exercising) to accommodate subsequent eating.

Delayed eating: Postponing eating as a means of weight control or resisting binge eating.

Dietary guidelines: General dietary objectives that are flexible in nature.

Driven exercising: A particular form of excessive exercising in which there is a subjective sense of being driven or compelled to exercise; the giving of exercise precedence over other activities and exercising when it might do physical harm.

Excessive exercising: Exercising to an undue extent, either in terms of physical health or psychosocial adjustment or both.

Purging: A collective noun used to denote self-induced vomiting or the misuse of laxatives or diuretics.

> *Compensatory purging*: Episodes of purging designed to compensate for specific episodes of perceived or actual overeating.

> *Noncompensatory purging*: Episodes of purging that are not in response to specific episodes of perceived or actual overeating.

(Adapted from Table 2.2, Fairburn, 2008)

one faces in identifying, designing, and implementing treatments for those with an underlying eating disorder. Some specific challenges often include the secrecy associated with disordered eating behaviors and the ego-syntonic nature, or satisfaction, many experience regarding these behaviors (e.g., restricting and purging) when they are perceived to be successful in achieving the desired weight loss or maintenance of an unhealthy weight (Bankoff, Karpel, Forbes, & Pantalone, 2003). As such, a careful medical and psychosocial assessment for an underlying eating disorder is imperative for both underweight and overweight individuals, or those sus-pected of having disordered eating behavior.

EATING DISORDERS AND LGBT POPULATIONS

Medical knowledge around eating disorders in lesbian, gay, bisexual, and transgender (LGBT) populations has been slowly evolving since the first theories of how sexual orientation affects body image ideals were pub-lished in the late 1980s (Ray, 2007). Early hypotheses suggested that lesbi-ans do not struggle with body image concerns to the same degree as heterosexual women and are therefore less vulnerable to develop disor-dered eating (Brown, 1987). By contrast, gay men were thought to be at relatively increased risk of developing an eating disorder because of the heightened importance they supposedly place on physical attractiveness when selecting a partner (Russell & Keel, 2002). While certain aspects of these theories may prove to be accurate, there is little conclusive evidence to be found in the currently available literature. With so much conflicting information surrounding differences in risk and disease prevalence between homosexual and heterosexual men and women, the only conclu-sion that can be reached at this time is that far more research is needed in this area.

Interest in studying eating disorders in men arose, in part, out of a desire to better characterize their etiology in women. At a time when it was commonly accepted that a complex combination of psycho-cultural factors led to the development of anorexia nervosa (AN) and bulimia ner-vosa (BN), some researchers sought to prove a more simplified biologic explanation. To this end, if it were found that men with eating disorders had similar characteristics to women with EDs, it might support the hypothesis of a homogenous disease entity (Pope & Hudson, 1988). One of the first studies examining eating disorders in a large group of men came out of the Massachusetts General Hospital's Eating Disorders Unit in 1997 (Carlat, Camargo, & Herzog, 1997). They retrospectively examined the medical records of the 135 men treated at MGH between 1980 and 1994 who were confirmed to meet DSM-IV diagnostic criteria for an eating dis-order. The most common DSM-IV diagnosis was BN (46 percent of the study subjects), followed by EDNOS (32 percent), and then AN (22 per-cent). In addition to the finding of other psychiatric disorders that co-occur (more than half of the men met criteria for major depressive disorder, and over one-third struggled with substance abuse), homosexuality/bisexuality was found to be a "specific risk factor" for disordered eating. Patients' self-reported sexual orientation was ascertained for 122 (90 per-cent) of the men in the study population, 27 percent of whom identified as homosexual or bisexual (the two categories were combined in the statistical analysis). Most significant, 42 percent of the men with BN identified as homosexual/bisexual.

The authors of the above study noted, "Many subjects reported that their sexuality played an important role in the development of their eating disorder, and five homosexual men explicitly stated that their eating disorder began in response to pressures toward thinness in the gay subculture." This perspective seemed to be confirmed by a handful of available studies comparing survey results of homosexual and heterosexual men. Their data revealed common findings, such as relatively more body dissatisfaction among gay men and a greater emphasis on physical appearance as a component to their "sense of self" (Silberstein, Mishkind, Striegel-Moore, Timko, & Rodin, 1989). Another study found a positive association between adult gay men's extent of involvement in gay community activities or organizations and their rates of body dissatisfaction (Beren, Hayden, Wilfley, & Grilo, 1996).

Consistent with these findings, a 2004 analysis of 4,374 adolescent boys participating in a longitudinal cohort study called the Growing Up Today Study (GUTS) found that self-identified gay or bisexual boys made more effort to look like men in the media and also binged more than their heterosexual peers (Austin et al., 2004). Yet, as Striegel-Moore and Bulik note in their 2007 review of evidence-based risk factors for eating disorders, these findings do not confirm a definitive causal connection between homosexuality and the development of an eating disorder, especially given the young age (mean age was 14.3 years old) of the sample (Striegel-Moore & Bulik, 2007). It is also possible to find data that suggests that even if differences in gay subculture and their related social influences do exist, they do not clearly create a vulnerability to disordered eating in gay men. A case control study comparing men aged 18 to 25 who met DSM-IV criteria for an eating disorder with an age-matched cohort of men without symptoms of disordered eating found no significant differences in the rate of homosexuality between the two groups (Olivardia, Pope, Mangweth, & Hudson, 1995).

Evidence of the role that homosexuality plays in women's development of eating disorders is remarkably inconsistent, especially when compared to the available literature on gay men. Survey data, which began to appear in peer-reviewed publications in the 1990s, seemed to support contemporary anthropologic views of lesbians as essentially "opposite" heterosexual women in their susceptibility to societal pressures to be thin. For example, the same study that found men's affiliation with the gay community was associated with body dissatisfaction did not find a similar relationship in lesbian women (Beren et al., 1996). Lower rates of dieting and disordered eating behaviors were cited as supporting evidence that lesbians are more likely to be accepting of their bodies (Moore & Keel, 2003). However, there is also a body of research that suggests that lesbians are exposed to and internalize societal body image ideals in the same way as their heterosexual counterparts. Study populations comparing women of different sexual orientations have found lesbians to display equivalent rates of frequent dieting, weight concerns, and disordered eating, including binging and purging (French, Story, Remafedi, Resnick, & Blum, 1996). In fact, some evidence points to lesbian women being at higher risk for binge eating and possessing a relatively stronger connection between self-esteem and satisfaction with their bodies (Striegel-Moore & Huydic, 1993).

While further research is needed to elucidate the mechanisms by which homosexuality potentially increases the risk for developing an ED, current clinical thinking suggests that young patients who are struggling with gender identity or who are coming out may be most predisposed to disordered eating. Advocacy groups, including the National Eating Disorders Association, recommend screening young LGBT patients for ED symptoms, especially those who appear to be at risk for comorbid mood disorders, post-traumatic stress disorders, or homelessness (National Eating Disorders Association, 2012). There is some research that provides hopeful results. A 2007 study utilizing DSM-IV criteria found that a "sense of connectedness to the gay community" is protective against developing an eating disorder (National Eating Disorders Association, 2012).

DIAGNOSIS AND CLINICAL FEATURES

Clinically, anorexia nervosa and bulimia nervosa remain disorders with broad clinical significance, and historically, these disorders have remained the focus of most disordered eating research.

Anorexia Nervosa (AN)

The term "anorexia" was first described as a "nervous loss of appetite" in the medical literature of the early 19th century and included extreme fasting and food refusal (Vandereycken, 2002) . It is currently believed that a central feature of AN is an intense fear of fatness that leads to a sustained and determined pursuit of weight loss, often through self-starvation and extreme forms of exercise. In many patients, other motivating psychological factors, including asceticism, competitiveness, and a desire for self-punishment lead to severely restrictive patterns of eating. Because the pursuit to maintain a low body weight is usually successful in patients with AN, their restrictive behavior is not often seen as a problem to them, resulting in very little motivation to change (Beaumont, 2002).

The current diagnostic criteria for AN, as presented in the DSM-5, stipulate that there is food restriction leading to a body weight that is below the least-expected or lowest norm for a person's age, gender, developmental stage, and health. The food-restrictive behavior is accompanied by a fear of—and interference with any action that might cause—weight gain. A person with AN, regardless of their below-average minimum weight and its potential health effects, nonetheless fears gaining weight or becoming "fat." People with this condition have a disturbed perception of their weight or physique, evaluate themselves primarily on this self-evaluation, and/or do not recognize the dangers of their low weight (American Psychiatric Association, 2013).

The DSM-5 further delineates two types of AN—the restricting type and the binge-eating/purging type. Those individuals with the restricting subtype predominantly attain their low body weights through restrictive eating and fasting. Those with the binge-eating/purging subtype typically engage in compensatory behaviors, including diuretic abuse, laxative abuse, self-induced vomiting, and/or excessive exercise (American Psychiatric Association, 2013).

Bulimia Nervosa (BN)

The main clinical feature that distinguishes BN from AN is that attempts to restrict food intake are punctuated by repeated binges (Fairburn & Harrison, 2003) . Following binges, compensatory behaviors are subsequently employed to avoid possible weight gain. Common compensatory behaviors in patients with BN include self-induced vomiting, fasting, laxative use, diuretic use, and/or excessive exercise.

The diagnostic criteria for BN include repeated periods of binge eating and purging, at least one day each week for at least three months. During a binge, the person loses control and cannot stop eating, taking in much more food than what is average for most people in a similar situation and time frame. Afterward, to prevent weight gain, the person engages in unhealthy behaviors that can include forced vomiting or the ingestion of laxatives, diuretics, or drugs. Another behavior to avoid weight gain may be exercise for durations and intensities beyond the norm. Like people with AN, those with BN also primarily base their self-perception on their weight and physique. Their binging and purging, however, occurs even when there is no low body weight, as in AN (American Psychiatric Association, 2013).

Binge-Eating Disorder (BED)

This classification is intended for individuals who experience recurrent episodes of binge eating in the absence of extreme methods of weight control seen in BN and AN. To date, studies have suggested that less than 10 percent of adult eating disorder cases meet diagnostic criteria for BED and BED has yet to be fully clinically characterized.

The DSM-5 diagnostic criteria for binge-eating disorder include repeated periods of binge eating, with marked distress over the behavior when it occurs. At least three of five binge behaviors must be present: eating a lot when not physically hungry, eating uncharacteristically fast, eating alone so no one will see, feeling uncomfortably full or sick afterward, then feeling guilt, depression, or self-disgust. Unlike those affected by BN, people affected by BED do not compensate for the overeating episodes with forced vomiting, medications such as laxatives, or excessive exercise. BED occurs outside any AN or BN episodes (American Psychiatric Association, 2013).

Eating Disorder NOS (EDNOS)

As previously discussed, EDNOS has been the most common eating disorder encountered in clinical practice across clinical and community samples. In the DSM-IV, it is essentially reserved for eating disorders of clinical severity that do not meet strict diagnostic criteria for either AN or BN. As such, most cases of EDNOS have clinical features that resemble those seen in either AN or BN, though at slightly different combinations or levels (Fairburn & Bohn, 2005). DSM-5's Other Specified Feeding or Eating Disorders category is an alternative to the EDNOS category that permits a disordered eating diagnosis for those individuals with disordered eating that resembles AN or BN, but does not meet full DSM-5 diagnostic criteria (American Psychiatric Association, 2012).

PATHOGENESIS

Research to date on eating disorders has mainly centered on anorexia nervosa and bulimia nervosa. The etiologies of both disorders are complex and multifactorial and are currently thought to include biologic (genetic and biological), psychological, and environmental components. Of note, little is known about the individual causal processes involved or about their interactions across these disorders.

Genetic

In studies of twins, clinic subjects show concordance for AN around 55 percent in monozygotic twins and 5 percent in dizygotic twins, with the analogous figures for BN being 35 percent and 30 percent, respectively (Treasure, 1989). These figures suggest that AN is more significantly heritable than BN. In addition, eating disorders occur more frequently in patients who have a family history of eating disorders, obesity, and mood disorders (Goldstein et al., 2011).

Molecular genetic studies on eating disorders to date have not yielded conclusive findings. For AN, linkage analyses have discovered several regions of interest on chromosomes 1, 2, 4, and 13, which are genes involved in the serotonin and cannabinoid systems. For BN, there is evidence of a susceptibility locus on chromosome 10p, which has already been associated with genome scans for obesity (Herpertz-Dahlmann, Holtkamp, & Konrad, 2012).

Neurobiological Findings

The past decade has seen an exponential increase in the number of studies devoted to elucidating the neurobiological underpinnings of eating disorders (Kaye, 2008). Most of the work has centered on neuropeptide and monoamine systems involved in the physiology of eating and weight regulation. Most studies have postulated that altered brain serotonin (5-HT) function contributes to dysregulation of appetite, mood, and impulse control in both AN and BN (Fairburn & Harrison, 2003). Though the studies have had small sample sizes, imaging studies have revealed disturbances in 5-HT function when patients with eating disorders are acutely ill. Interestingly, some of these disturbances persist after recovery, which has led to the development of theories that suggest a trait monoamine abnormality that might predispose some individuals to the development of eating disorders or to associated characteristics.

Psychological

Cognitive-behavioral models of AN have proposed that it is the intense fear of weight gain and degree of body image disturbance that lead to the motivation of afflicted individuals to engage in compensatory behaviors that maintain emaciated body states. Because these behaviors, including restrictive eating, fasting, and/or excessive exercise, are often accompanied by a reduction in the anxiety or stress associated with the fear of weight gain, these behaviors are reinforced, thereby maintaining the disorder (Williamson, White, York-Crowe, & Stewart, 2004b).

Cognitive-behavioral models have also been proposed for BN. Though it appears that binges might be at odds with one's intense fear of weight gain and desire to restrict caloric intake, it has been postulated that binges are a product of dietary restraint. According to Fairburn's cognitive-behavioral theory of eating disorders, patients who binge try to strictly adhere to multiple demanding and highly specific dietary rules instead of adopting general guidelines about how they should eat. Because breaking such strict rules is nearly inevitable, minor dietary slips are handled in an extreme and negative fashion and are usually viewed as evidence of a lack of self-control. As such, these patients respond to such dietary slips by temporarily abandoning their dietary restraint and succumbing to the urge to eat that arises from the restraint itself (Fairburn, 2008).

EPIDEMIOLOGY AND DISTRIBUTION

In general, epidemiological studies provide information about the occurrence of disorders and trends in the frequency of disorders over time. Because eating disorders are relatively rare among the general population and those afflicted with an eating disorder deny or conceal their illness, thereby avoiding professional help, there are a number of methodological issues that make epidemiological studies in this area quite challenging to interpret (Smink et al., 2012). As a result, these factors necessitate that studies use large numbers of subjects from the general population to achieve enough differential power for the cases, which can be quite time-consuming, ineffective, and cost-intensive (Hoek & van Hoeken, 2003). As such, most epidemiological studies on eating disorders use psychiatric case registers or medical records from hospitals in any given area to collect their data. Such studies may therefore underestimate the occurrence of eating disorders in the general population, as many of the afflicted never present to formal medical or psychiatric care. In addition, differences in rates over time could be due to improved diagnostic acumen by clinicians or earlier detection due to increased public awareness instead of a true occurrence.

As previously discussed, the eating disorders section in the DSM-IV comprised the diagnoses of anorexia nervosa, bulimia nervosa, and EDNOS, with EDNOS being the most common in the general population (van Son, van Hoeken, Bartelds, van Furth, & Hoek, 2006). In the DSM-5, the goals of the new section include reducing the size of the EDNOS by broadening the criteria for AN and BN and adding binge-eating disorder as a specific eating disorder in the hopes of accurately diagnosing individuals (Wilson & Sysko, 2009). These DSM-5 changes will alter the coverage and frequency of the disorders as discussed below. The data below are all from DSM-IV criteria, unless otherwise specified.

Incidence and prevalence rates are epidemiologic terms that are the basic measures of disease frequency. The incidence of disease represents the rate of occurrence of new cases arising in a given period in a specified population, while prevalence is the total number of existing cases in the population (Bonita, 2006). The incidence of eating disorders is most often expressed in terms of the number of new cases per 100,000 persons per year (person-years). The study of incidence provides clues to etiology as it relates to new cases of eating disorders. Prevalence can be expressed in a number of ways, including point prevalence (prevalence at a specific point in time), one-year prevalence rate (point prevalence plus annual incidence rate, or number of new cases in the following year), and the lifetime prevalence (proportion of people who had the disorder at any point in their lives). A two-stage screening approach is the standard procedure to estimate the prevalence of eating disorders. In the first stage, a large population is screened for the likelihood of an eating disorder through the use of a screening questionnaire that identifies an at-risk group. In the second stage, definite cases are established on the basis of a personal interview in the at-risk group. The study of prevalence is most useful in planning health care facilities, as it indicates demands of care (Hoek, 2006). Methodological problems in these types of studies include poor response rates, low sensitivity and specificity of screening instruments, and small size of the groups interviewed (Fairburn & Beglin, 1990).

Anorexia Nervosa

Incidence

The highest documented age- and sex-adjusted incidence rate of DSM-IV's AN was 8.3 per 100,000 person-years in Rochester, Minnesota, during a study period that spanned more than 50 years between 1935 and 1989 (Lucas, Crowson, O'Fallon, & Melton, 1999). This study employed an extensive case-finding method that included all medical records of health care providers, general practitioners, and specialists in Rochester. Incident rates derived solely from general practices represent eating disorders at the earliest stage of detection (Smink et al., 2012). In a study performed in the United Kingdom that searched the General Practice Research Database there for new cases of AN between 1994 and 2000 and compared its data with findings from similar studies performed between 1988 and 1993, the age- and sex-adjusted incidence rates of AN were relatively stable between both study periods, yielding a rate of 4.7 per 100,000 person-years in 2000 and 4.2 per 100,000 person-years in 1993 (Currin, Schmidt, Treasure, & Jick, 2005; Turnbull, Ward, Treasure, Jick, & Derby, 1996).

Incidence rates for DSM-IV's AN are highest among females between the ages of 15 and 19 and represent approximately 40 percent of all cases (Hoek, 2006; Hoek & van Hoeken, 2003). One study found an incidence rate of 109.2 per 100,000 15-to-19-year-old females per year between the years 1995 and 1999 (van Son et al., 2006). Though AN also occurs in males, there are few studies that report incidence rate for males. Based on the few studies available, however, it appears as though the incidence of AN among males is below 1.0 per 100,000 persons per year (Hoek, 2006).

Prevalence

In studies of individuals diagnosed with AN using the DSM-IV criteria, prevalence rates of AN have varied between 0 and 0.9 percent, with an average point prevalence rate of 0.29 percent in young females (Hoek & van Hoeken, 2003). The prevalence rate of AN has been found to be approximately 0.3 percent in men (Goldstein et al., 2011). Of note, some studies have found slightly higher prevalence rates for those individuals with partial syndromes of AN.

Bulimia Nervosa

Incidence

Few incidence studies have been conducted since BN was distinguished as a clinical entity separate from AN in 1979. An annual incidence of BN of 13.5 per 100,000 person-years was found in a study conducted in Rochester, Minnesota, between 1980 and 1990, and a similar prevalence rate of 11.5 per 100,000 person-years between 1985 and 1989 (Hoek et al., 1995; Soundy, Lucas, Suman, & Melton, 1995). It is interesting to note that several studies suggest that the age of onset of BN is decreasing. In an Italian study of 793 patients referred to an outpatient unit for eating disorders between 1985 and 2008, subjects born between 1970 and 1972 had a mean age of onset of 18.5 years, compared to a mean age of onset of 17.1 years in patients born between 1979 and 1981 (Favaro, Caregaro, Tenconi, Bosello, & Santonastaso, 2009). In a primary care study done in Holland, the high risk group of BN shifted from females ages 25 to 29 between 1985 and 1989 to females ages 15 to 24 between 1995 and 1999 (van Son et al., 2006). These figures may reflect earlier detection of BN instead of a true earlier age of onset.

Prevalence

The generally accepted point prevalence of DSM-IV's BN is approximately 1 percent in young females. In a large-scale two-stage study done in the United States, however, the lifetime prevalence of BN varied between

0.9 and 1.5 percent among women and between 0.1 and 0.5 percent among men (Hudson, Hiripi, Pope, & Kessler, 2007).

Eating Disorder NOS

Because of the heterogeneity of DSM-IV's EDNOS as detailed above, there are very few epidemiological studies detailing this disorder, though in outpatient settings, EDNOS cases account for an average of 60 percent of all ED cases, as compared with 14.5 percent for AN and 25.5 percent for BN (Hoek, 2006). The prevalence of EDNOS has been estimated to be 3.5 percent in women and 2 percent in men (Hudson et al., 2007).

Distribution of Eating Disorders

Recent data suggest that the incidence and prevalence of eating disorders have increased over recent decades. Though this may be true, greater help-seeking and improved diagnostic acumen may be responsible for this trend (Smink et al., 2012). Table 2.2, adapted from Fairburn, is a summary of what is known to date about the distribution of eating disorders.

Table 2.2   Distribution of Eating Disorders

	Anorexia Nervosa	Bulimia Nervosa
Worldwide distribution	Predominantly Western societies	Predominantly Western societies
Ethnic origin	Mainly Caucasians	Mainly Caucasians
Sex	Mostly female (~90%)	Mostly female (unknown proportion)
Age	Adolescents	Young adults
Social class	Possible excess in higher social classes	Even distribution
Prevalence	0.7% (in teenage girls)	1–2% (in 16- to 35-year-old females)
Incidence (per 100,000 per year)	19 in females, 2 in males	29 in females, 1 in males
Change in prevalence	Possible increase	Likely increase

(Adapted from Panel 2, Fairburn, 2003)

RISK FACTORS

The individual risk of developing an eating disorder may be influenced by a host of epidemiologic, biologic, and genetic factors. Some of these have been described above. For example, the disproportionate prevalence of DSM-IV's AN and BN among adolescent and young adult women suggests that these age and gender characteristics increase the risk of developing these disorders. It appears that there is a heritable component to risk, though the specific genes that cause susceptibility have yet to be confirmed (Grilo & Mitchell, 2010). Evidence of this link has been demonstrated by multiple twin studies that show that identical twins have significantly more risk of developing AN or BN than fraternal twins (Bulik, Sullivan, Wade, & Kendler, 2000; Treasure, 1989). Predisposition for an eating disorder may also be conferred during fetal development. A study comparing outcomes of same-sex twins versus opposite-sex twins found that exposure to testosterone during pregnancy may have a possible protective effect on the risk of eventual development of disordered eating (Culbert, Breedlove, Burt, & Klump, 2007). Additionally, a 2006 study found an inverse relationship between the number of perinatal obstetric complications (including maternal anemia, gestational diabetes, and preeclampsia) and the age of onset of AN (Favaro, Tenconi, & Santonastaso, 2008). Early childhood eating and gastrointestinal problems, as well as other developmental events, such as physical and sexual abuse in childhood, have been found to predispose children to the later development of an eating disorder (Jacobi, Hayward, de Zwaan, Kraemer, & Agras, 2004; Wonderlich, Brewerton, Jocic, Dansky, & Abbott, 1997). These aspects of a patient's history may complicate treatment and clinical course because of the increased risk of related comorbid conditions, including depression, posttraumatic stress disorder, and substance abuse.

The role that gender or any of the above characteristics play as risk factors for the development of disordered eating likely extends beyond biological explanations. Psychological, social, and cultural influences have long appeared to be principal determinants of risk. The classic example found throughout the literature is the theory that body image ideals predominant among women in Western cultures emphasize thinness, which perpetuates a fear of gaining weight or becoming fat (Grilo & Mitchell, 2010). However, the majority of women do not develop an eating disorder, despite exposure to the same cultural climate, leading to the identification of additional variables which may amplify or mitigate against risk arising from the thin beauty ideal (Striegel-Moore & Bulik, 2007). (See Table 2.3.)

One particular social group demonstrated to be at higher risk of developing an eating disorder is athletes. Both male and female athletes can be affected, with prevalence estimates for disordered eating ranging as

Table 2.3   **Psychosocial Risk Factors**

Risk Factor	Psychological Implication
High social class	More attention paid to, and more resources available for, working toward the beauty ideal
Personality traits such as "perfectionism"	One is more eager to comply with social norms
High social anxiety	Increasing one's susceptibility to social feedback
Elevated weight or obesity	Moving one's body further away from the ideal
High "impulsivity"	Making maintenance of restrictive eating more challenging and amplifying risk for binge eating

(Adapted from Striegel-Moore and Bulik, 2007)

high as 62 percent among female athletes and 33 percent among male athletes (Bonci et al., 2008). The percentage of athletes who actually meet criteria for a diagnosable eating disorder is likely significantly lower, but definitive evidence is limited by confounding factors, such as an athlete's rare likelihood of reporting his or her symptoms and greater resistance to starting treatment.

COURSE AND MEDICAL COMPLICATIONS

Eating disorders can cause considerable morbidity, manifested in myriad ways, from severe medical complications to diminished quality of life. Because they often arise at critical times of physical and social development, in adolescence and early adulthood, eating disorders have the potential to greatly influence one's overall life trajectory. Despite engagement in treatment, a significant percentage of patients with an ED, especially AN, succumb to their disease.

Anorexia Nervosa

The clinical course and prognosis for an individual diagnosed with AN is remarkably variable. Outcome studies suggest that less than half of patients with AN achieve total recovery with full resolution of symptoms (Williamson et al., 2004a). Only one-third of all cases achieve even a temporary remission of symptoms, with a further 20 percent of patients most accurately described as chronically ill (Williamson et al., 2004a). Within 10 years of diagnosis, it is estimated that up to 10 percent of patients with AN will die due to complications of chronic starvation, infection, or suicide (Patrick, 2002). This makes AN the leading cause of death in young women aged 15 to 24 and, statistically, the most lethal of any psychiatric diagnosis (Patrick, 2002).

The medical complications that develop from AN can affect every organ system and, depending on extent and severity, may require immediate intervention—at times, against a patient's will. The most obvious outward signs of significant physical changes secondary to AN include symptoms of starvation, and skin abnormalities such as thinning hair. Lanugo, a fine, downy hair, can be seen to develop on the face, neck, and back. Other dermatologic abnormalities include carotodermia, a yellowish tinge to the skin that occurs secondary to excess ingestion of vegetables (Fairburn & Harrison, 2003). Patients may notably try to hide their thinning frames or skin changes by wearing baggy clothing, using makeup, and grooming carefully. However, once these physical signs are present, other more serious underlying pathology may be found on physical exam or laboratory analysis. A careful history may reveal other common (and concerning) symptoms such as sensitivity to cold, bloating, dizziness or syncope, and loss of menstruation (Fairburn & Harrison, 2003).

A detailed physical exam is an essential part of the initial workup in a patient with a suspected eating disorder, especially if they are reporting any of the symptoms above. In addition to emaciation and characteristic skin changes, signs to look for include:

- Cold hands and feet; low body temperature
- Low heart rate; low blood pressure; heart rhythm problems (especially in underweight patients and those with electrolyte abnormalities)
- Swelling in the hands and feet (complicating assessment of body weight)
- Weaker muscles in the torso, pelvis, and upper legs (elicited as difficulty rising from a squatting position) (Fairburn & Harrison, 2003)

The presence of these exam findings may warrant laboratory investigations to check for electrolyte abnormalities and other signs of organ damage (electrocardiograms) to assess for the presence of abnormal heart rhythm, and urine and stool studies. Table 2.4 outlines the range of physical problems that may be uncovered.

Because the medical complications of AN can be life-threatening, patients may be compelled to undergo treatment, even against their will. The criteria that have been proposed to determine when it is appropriate to begin involuntary administration of fluids and nutrients will be reviewed in the following Treatment section. However, it is important to note that one of the common and most severe complications of AN that occurs as a consequence of treatment is "refeeding syndrome." Resulting from a complex process of fluid and electrolyte shifts throughout the body, sudden and potentially fatal drops in serum phosphate, potassium, and magnesium levels can occur in the setting of oral or parenteral nutritional

Table 2.4   Clinical Abnormalities in Anorexia Nervosa

Organ System	Physical Finding
Endocrine	Low luteinizing hormone, follicle-stimulating hormone
	Low T3 syndrome (low T3 and low-to-normal T4 w/normal TSH)
	Mildly elevated plasma cortisol
	Elevated growth hormone concentration
	Severe hypoglycemia (rare)
Cardiovascular	ECG abnormalities (especially in those with electrolyte disturbances)
	Slow heart rate
	Conduction defects
	Q-T interval prolongation
Gastrointestinal	Slow stomach emptying
	Decreased colon motility (secondary to chronic laxative misuse)
	Acute stomach enlargement (rare; secondary to binge eating or excessive refeeding)
Hematological	Moderate normocytic normochromic anemia
	Mild leukopenia with relative lymphocytosis
	Thrombocytopenia
Electrolyte and metabolic abnormalities	Hypercholesterolemia
	Raised serum carotene
	Hypophosphatemia (exaggerated during refeeding)
	Dehydration
	Metabolic alkalosis
	Hypokalemia (secondary to vomiting)
	Metabolic acidosis
	Hyponatremia (secondary to laxative abuse)
Musculoskeletal	Osteopenia and osteoporosis (with heightened fracture risk)
Central nervous system	Enlarged cerebral ventricles and external cerebrospinal fluid spaces (pseudoatrophy)

(Adapted from Panel 5, Fairburn, 2003)

replacement in the severely starved anorexic patient. Clinical warning signs include respiratory distress, signs of pneumonia, heart failure, muscle problems, and neuropathy (Patrick, 2002). Strategies to prevent refeeding syndrome include following clinical guidelines to help identify patients who are at greatest risk of developing this complication and using electrolyte supplementation to prevent low phosphate levels (Terlevich et al., 2003).

Bulimia Nervosa

The clinical course of bulimia is even more variable than that of AN because of the nature of the disorder. Although BN has a slightly later age of onset, the disordered eating often begins with a restricting pattern that is similar (and often meets criteria) for AN (Fairburn & Harrison, 2003). Over time, patients develop binge-eating behavior, which leads to a stabilization of their weight but also compensatory purging behaviors (Fairburn, Cooper, Doll, Norman, & O'Connor, 2000). This cycle leads to a self-perpetuating pattern of disordered eating that can continue in various forms without the obvious clinical consequences of extended restricting seen with AN. The mortality rate for BN is significantly lower than the rate for AN, though the actual lethality of BN is likely worse than the numbers suggest. Within 10 years of diagnosis, 1 to 2 percent of patients with BN will likely die (Patrick, 2002). However, this statistic does not capture the 50 percent of patients with AN who become bulimic during the course of their illness (Patrick, 2002). About half of patients with BN have no clinical symptoms after five years, compared to 20 percent who continue to fulfill DSM criteria for the disorder (Fairburn et al., 2000).

Patients with BN may develop any of the medical complications outlined above for AN, especially if they display significant weight loss and emaciation. However, many patients with BN develop only minor physical consequences, enabling their disordered eating to continue undetected (Hoek et al., 1995). There are a few notable patterns of medical complications that occur secondary to BN, the most severe of which are electrolyte abnormalities. Periods of extended or frequent vomiting result in lowering of blood pressure, changes in electrolytes, and heart rhythm abnormalities (Patrick, 2002). Frequent laxative or diuretic misuse can lead to low blood sodium and metabolic problems, placing a patient at risk of mental status changes and seizures (Fairburn & Harrison, 2003). Characteristic physical exam findings in patients with frequent vomiting include poor dentition or obvious damage to the teeth, including the erosion of the inner surface of front teeth (Fairburn & Harrison, 2003). Bulimic patients who frequently vomit may also demonstrate conspicuous swelling of salivary glands.

Binge-Eating Disorder and Eating Disorder NOS

There is limited evidence currently available to definitively characterize the clinical courses of BED and EDNOS (Fairburn et al., 2000). Some generally established aspects of the natural history of BED include relatively later onset than other eating disorders (patients are often in their 40s) and many years of self-reported overeating, often in response to stress (Fairburn & Harrison, 2003). Patients with BED are thought to have a relatively high likelihood of achieving symptom reduction and even clinical remission, even spontaneously, without any treatment intervention (Fairburn et al., 2000). The only clearly defined medical complication of BED is fairly obvious. Recurrent binge episodes without the presence of compensatory mechanisms to counter the excess caloric intake, such as those present in bulimia, often lead to obesity (Fairburn et al., 2000). By extension, patients are at risk for developing all of the chronic comorbidities commonly associated with obesity, including hypertension, diabetes, and coronary and peripheral vascular disease.

TREATMENT

The approach to treating a patient with an eating disorder is complex, often employing many modalities of treatment, and requires a multidisciplinary team of medical and psychiatric specialists. The first essential goal of treatment is to establish a patient's safety and assess the need for medical and nutritional stabilization. Although the majority of severely medically ill patients will be those with dangerously low weights secondary to anorexia, the electrolyte abnormalities that can be associated with vomiting, laxative, and diuretic misuse found in bulimia should not be overlooked. Regarding long-term treatment, there is a relative abundance of evidence-based therapeutic interventions to guide the management of patients with BN. This is in comparison to very few published randomized controlled trials examining the long-term effectiveness of treatment in AN (Berkman et al., 2006). Current research efforts are focused on building greater evidence to guide the treatment of AN, creating therapeutic interventions specific for BED, and obtaining long-term outcome data for all classes of eating disorders (Fairburn & Bohn, 2005).

Anorexia Nervosa

The initial approach to a patient suspected of having AN includes a comprehensive medical evaluation, including assessment of vital signs, blood chemical analysis, and heart rhythm check (electrocardiogram, or ECG) (Attia & Walsh, 2009). The American Psychiatric Association (APA) has published recommendations that guide emergent treatment. Patients meet criteria for inpatient hospitalization if they are 75 percent of their ideal body weight (or any adult with a body mass index (BMI) less than or equal to 16.5), are found to have any significant medical complications

(such as electrolyte abnormalities, end organ damage, or unstable or compromised vital signs), are at risk for suicide, or are placing a pregnancy at
risk (Berkman et al., 2006). Hospitalization, such as partial hospitalization
or an outpatient program, is also indicated for patients who have failed
lower levels of care or those who are unlikely to be successfully managed in
less contained treatment environments because of psychiatric comorbidity
or limited social support. An analysis of insurance databases found that
the average length of stay for inpatient treatment in the United States is 26
days, which is remarkably shorter compared to treatment averages across
Europe, which range from 40.6 days in Finland to 135.8 days in Switzerland (Berkman et al., 2006).

For patients who are not so medically compromised that they necessitate admission to a hospital, treatment interventions can be provided in a
variety of settings, from structured residential programs to outpatient
care. Best-practice guidelines from organizations such as the APA and the
American Academy of Pediatrics suggest that patients receive their care
from a multidisciplinary treatment team of psychiatrists, psychologists,
social workers, nutritionists, and primary care pediatricians or internists
(Attia & Walsh, 2009). The treatment of AN is based on widely accepted
clinical experience rather than evidence-based research. A 2007 systematic review of the currently available literature on the treatment of AN
found that "the literature on medication treatments and behavioral treatments for adults with anorexia nervosa is sparse and inconclusive" (Bulik,
Berkman, Brownley, Sedway, & Lohr, 2007). Despite reviewing 32 published studies, the authors concluded that "evidence for AN treatment is
weak; evidence for treatment-related harms and factors associated with
efficacy of treatment are weak; and evidence for differential outcome by
sociodemographic factors is nonexistent" (Bulik et al., 2007).

Common approaches to treating AN include various modalities of individual and group psychotherapy (cognitive behavioral, interpersonal, and
psychodynamic), family therapy, psychological and nutritional education,
and medications. Both inpatient and outpatient treatment centers are
likely to use a structured behavioral program that focuses on refeeding for
weight restoration, reinstating normal eating behavior, and ultimately
instilling skills for relapse prevention (Attia & Walsh, 2009). Data suggest
that cognitive behavioral psychotherapy may reduce the risk of relapse, and
it has been demonstrated that it is more likely to achieve a better outcome
when combined with concomitant antidepressant medication (Pike,
Walsh, Vitousek, Wilson, & Bauer, 2003). Medications that have been
studied in this population include antidepressants, nutritional supplementation (e.g., zinc), and hormonal treatment with testosterone, growth hormone, and estrogen/progesterone (Bulik et al., 2007). More recently, treatment
with atypical antipsychotics, notably olanzapine, has been found to result

in increased rate of weight gain and improved obsessional symptoms (Attia & Walsh, 2009). For adolescent patients, some form of family therapy is often strongly recommended, and there are differing schools of thought around how this should be structured. For example, one well-known and widely practiced approach is the Maudsley Method, in which the family is treated together as a unit and parents are supported in initially refeeding their child and then turning that responsibility over to the adolescent.

Bulimia Nervosa

Similar to the treatment for anorexia, the initial approach to a patient with BN includes a comprehensive medical evaluation (Berkman et al., 2006). Also similar to AN, guidelines suggest that patients with BN who develop significant medical complications, those who are pregnant, and patients who are unable to control a binge-purge cycle in outpatient treatment or in a partial hospitalization setting warrant inpatient admission (Berkman et al., 2006). A robust body of evidence (over 50 positive randomized studies) has proven that a specific type of cognitive behavioral therapy developed by Christopher Fairburn beginning in the 1980s is the most effective treatment for BN (Fairburn & Harrison, 2003). Fairburn's model of cognitive behavioral psychotherapy for BN typically involves 20 sessions over five months and focuses on modifying the specific behaviors and thought patterns that maintain the disordered eating behavior (Fairburn & Harrison, 2003). More recent studies have suggested that interpersonal therapy may be as effective as cognitive behavioral psychotherapy (Shapiro et al., 2007). The current standard of care for treating BN includes both psychotherapy and pharmacotherapy. Positive medication trials have demonstrated the antidepressant fluoxetine (60 mg/day) to effectively reduce symptoms of both binging and purging over an 8-to-16-week period (Berkman, Lohr, & Bulik, 2007). This led to the FDA approving fluoxetine for the treatment of BN in 1996, making it the only medication with an approved indication for an eating disorder. However, studies are essentially limited to only relatively short-term follow-up periods, leaving a need for further research into the optimal duration of medication treatment.

Binge Eating Disorder and Eating Disorder NOS

The treatment for BED has, generally, been a direct extension of interventions that had been found to be efficacious for binge eating symptoms in bulimia. Recently there has been a greater focus on finding evidence to support treatments specifically for BED. In general, the primary targets for treatment in BED are decreasing the extent and frequency of binge eating behavior and those that lead to reductions in weight in overweight and obese patients (Berkman et al., 2006). Similar to the available evidence for BN, there are positive studies that show antidepressants have a short term benefit in terms of symptom reduction, but there is no definitive evidence to confirm which medications work best, or that any have efficacy for long term abstinence from binging or maintained weight loss (Brownley, Berkman, Sedway, Lohr, & Bulik, 2007). Although some studies suggest that cognitive behavioral psychotherapy for BED results in decreased rates of binging, there is no definitive evidence that it results in significant weight reduction. This has led some to theorize that cognitive behavioral psychotherapy leads to decreased reporting of binging behavior without clinically meaningful reductions in symptoms (Brownley et al., 2007).

REFERENCES

Academy for Eating Disorders. (2011). Prevalence of eating disorders. Retrieved from https://www.aedweb.org/prevalence_of_ed.html

American Psychiatric Association. (2012). DSM-5 development: Binge eating disorder. Retrieved from http://www.dsm5.org/ProposedRevisions/Pages/proposedrevision.aspx?rid=372

American Psychiatric Association. (2013). *Diagnostic and statistical manual of mental disorders* (5th ed.). Arlington, VA: Author.

Attia, E., & Walsh, B. T. (2009). Behavioral management for anorexia nervosa. *The New England Journal of Medicine, 360*(5), 500–506.

Austin, S. B., Ziyadeh, N., Kahn, J. A., Camargo, C. A. J., Colditz, G. A., & Field, A. E. (2004). Sexual orientation, weight concerns, and eating-disordered behaviors in adolescent girls and boys. *Journal of the American Academy Child and Adolescent Psychiatry, 43*(9), 1115–1123.

Bankoff, S. M., Karpel, M. G., Forbes, H. E., & Pantalone, D. W. (2003). A systematic review of dialectical behavior therapy for the treatment of eating disorders. *Eating Disorders, 20*(3), 196–215.

Beaumont, P. J. V. (2002). Clinical presentation of anorexia nervosa and bulimia nervosa. In C. G. Fairburn & K. D. Brownell (Eds.), *Eating disorders and obesity: A comprehensive handbook* (pp. 162–170). New York: Guilford Press.

Beren, S. E., Hayden, H. A., Wilfley, D. E., & Grilo, C. M. (1996). The influence of sexual orientation on body dissatisfaction in adult men and women. *The International Journal of Eating Disorders, 20*(2), 135–141.

Berkman, N. D., Bulik, C. M., Brownley, K. A., Lohr, K. N., Sedway, J. A., Rooks, A., & Gartlehner, G. (2006). *Management of eating disorders. Evidence report/technology assessment No. 135. (Prepared by the RTI International-University of North Carolina Evidence-Based Practice Center under Contract No. 290-02-0016.) AHRQ Publication No. 06-E010.* Rockville, MD: Agency for Healthcare Research and Quality.

Berkman, N. D., Lohr, K. N., & Bulik, C. M. (2007). Outcomes of eating disorders: A systematic review of the literature. *The International Journal of Eating Disorders, 40*(4), 293–309.

Bonci, C. M., Bonci, L. J., Granger, L. R., Johnson, C. L., Malina, R. M., Milne, L. W., . . . Vanderbunt, E. M. (2008). National athletic trainers' association position statement: Preventing, detecting, and managing disordered eating in athletes. *Journal of Athletic Training, 43*(1), 80–108.

Bonita, R. (2006). *Basic Epidemiology* (2nd ed.). Geneva: World Health Organization.

Brown, L. S. (1987). Lesbians, weight and eating: New analyses and perspectives. In Boston lesbian psychologies collective (Ed.), *Lesbian psychologies: Explorations and challenges* (pp. 298–310). Chicago: University of Illinois Press.

Brownley, K. A., Berkman, N. D., Sedway, J. A., Lohr, K. N., & Bulik, C. M. (2007). Binge eating disorder treatment: A systematic review of randomized controlled trials. *The International Journal of Eating Disorders, 40*(4), 337–348.

Bulik, C. M., Berkman, N. D., Brownley, K. A., Sedway, J. A., & Lohr, K. N. (2007). Anorexia nervosa treatment: A systematic review of randomized controlled trials. *The International Journal of Eating Disorders, 40*(4), 310–320.

Bulik, C. M., Sullivan, P. F., Wade, T. D., & Kendler, K. S. (2000). Twin studies of eating disorders: A review. *The International Journal of Eating Disorders, 27*(1), 1–20.

Carlat, D. J., Camargo, C. A., & Herzog, D. B. (1997). Eating disorders in males: A report on 135 patients. *The American Journal of Psychiatry, 154*(8), 1127–1132.

Culbert, K. M., Breedlove, S. M., Burt, S. A., & Klump, K. L. (2007). Prenatal hormone exposure and risk for eating disorders: A comparison of opposite-sex and same-sex twins. *Archves of General Psychiatry, 65*(3), 329–336.

Currin, L., Schmidt, U., Treasure, J., & Jick, H. (2005). Time trends in eating disorder incidence. *The British Journal of Psychiatry, 186*, 132–135.

Fairburn, C. (2008). *Cognitive behavior therapy and eating disorders.* New York: The Guilford Press.

Fairburn, C. G., & Beglin, S. J. (1990). Studies of the epidemiology of bulimia nervosa. *The American Journal of Psychiatry, 147*(4), 401–408.

Fairburn, C. G., & Bohn, K. (2005). Eating disorder NOS (EDNOS): An example of the troublesome "not otherwise specified" (NOS) category in DSM-IV. *Behavior Research and Therapy, 43*(6), 691–701.

Fairburn, C. G., & Cooper, Z. (2007). Thinking afresh about the classification of eating disorders. *The International Journal of Eating Disorders, 40*(3), 107–110.

Fairburn, C. G., Cooper, Z., Doll, H. A., Norman, P., & O'Connor, M. (2000). The natural course of bulimia nervosa and binge eating disorder in young women. *Archves of General Psychiatry, 57*(7), 659–665.

Fairburn, C. G., & Harrison, P. J. (2003). Eating disorders. *Lancet, 361*(9355), 407–416.

Favaro, A., Caregaro, L., Tenconi, E., Bosello, R., & Santonastaso, P. (2009). Time trends in age at onset of anorexia nervosa and bulimia nervosa. *The Journal of Clinical Psychiatry, 70*(12), 1715–1721.

Favaro, A., Tenconi, E., & Santonastaso, P. (2008). Prenatal hormone exposure and risk for eating disorders: a comparison of opposite-sex and same-sex twins. *Archives of General Psychiatry, 63*(1), 82–88.

French, S. A., Story, M., Remafedi, G., Resnick, M. D., & Blum, R. W. (1996). Sexual orientation and prevalence of body dissatisfaction and eating disordered behaviors: A population-based study of adolescents. *The International Journal of Eating Disorders, 19*(2), 119–126.

Goldstein, M. A., Dechant, E. J., & Beresin, E. V. (2011). Eating disorders. *Pediatrcian Review, 32*(12), 508–521.

Grilo, C. M., & Mitchell, J. E. (Eds). (2010). *The treatment of eating disorders—A clinical handbook.* New York: The Guilford Press.

Herpertz-Dahlmann, B., Holtkamp, K., & Konrad, K. (2012). Eating disorders: Anorexia and bulimia nervosa. *Handbook of Clinical Neurology, 106*(3), 447–462.

Hoek, H. W. (2006). Incidence, prevalence and mortality of anorexia nervosa and other eating disorders. *Current Opinion in Psychiatry, 19*(4), 389–394.

Hoek, H. W., Bartelds, A. I., Bosveld, J. J., van der Graaf, Y., Limpens, V. E., Maiwald, M., & Spaaij, C. J. (1995). Impact of urbanization on detection rates of eating disorders. *The American Journal of Psychiatry, 152*(9), 1272–1278.

Hoek, H. W., & van Hoeken, D. (2003). Review of the prevalence and incidence of eating disorders. *International Journal of Eating Disorders, 44*(4), 383–396.

Hudson, J. I., Hiripi, E., Pope, H. G. J., & Kessler, R. C. (2007). The prevalence and correlates of eating disorders in the National Comorbidity Survey Replication. *Biological Psychiatry, 16*(3), 348–358.

Jacobi, C., Hayward, C., de Zwaan, M., Kraemer, H. C., & Agras, W. S. (2004). Coming to terms with risk factors for eating disorders: Application of risk terminology and suggestions for a general taxonomy. *Psychological Bulletin, 130*(1), 19–65.

Kaye, W. (2008). Neurobiology of anorexia and bulimia nervosa. *Physiology Behavior, 94*(1), 121–135.

Lucas, A. R., Crowson, C. S., O'Fallon, W. M., & Melton, L. J. (1999). The ups and downs of anorexia nervosa. *The International Journal of Eating Disorders, 26*(4), 397–405.

The Massachusetts General Hospital. (2010). *McLean Hospital residency handbook of psychiatry.* Philadelphia: Lippincott Williams and Wilkins.

Moore, F., & Keel, P. E. (2003). Influence of sexual orientation and age on disordered eating attitudes and behaviors in women. *The International Journal of Eating Disorders, 34*(3), 370–374.

National Eating Disorders Association. (2012). Eating disorders and LGBT populations. Retrieved from https://www.nationaleatingdisorders.org/eating-disorders-lgbt-populations

Olivardia, R., Pope, H. G. J., Mangweth, B., & Hudson, J. I. (1995). Eating disorders in college men. *The American Journal of Psychiatry, 152*(9), 1279–1285.

Patrick, L. (2002). Eating disorders: A review of the literature with emphasis on medical complications and clinical nutrition. *Alternative Medicine Review, 7*(3), 184–202.

Pike, K. M., Walsh, B. T., Vitousek, K., Wilson, G. T., & Bauer, J. (2003). Cognitive behavior therapy in the posthospitalization treatment of anorexia nervosa. *The American Journal of Psychiatry, 160*(11), 2046–2049.

Pope, H. G. J., & Hudson, J. I. (1988). Is bulimia nervosa a heterogeneous disorder? Lessons from the history of medicine. *The International Journal of Eating Disorders, 7*(2), 155–166.

Ray, N. (2007). *Lesbian, bisexual and transgender youth: An epidemic of homelessness.* New York: National Gay and Lesbian Task Force Policy Institute and the National Coalition for the Homeless.

Russell, C. J., & Keel, P. K. (2002). Homosexuality as a specific risk factor for eating disorders in men. *The International Journal of Eating Disorders, 31*(3), 300–306.

Shapiro, J. R., Berkman, N. D., Brownley, K. A., Sedway, J. A., Lohr, K. N., & Bulik, C. M. (2007). Bulimia nervosa treatment: A systematic review of randomized controlled trials. *The International Journal of Eating Disorders, 40*(4), 321–336.

Silberstein, L. R., Mishkind, M. E., Striegel-Moore, R. H., Timko, C., & Rodin, J. (1989). Men and their bodies: A comparison of homosexual and heterosexual men. *Psychosomatic Medicine, 51*(3), 337–346.

Smink, F. R., van Hoeken, D., & Hoek, H. W. (2012). Epidemiology of eating disorders: Incidence, prevalence and mortality rates. *Current Psychiatry Report, 14*(4), 406–414.

Soundy, T. J., Lucas, A. R., Suman, V. J., & Melton, L. J. (1995). Bulimia nervosa in Rochester, Minnesota from 1980 to 1990. *Psychology Medicine, 25*(5), 1065–1071.

Striegel-Moore, R. H., & Bulik, C. M. (2007). Risk factors for eating disorders. *The American Journal of Psychiatry, 62*(3), 181–198.

Striegel-Moore, R. H., & Huydic, E. S. (1993). Problem drinking and symptoms of disordered eating in female high school students. *The International Journal of Eating Disorders, 14*(4), 417–425.

Terlevich, A., Hearing, S. D., Woltersdorf, W. W., Smyth, C., Reid, D., McCullagh, E., . . . Probert, C. S. (2003). Refeeding syndrome: effective and safe treatment with Phosphates Polyfusor. *Alimentary Pharmacology and Therapeutics, 17*(10), 1325–1329.

Treasure, J. (1989). Genetic vulnerability to eating disorders: Evidence from twin and family studies. In H. Remschmidt (Ed.), *Child and youth psychiatry: European perspective* (pp. 59–68). New York: Hogrefe and Huber.

Turnbull, S., Ward, A., Treasure, J., Jick, H., & Derby, L. (1996). The demand for eating disorder care. An epidemiological study using the general practice research database. *The British Journal of Psychiatry, 169*(6), 705–712.

van Son, G. E., van Hoeken, D., Bartelds, A., van Furth, E. F., & Hoek, H. W. (2006). Time trends in the incidence of eating disorders: A primary care study in the Netherlands. *The International Journal of Eating Disorders, 39*(7), 565–569.

Vandereycken, W. (2002). History of anorexia nervosa and bulimia nervosa. In C. G. Fairburn & K. D. Brownell (Eds.), *Eating disorders and obesity: A comprehensive handbook* (pp. 151–155). New York: Guilford Press.

Williamson, D. A., Martin, C. K., & Stewart, T. (2004a). Psychological aspects of eating disorders. *Best Practice & Research: Clinical Gastroenterology, 18*(6), 1073–1088.

Williamson, D. A., White, M. A., York-Crowe, E., & Stewart, T. M. (2004b). Cognitive-behavioral theories of eating disorders. *Behavior Modification, 28*(6), 711–738.

Williamson, D. A., Womble, L. G., Smeets, M. A., Netemeyer, R. G., Thaw, J. M., Kutlesic, V., & Gleaves, D. H. (2002). Latent structure of eating disorder symptoms: A factor analytic and taxometric investigation. *The American Journal of Psychiatry, 159*(3), 412–418.

Wilson, G. T., & Sysko, R. (2009). Frequency of binge eating episodes in bulimia nervosa and binge eating disorder: Diagnostic considerations. *The International Journal of Eating Disorders, 42*(7), 603–610.

Wonderlich, S. A., Brewerton, T. D., Jocic, Z., Dansky, B. S., & Abbott, D. W. (1997). Relationship of childhood sexual abuse and eating disorders. *Journal of the American Academy Child and Adolescent Psychiatry, 36*(8), 1107–1115.

3

Substance Use and Abuse among LGBT Populations

Faye Chao and Elie G. Aoun

Substance use disorders (SUDs) are common among LGBT people, and substance use plays a significant role in the lives of many. The Institute of Medicine report (Institute of Medicine Committee on Lesbian, Gay, Bisexual, and Transgender Health Issues and Research Gaps and Opportunities, 2011), as well as GLMA's companion document to the surgeon general's Healthy People 2020 report (Gay and Lesbian Medical Association & U.S. Department of Health and Human Services, 2001), discuss the limited state of research studies addressing health disparities for the LGBT population in general, but in particular for LGBT subpopulations such as transgender people and certain racial/ethnic groups. Most available research indicates a higher prevalence of SUDs in LGBT people compared to heterosexual cisgender individuals. Studies also highlight increased rates of club or party drug use among gay men. In addition, high-risk behaviors such as unprotected anal intercourse and sharing of needles often occur under the influence of substances.

Understanding specificities of SUDs in LGBT populations, such as minority stress, resiliency, risky behaviors, and specific substances used, as well as the intricacies of the interplay between sexual orientation and gender identity, substance use, and societal pressure, is important for providing adequate services that meet the needs of this population. Concerns for internalized homophobia and societal antigay bias are common, guide specific considerations in treatment, and define prognosis and clinical and social outcomes.

In this chapter, we review the limited research available on substance use in LGBT populations. We discuss the role of drugs and alcohol in supporting maladaptive coping mechanisms such as denial, suppression, and repression, and how this leads to high-risk behaviors, in the hopes that better understanding this interplay can shed light on treatment considerations.

OVERVIEW OF SUBSTANCE USE DISORDERS IN THE LGBT POPULATION

Terminology

Not unlike LGBT terminology, SUD "jargon" can be complicated by nuances that can influence how information is communicated and sometimes carry affect, judgment, or historical context. As such, it is important to review some of the language and definitions used in the field of addictions.

Abstinence: Refraining from using the substance that a person has become dependent on.

Abuse (Substance Abuse): Nonspecific term referring to a maladaptive pattern of excessive use of a substance, use in a way other than what it was intended for, or use of a drug not as prescribed. Substance abuse is listed as a clinical diagnosis in the DSM-IV, commonly referring to less severe substance use patterns than substance dependence, but both diagnoses were dropped in the DSM-5 and replaced with the broader diagnosis of SUD.

Addict: A stigmatizing term used to refer to people with a SUD and carrying moral, health, safety, and social undertones (also commonly used in self-help groups to remind a person that they have a problem).

Addiction: A chronic neurobiological disease with genetic and psychosocial influences causing the compulsive and repetitive seeking of a substance or behavior that is often associated with physical dependence, withdrawal, and tolerance. The term is frequently used interchangeably with SUD or dependence.

Adult Children of Alcoholics (ACOA): A support group for the adult children of people with an alcohol use disorder (AUD). May also be used to refer to common behavioral and cognitive traits shared by children of parents with AUD.

Al-Anon: A self-help group for those with a family member with a SUD.

Alcoholics Anonymous (AA): A self-help group helping those with AUD with recovery and continued sobriety using a 12-step treatment model.

Agonist: In the context of SUD, an agonist is a drug of abuse or medication that binds to and activates a receptor mimicking the effects of natural (in the case of drugs of abuse) or abused substances (in the case of treatment medications). For example, heroin is an agonist at the brain opioid receptors, mimicking the effects of natural opioids produced by the brain, and methadone used in the treatment of opioid use disorder (OUD) mimics the effects of heroin.

Antagonist: In the context of SUD, an antagonist is a chemical that binds to a receptor to block or reverse its activation and the response that would have followed. For example, in the case of opioid overdoses, naloxone is administered to reverse the activation of opioid receptors, thus reversing the opioid's effects.

Benzodiazepines (benzos): A prescribed medication used to relieve acute anxiety (among other indications) with significant potential for dependence.

Buprenorphine: A prescribed, highly controlled medication that is a long-acting opioid partial agonist. It binds to the same receptors as a full agonist but activates it only partially and is used for the maintenance treatment of OUD. It is most commonly formulated with naloxone (an opioid antagonist) to prevent intravenous misuse of the medication.

Comorbidity (dual diagnosis): In the context of SUD, refers to having a SUD as well as a co-occurring psychiatric illness.

Compulsion: Repetitive behaviors driven by obsessive thoughts or urges that are aimed at reducing distress or preventing a real or imagined negative consequence of not engaging in the behavior.

Craving (urges): A strong desire or an overpowering urge for a substance or a behavior.

Dependence (substance dependence): A clinical diagnosis from the DSM-IV referring to SUD that was removed from the DSM-5. It is also used in the context of physical dependence (referring to the development of withdrawal and tolerance) or psychological dependence (the compulsion to use a substance for its pleasurable effects or to alleviate the fear of its withdrawal effects).

Detoxification (detox): The process of clearing a substance from the body. Withdrawal symptoms emerge during this time. Detox may take place under medical supervision (in an inpatient or an ambulatory setting) or not.

Dopamine: A neurotransmitter (brain chemical) that drives the reward pathway, commonly thought of as the underlying neurobiological mechanism behind SUD.

Enabling: The psychological effects of one's substance use on family members and friends. It typically involves helping the patient to avoid the consequences of their use and leads to guilt, relationship problems, and functional decline.

Harm reduction: A model that guides treatment and public policy for SUD, aiming at reducing adverse health, social, and economic consequences of substance use. It contrasts with the abstinence-only model.

Maintenance: The concept of stabilizing a patient on a long-term medication regimen. In the context of OUD, it often refers to the long-term prescribing of opioid agonist medications such as buprenorphine or methadone.

Narcotics Anonymous (NA): A self-help group helping those with OUD with recovery and continued sobriety using a 12-step treatment model.

Opioid-Induced Hyperalgesia: The increased pain sensitivity in persons with OUD.

Partial Agonist: In the context of SUD, a chemical possessing properties of agonists at lower doses and antagonists at higher doses. Buprenorphine is one such compound.

Post-Acute Withdrawal Syndrome (PAWS): Symptoms of withdrawal that continue after the initial acute withdrawal syndrome resolves. It frequently leads to relapses in the months following the discontinuation of substance use.

Recovery: The change in attitudes and behaviors that often accompanies abstinence from substance use. For many, it can be synonymous with a way of living in sobriety.

Sobriety: Refers to abstaining from substance use but, in contrast to recovery, does not necessarily imply a change in attitude.

Substance Use Disorder: The DSM-5 term referring to maladaptive substance use. It replaces older DSM-IV terms, including substance abuse and substance dependence.

Tolerance: The condition whereby higher doses of the same substance are required to achieve the same effect.

Withdrawal: Physical and emotional symptoms that occur following the discontinuation of substance use, typically consisting of symptoms that are opposite to the desired effects of the substance used.

Epidemiology of Substance Use and Substance Use Disorders in LGBT Populations

A relatively limited scientific literature, with significant methodological limitations, has been published over the past three decades examining patterns of substance use among the LGB population. Even less is known about transgender people and substance abuse. Most available studies seem to report that rates of SUD are higher in LGB individuals than heterosexual people and that these higher rates may hold true across age groups. Estimates of overall SUD prevalence among LGB populations are thought to range between 28 and 35 percent, roughly threefold that of the general population (Cabaj, 1997; Gillespie & Blackwell, 2009; Green & Feinstein, 2012). Using data from the 1996 National Household Interview Survey, Cochran et al. documented that homosexual or bisexual individuals were more than twice as likely as heterosexual individuals to report maladaptive drug use (16 percent vs. 7.7 percent for men and 14 percent vs. 3.8 percent for women) or SUD (5.7 percent vs. 2.8 percent for men and 5 percent vs. 1.3 percent for women) (Cochran, Ackerman, Mays, & Ross, 2004).

Gay men are the most studied group. One large survey found that using any substance except for alcohol was 3.6 times higher among men who have sex with men (MSM) compared with the national household survey. Most striking was the relative risk for nitrites (21.6), sedatives (6.98), hallucinogens (6.14), tranquilizers (4.99), and stimulants (4.47) (Stall & Purcell, 2000). The 2001 Urban Men's Health Study, looking at a large sample of MSM from four major urban centers, reported that 85 percent used alcohol and 52 percent used drugs recreationally. As many as 12 percent had three or more alcohol-related problems, 18 percent reported multiple drug use, 19 percent frequent drug use, and 8 percent frequent heavy alcohol use (Stall et al., 2001). Another study looking at substance use patterns among MSM in seven major U.S. urban areas reported that, in the past six months, 88 percent had used alcohol, 5 percent drank on four or more occasions weekly, two-thirds had used illegal drugs, 29 percent used drugs weekly or more frequently, and 28 percent used three or more drugs (Thiede et al., 2006). The most commonly used drugs were marijuana (59 percent), cocaine (21 percent), amphetamines (20 percent), ecstasy (19 percent), hallucinogens (19 percent), and nitrite inhalants (14 percent). African American, Asian/Pacific Islander, and Hispanic MSM were less likely than whites to report drug use. Such numbers represent a striking comparison to an age-matched sample from the 2014 national household survey, where 36.1 percent of young adults aged 18 to 25 years reported using drugs and 76.5 percent reported using alcohol in the past year (Center for Behavioral Health Statistics and Quality, 2015). Such results have been replicated in several similar studies (Greenwood et al., 2001; Sullivan, Nakashima, Purcell, Ward, & the Supplement to HIV/AIDS Surveillance Study Group, 1998; Kann et al., 1999). Methamphetamine and club drug use has increased significantly since the late 1980s, as they are popular at circuit parties and may lead to improved self-esteem, decreased social awkwardness, increased sexual activity (sexual encounters lasting up to several hours, with multiple sexual partners) and heightened sexual experience (Green & Halkitis, 2006; Kelly, Parsons, & Wells, 2006; Wainberg, Kolodny, & Drescher, 2006). Methamphetamine use is even more common among MSM who are HIV positive (Semple, Strathdee, Zians, & Patterson, 2012).

Not unlike gay men, lesbians have also been reported to have an increased prevalence of SUD, albeit with a significantly smaller number of studies examining this subject. Alcohol is used more commonly across the life span than drugs in this population. Two surveys have identified lesbians as having an increased prevalence of risk factors for AUD, including family history of AUD, rape and childhood sexual abuse, and a history of suicide attempts (Roberts, Grindel, Patsdaughter, DeMarco, & Tarmina, 2004; Hughes, 2003). Unlike studies of alcohol use in the general population, where alcohol use tends to decrease with age, no such trends were identified in lesbians, where older lesbians were found particularly vulnerable (Hughes et al., 2006).

While very few studies have looked exclusively at the bisexual subpopulation, it appears that those who self-identify as bisexual have a higher prevalence of alcohol and drug use compared to those who identify as homosexual or heterosexual (Thiede et al., 2003; Marshal et al., 2008).

There has been a renewed interest over the past decade in psychosocial research into transgender populations. Studies indicate that rates of SUD are particularly elevated (Santos et al., 2014). While the majority of available data comes from convenience samples, research demonstrates that transgender women are more likely to use than transgender men. Among transgender women, 69 percent reported using any drug in the previous six months, 82 percent reported using alcohol (Rowe et al., 2015), 18 to 30 percent reported using injection drugs (Clements-Nolle et al., 2001; Sevelius, Reznick, Hart, & Schwarcz, 2009), and 27 to 51 percent reported binge drinking (Rowe et al., 2015; Sevelius et al., 2009). Thirty-four percent have used injection drugs at any point in their lifetime (Clements-Nolle et al., 2001). For transgender men, 4 percent reported using injectable drugs in the previous six months and 18 percent in their lifetime (Clements-Nolle et al., 2001).

The vast majority of the data discussed above comes from cross-sectional studies of adult LGBT individuals. It appears that the trends discussed above are not limited to the adult population, suggesting that the higher prevalence of SUD may manifest in early adolescence. In fact, Marshal et al. (2008) published a meta-analysis looking at 18 studies concerning SUD in LGBT youth and reported that substance use in this population is 190 percent higher than for heterosexual youth (and, strikingly, 340 percent higher for bisexual youth and 400 percent higher for female LGB individuals). This is corroborated with similar trends from studies outside the United States, including Canada (Saewyc et al., 2006),

Australia (Smith, Lindsay, & Rosenthal, 1999), New Zealand (Fergusson, Horwood, & Beautrais, 1999), and Thailand (Van Griensven et al., 2004).

RISK FACTORS FOR SUBSTANCE USE IN THE LGBT POPULATION

Understanding the fixed as well as the modifiable risk factors and social determinants of SUD in the LGBT population serves an important clinical function not only to prevent and manage health and psychosocial conse-quences of substance use but also as a broad strategy to address and pre-vent high-risk behaviors, promote safer sex practices, and limit the spread of HIV and other sexually transmitted diseases. In fact, most LGBT indi-viduals are familiar with safer sex but fail to practice it while under the influence of alcohol or other substances (Choi et al., 2005). It is hypothe-sized that such behavior is complex and mediated by a combination of dir-ect and indirect effects of substances. Substances may directly affect risk-taking behavior by leading to increased libido and an increased inten-sity of the sexual act. They may also indirectly affect behavior by decreas-ing the cognitive awareness of the risks associated with unsafe sex. There may also be a common underlying vulnerability where certain charactero-logic traits, including compulsivity or risk taking, can lead to both sub-stance use and high-risk sexual behaviors (Stall, McKusick, Wiley, Coates, & Ostrow, 1986).

Psychosocial Determinants of Mental Health

Many of the risk factors for SUD in the general population, such as mood disorders, single-parent household, lack of parental supervision, or a family history of SUD, also apply to LGBT populations (Thiede et al., 2003; Kecojevic et al., 2012). Within the LGBT community, a personal history of physical or sexual abuse is associated with an increased risk for substance use, in particular for stimulants (associated with physical abuse) and tran-quilizers (associated with sexual abuse), and emotional abuse is suggested to carry similar risks (Kecojevic et al., 2012). Similarly, LGBT identity has been found to be associated with earlier initiation of sedative and opioid use but not stimulants (Kecojevic et al., 2012), and earlier initiation has been shown to lead to an increased prevalence and a more rapid progres-sion to SUD (Clark, Kirisci, &Tatar, 1998; Kandel, Yamaguchi, & Chen, 1992).

It also appears that the prevalence of substance use is highest among bisexuals and those who are "out" or self-identify as LGBT, and these asso-ciations are strongest for "harder" drugs such as cocaine and injection drugs (Thiede et al., 2003; Marshal et al., 2008). In fact, multiple substance use has been found to correlate with being "out" to a higher percentage of people (Thiede et al., 2003). This may be an indicator of the need to "self-medicate" the anxiety stemming from the actual or anticipated fear of social victimization (stigmatizing or denigrating nonheterosexual or non-gender-conforming identities, affecting housing, employment, and inter-personal relationships among others) associated with dealing with one's sexual identity and disclosure. Impaired self-esteem, identity-related shame, and internalized homophobia can lead to substance use as well as high-risk sexual behaviors (Cabaj, 1998; TolouShams et al., 2013). Substance use may provide "emotional security" allowing individuals to be comfortable with their LGBT identity and engage in sexual encounters that others disapprove of and consider shameful. This manifests most clearly with many gay men who see sex and emotional intimacy as two separate, nonintersecting concepts, and using substances may serve the purpose of maintaining this dissociation. Indeed, drugs and alcohol may heighten the intensity of sexual experiences, provide instant gratification, and relieve physical desires but hinder emotional intimacy and love.

Psychoanalysts and psychodynamic theorists suggest that the impetus for substance use in the LGBT community is best understood by thinking about the unconscious or preconscious motivation to defend oneself from intolerable thoughts or emotions. The assumption of an LGBT identity comes with external and internal stressors, the struggle to be accepted by family and friends, and the struggle for self-acceptance combined with the quest to "fit in" with the LGBT community (ageism and expectations of physical appearance at bars, circuit parties, and other LGBT venues tradi-tionally supportive of drug and alcohol use) (Ostrow & Shelby, 2000). These factors lead to anxiety, distress, unprotected vulnerabilities, and feelings of inadequacy, leading to social inhibition. As such, substance use can serve as a vehicle for primitive defenses, including repression and sup-pression, to undo such inhibition, mediate the desires to express sexual fantasies, or allow one to disavow unacceptable aspects of reality, manage distress, and cope with the fear of being alienated (Ostrow & Shelby, 2000).

Minority Stress

Stress is defined as external circumstances that are expected to be strenuous beyond what one is equipped to tolerate, instigating the activa-tion of defenses and other adaptive mechanisms. Stress may lead to emo-tional or somatic symptoms, increasing one's susceptibility to illness and disease. While social stress theory applies to the general experience of an individual maneuvering the challenges of living in a particular society, minority stress relates specifically to those stressors defined by identified differences from the majority (resulting in prejudice and stigma) facing members of a minority group. Minority stress is thought to compromise the person's health and functional status (Meyer, 2003). One's sense of self and well-being is typically developed based on an interpersonal interactions framework and grows by comparing oneself to others. In a society where the majority's values and norms are dominant, minority individuals experience alienation and an impaired sense of belonging and may lack social control, leading to a poorer overall health profile (Meyer, 2003).

In the case of LGBT individuals, their sexual minority status serves as a chronic stressor. As such, they may be subjected to external stressors stemming from stigma and prejudice (violence, discrimination), as well as internal stressors relating to their internal experience of external stressors. The latter can manifest as hypervigilance, fear of rejection, concealment of one's sexual and gender identity, and internalized homophobia. Such processes may be rooted in the early psychosocial development of LGBT individuals. In addition to the challenges of puberty (physical, social, and emotional changes, the exploration of one's individualization, sex, and intimacy) that heterosexual youth have to maneuver through, LGBT youth face additional stressors of nonconforming sexual orientation and/or gender identity. This is particularly challenging as coping mechanisms and resilience skills are typically underdeveloped in adolescence. As such, LGBT youth are often subjected to explicit/personal (including possible devastating parental rejection) or implicit/societal harassment and victimization (although not all LGBT individuals experience the same degree of difficulty) and frequently opt to conceal their LGBT identity from family members, depriving them of parental support and protection from bullying (D'Augelli, 2002). LGBT youth are reported to have higher rates of childhood abuse and, in turn, depression, anxiety, and SUD, as well as increased risk-taking behaviors later in life (Kecojevic et al., 2012; Friedman et al., 2011; Huebner, Rebchook, & Kegeles, 2004). The effects of drugs and alcohol may also be reminiscent of the emotional dissociation state that may LGBT youth adopt to fight (or ignore) the effects of external and internalized homophobia (Cabaj, 2014). According to the minority stress model, substance use reflects a maladaptive mechanism to cope with distress, rapidly relieving intrapersonal and intrapsychic conflict and alleviating self-hatred. As such, substance use may "allow" the individual to feel disinhibited and engage in what sexual behaviors they have grown to believe are unacceptable within societal norms. In some cases, even socializing for an LGBT individual feels "forbidden" unless they use drugs or alcohol.

Minority stress may also lead to the development of a "ghetto mentality," causing many LGBT individuals to create, live, and socialize in LGBT-friendly neighborhoods and cities, bars, and organized parties known as "circuit parties" where substance use is common (particularly methamphetamine and other stimulants, gamma hydroxyl-butyrate [GHB], inhaled nitrites such as poppers, and certain hallucinogens) (Cabaj, 2014).

Transgender individuals may be affected by minority stress even more so than LGB people. They commonly experience discrimination, victimization, and violence both physically and sexually (Hendricks & Testa, 2012). They are also more likely to face violent or lethal police encounters than the general population. There is growing evidence that they also face discrimination based on their gender identity in medical settings, often being denied comprehensive health care or provided with suboptimal services due to bias or unfamiliarity of providers with the specific needs of this community (Stroumsa, 2014). As predicted by the minority stress model, transgender populations have worse mental health outcomes including a higher prevalence of mood, adjustment, and anxiety disorders; suicidal behaviors; and SUD (Polak, Haug, Drachenberg, & Svikis, 2015).

The minority stress model provides a framework for understanding the strained interactions between LGBT individuals and the health care system. In fact, many choose to conceal their LGBT identity from health care providers to prevent actual or anticipated discrimination. Many worry that disclosure could lead to loss of privacy, such as their sexual or gender minority status being revealed to their health insurance providers, employers, or families. In the context of SUD, when seeking treatment, many experience—or worry that they will experience—providers focusing on their LGBT status rather than treating their SUD (Silvestre, Beatty, & Friedman, 2013).

Resiliency

While acknowledging the immense impact of minority stress processes, it is of great clinical and psychosocial significance to appreciate that most LGBT individuals do not develop functionally impairing conditions. In fact, despite victimization and discrimination against LGBT people, most do not engage in unprotected sex and are HIV negative (Stall, Friedman, & Catania, 2008) and, despite the high prevalence of drug use, most manage to avoid developing SUD. As important as identifying risk factors for individuals is recognizing that most go on unaffected despite dealing with difficult psychosocial circumstances. Examining predictors of abstinence and nonproblematic use should be used to develop prevention strategies and intervention programs promoting health for LGBT communities.

It has been postulated that minority status is associated with protective individual and group resources that counteract the effects of minority stress. The concept of resilience has been studied in LGBT populations in an attempt to understand the human capacity for adaptation and harness those coping skills. LGBT persons offset minority stress by developing alternative mechanisms and values, and it appears that the interaction between stress and resilience is the best predictor of mental health outcomes and SUD (Meyer, 2003). Anti-LGBT violence, coming out, and other stressors that could potentially lead to psychiatric symptoms associated with LGBT identity are "opportunities for subsequent growth" where LGBT people learn to manage and overcome the effects of minority stress (Garnets, Herek, & Levy, 1990). Resilience can provide LGBT people with mechanisms to manage bullying, marginalization, and institutional homophobia. These mechanisms could include self-acceptance, rallying family and community support, endurance, developing institutional programs such as gay/straight alliances or Parents and Friends of Lesbians and Gays (PFLAG), cohesiveness, and embracing a sense of community where LGBT persons are able to identify and compare themselves with others.

The theory of resilience has been applied to MSM in particular to develop a framework to promote health, reduce risk-taking behaviors, and prevent HIV infection by channeling prevention resources into strengths-based activities (Herrick et al., 2011). This can be adapted to SUD in the LGBT community. As such, resilience can lead to shamelessness (aka pride); and addressing the consequences of homophobia, both overt and internalized; disrupting the progression of the classical effects of minority stress and its effects on substance use. Social creativity can be used as a protective mechanism against loneliness and social isolation to promote social support, offer alternative and safe community spaces to encourage organic socialization, and manage high-risk situations that may be triggering for alcohol and drug use. Altruism and social activism address social and cultural vulnerability as well as victimization and violence. Self-monitoring promotes empowerment, personal responsibility, and one's control of one's own fate. Finally, social support combats solitude, social isolation, and detrimental interpersonal relationships. In theory, managing these consequences of minority stress would reverse its adverse health consequences, improve mental health outcomes, and help individuals struggling with SUD to preclude the need for self-medicating and achieve and maintain sobriety.

INTERSECTIONALITY, LGBT POPULATIONS, AND SUBSTANCE USE DISORDERS: CO-OCCURRING PSYCHIATRIC, MEDICAL, AND SUBSTANCE USE DISORDERS

Addiction often does not occur in isolation. Certain mental and medical illnesses commonly co-occur with substance use disorders, and it is important to recognize and screen for these comorbidities as treatment of all aspects of an individual's health is necessary for the best outcomes.

Several large epidemiologic studies have been conducted over the past 25 years that have contributed significantly to the body of literature examining the co-occurrence of substance use disorders and other psychiatric illnesses. Three of the largest are the National Comorbidity Survey (NCS), the National Epidemiologic Study of Alcohol and Related Conditions (NESARC), and the National Survey on Drug Use and Health (NSDUH). Of these, the NSDUH is the only one to be updated annually, and the NESARC was the only one to collect sexual orientation data. These surveys give a good overview of the rates of co-occurring mental illnesses in the addicted population, but for data regarding the LGBT population, other studies must be considered. Major depression is the most common psychiatric disorder in patients presenting for treatment of SUD, with lifetime prevalence ranging from 15 to 50 percent in the addicted population (as opposed to 10 percent in the general population). Bipolar disorder and PTSD, though less prevalent overall, increase the likelihood of an SUD by factors of two to four and higher (particularly for patients with bipolar disorder). The rate of PTSD in the general population is about 7 percent, while in the population seeking treatment for SUD, the rate increases to about 25 to 30 percent (Brown, Recupero, & Stout, 1995).

Many studies suggest that LGBT populations have higher incidences of mental illness, with rates around 2.5 times that of the heterosexual cisgender population (Cochran, Sullivan, & Mays, 2003). In a summary of several studies (Cochran, 2001), it was found that there were higher rates of major depression and generalized anxiety disorder in lesbian and gay youth and higher rates of recurrent major depression among gay men. The same report also showed higher rates of anxiety, mood, and substance use disorders, and suicidal thoughts among people ages 15 to 54 with same-sex partners and higher use of mental health services in men and women reporting same-sex partners. Cochran and Cauce used data from the Treatment and Assessment Report Generation Tool (TARGET) database to determine characteristics of persons who identified as LGBT and had sought publicly funded treatment in the state of Washington (Cochran & Cauce, 2006). They found that LGBT individuals had sought prior mental health treatment more frequently, had more recent psychiatric hospitalizations, and were more likely to be taking psychotropic medications than heterosexual cisgender individuals.

There are several implications to these findings. First, people with untreated co-occurring psychiatric illness have poorer outcomes, including more disability overall, frequent hospital visits and hospitalizations, more difficulty maintaining sobriety, and less treatment retention. Second, there are changes in neurobiology related to chronic substance use that can exacerbate co-occurring psychiatric illness, and vice versa. For example, previous traumatic experiences and post-traumatic stress disorder

(PTSD) symptoms are common in LGBT populations; chronic alcohol consumption leads to increased stress sensitivity and reactivity, which can significantly worsen these PTSD symptoms. Finally, the presence of a co-occurring psychiatric illness along with a substance use disorder can affect choice of treatment modality or management. Again, using PTSD as an example, studies show that treating PTSD and substance use disorder concurrently rather than sequentially leads to better outcomes for both illnesses (McGovern, Lambert-Harris, Alterman, Haiyi, & Meier, 2011; Hien, Cohen, Miele, Litt, & Capstick, 2004). Seeking Safety (Najavits, 2002) is a type of therapy specifically created to treat individuals who have both illnesses and is very effective in reducing PTSD symptoms and decreasing substance use. Clinicians should be mindful to assess and properly diagnose co-occurring psychiatric illnesses in order to provide the most comprehensive treatment.

In addition to co-occurring mental health disorders, there are some medical illnesses that substance abusing populations are more vulnerable to. Needle use exposes users to infectious diseases, particularly HIV and hepatitis C, as well as soft-tissue infections such as cellulitis and abscesses. Heavy alcohol use can affect a number of organs, including the liver (alcoholic hepatitis, fatty liver, cirrhosis), stomach (gastritis, reflux), and heart (cardiomyopathy). These medical illnesses are not specific to the substance-using LGBT population, but there are a few instances where medical illnesses are more prevalent in certain LGBT groups. There is an increased rate of the use of certain "club drugs" among MSM. The use of these substances, which include crystal methamphetamine, MDMA, and GHB, is correlated with increased sexual risk-taking behaviors, which itself is associated with higher rates of HIV and sexually transmitted illnesses (STIs). There also is a positive correlation between the use of crystal methamphetamine and HIV in MSM ("CDC HIV/AIDS Fact Sheet," n.d.). In transgender people, health risks of hormone use (such as liver damage) can be exacerbated by concomitant substance use (e.g., alcohol).

TREATMENT OF SUBSTANCE USE DISORDERS IN LGBT POPULATIONS

Treatment Principles

Substance use disorders can be successfully treated with a number of different modalities and in a variety of different settings. Addiction treatment programs can be inpatient, outpatient, or residential, and most provide a combination of medication, individual, and group therapy to address the complex needs of the addicted population. Unfortunately, access to these specialized programs can be limited. In 2009, 23.5 million persons aged 12 or older needed treatment for a substance use problem (9.3 percent of the population of people 12 or older); of these, only 2.6 million—11.2 percent of those who needed treatment—received it at a specialty facility (Substance Abuse and Mental Health Services Administration, 2010). Compare this with mood disorders, which have a 12-month prevalence of 9.5 percent in the general population, with 50.9 percent of those requiring treatment receiving it over 12 months (Wang et al., 2005). The LGBT population has an even more difficult time accessing LGBT-sensitive or -affirming substance use treatment.

There are real barriers to treatment as well as the perception among the LGBT community of barriers that ultimately makes individuals reluctant to use mainstream health care services, and it is not uncommon for LGBT individuals to avoid seeking treatment altogether (Eliason, 1996). One reason for this could be past mistreatment by the medical community. In a survey conducted by GLMA in 1994, 52 percent of their members had observed the denial of care or the provision of suboptimal care to lesbian and gay patients, and 88 percent had heard colleagues make disparaging remarks about their lesbian and gay patients. Unsurprisingly, there is less compliance with treatments recommended by homophobic providers. Accessible treatment for transgender individuals is particularly sparse, and approximately 50 percent of transgender individuals delay or fail to seek addiction treatment because of anticipated maltreatment (Nuttbrock, 2012). When services are accessed, often LGBT persons do not disclose their sexual orientation or gender identity to their health care providers. Even if a provider is open and interested in providing LGBT-affirming treatment, lack of familiarity with the population can prove to be a treatment obstacle. For example, in one survey of 164 staff members from 36 alcohol treatment programs in New York City, 71 percent of respondents reported little to no training about lesbian and gay issues (Hellman, Stanton, Lee, Tytun, & Vachon, 1989). In another study, less than 5 percent of counselors and administrators in mainstream addiction treatment programs had received any formal education or on-the-job training specifically related to transgender identity (Rachlin, Green, & Lombardi, 2008). Yet another barrier is that LGBT individuals are less likely to be covered by health insurance than heterosexual individuals—one study found that while 82 percent of heterosexual adults had health insurance, 77 percent of lesbian/gay/bisexual adults and only 57 percent of transgender individuals did ("Center for American Progress," n.d.).

Despite a 2001 recommendation by the Substance Abuse and Mental Health Services Administration (SAMHSA) to increase access to LGBT-sensitive addiction treatment, specialized care continues to be lacking. A phone survey was conducted in 2007 to 854 agencies listed as providing specialized LGBT programs in the National Survey of Substance Abuse

Treatment services. Of these, only 62 (7.3 percent) indicated having specialized programming, and half of these agencies were located in New York or California (Cochran, Peavy, & Robohm, 2007). Educating providers about LGBT-specific issues and expanding access to LGBT-affirming treatment across the country is an ongoing process for many programs.

In places where LGBT-specific addiction treatment does exist, the question still remains as to whether outcomes differ from general addiction treatment. In other words, if treatment is easily accessed and is delivered in a skilled and empathic way, can LGBT individuals still benefit even if the treatment is not tailored to an LGBT population? There actually is very limited research into treatment outcomes in LGBT substance users, and what evidence does exist focuses primarily on gay males using illicit substances. For the most part, the studies do not find a significant difference in outcome between LGBT-specific treatment and general treatment. Shoptaw et al. randomized 162 methamphetamine-dependent gay and bisexual men into one of four treatment groups: standard cognitive behavioral therapy (CBT), contingency management (CM), combined CBT and CM (CBT/CM), and a culturally tailored gay-specific CBT (GS-CBT) (Shoptaw et al., 2005). All groups showed significant reductions in drug use and psychiatric subscales of the Addiction Severity Index, and there were no differences in rates of drug use between treatment groups at 12-month follow-up. Another study by the same group compared GS-CBT and gay-specific social support therapy (GS-SST) in a population of gay and bisexual men in a community health clinic (Shoptaw et al., 2008). Both groups showed significant reduction in the rates of alcohol and drug use at the end of the 16-week study and at one-year follow-up. Morgenstern et al. compared motivational interviewing (MI) with CBT in a group of 188 MSM with alcohol use disorder, with the result that both types of therapy led to decreases in the number of drinks per day during the 12-week treatment protocol and decreased negative consequences of drinking at 12-month follow-up (Morgenstern et al., 2008).

The outcomes of these studies suggest that treatment specifically identified as LGBT-affirming may not necessarily be prerequisite for treatment effectiveness. Until more research is conducted (particularly among sexual minority women and transgender populations) into the need for and the outcome of LGBT-specific treatment, the broad principles of substance use treatment for the general population will continue to be applied to the LGBT population.

Medication-Assisted Treatment of Substance Use Disorders

There is a relative dearth of medications available to treat substance use disorders. As of 2017, there are only 12 FDA-approved medications (not counting different formulations of the same drug) for any substance use disorder; in contrast, there are 14 approved medications for bipolar disorder alone. Medications are only available for treating alcohol, opioid, or nicotine use disorders, but there are several promising medications in development and undergoing study for other substance use disorders. Off-label usage of some medications is common practice, but in this section, only medications with FDA approval for the treatment of SUD will be reviewed.

Disulfiram and *acamprosate* are medications used to treat alcohol use disorder. Disulfiram works by blocking an enzyme involved in alcohol metabolism; this allows for the buildup of a toxic metabolite that causes unpleasant symptoms—flushing, sweating, palpitations, nausea and vomiting, and headache. This reaction only occurs if the patient ingests alcohol, and most people on disulfiram will be abstinent in order to avoid the reaction. This medication works very well if taken, but the difficulty is that one can easily choose to discontinue the medication and resume drinking. To reduce the risk of this, disulfiram is often given daily in a supervised setting (by a family member, partner, or treatment provider). The mechanism by which acamprosate works is unknown, but it may help stabilize one of the neurotransmitter systems that is disrupted with chronic alcohol consumption. The clinical effect is that it decreases cravings for alcohol. It is relatively well tolerated and is a good option for those with liver disease, as the other two medications approved for alcohol use disorder (disulfiram and naltrexone) both have the potential to worsen liver damage. Evidence for its efficacy has been strongest out of European countries and is somewhat more varied in the United States.

Naltrexone is a medication that is approved to treat both opioid use disorder and alcohol use disorder. It is an opioid *antagonist*; i.e., it occupies the opioid receptor without activating it. Naltrexone binds very tightly to this receptor and is unable to be displaced by the majority of opioids. For opioid users, naltrexone leads to abstinence by blocking any effect from opioids; therefore, abstinence is enforced as attempts to achieve euphoria from opioids are essentially futile. Naltrexone is also an effective medication for alcohol use disorder, although the mechanism is less clear. It likely works by decreasing the reward from drinking by affecting the endogenous opioid system. Subjectively, patients report a decrease in cravings for alcohol, and in clinical trials, naltrexone has been shown to increase time to relapse and decrease the severity of relapses (Anton et al., 2006). Naltrexone is available both as an oral tablet and as a long-acting injection that lasts for 28 days.

For opioid use disorder, there are two other options that are considered *maintenance* therapy: *methadone* and *buprenorphine*. Methadone is a long-acting opioid agonist that activates the same receptor as substances such as heroin and oxycodone; however, methadone builds up more gradually to a plateau in the body and lasts for about 24 hours. Thus, it may be dosed once a day and does not have the peaks of euphoria and valleys of withdrawal that shorter-acting agents have. Though methadone may be prescribed for chronic pain out of any physician's office, when it is given for the purpose of treating addiction, it must be dispensed through a licensed opioid treatment program (OTP) that is under tight federal regulation. Patients on methadone are dosed once a day at a licensed facility that is open six days a week. Patients receive a "take-home" dose for Sundays or holidays and can also earn take-homes if they appear clinically stable and have provided urine free of drugs for a period of time. Methadone maintenance significantly decreases negative outcomes associated with opioid use disorder, including rates of infectious disease (particularly HIV and hepatitis C) and rates of overdose death.

Buprenorphine is a long-acting opioid *partial agonist*. This binds to the same receptors as a full agonist but activates it only partially. Buprenorphine activates the opioid receptor to about 30 percent of the activity of full agonists; therefore, it tends to have a "ceiling effect" where escalation of dosage beyond a certain point does not lead to increased effect. This makes buprenorphine an effective medication for addressing opioid withdrawal and craving but relatively less reinforcing and relatively less lethal in overdose when compared to full opioid agonists. Buprenorphine may be dispensed in the same way as methadone in an OTP, or it can be prescribed out of a physician's office. A physician must obtain a special waiver from the DEA in order to be able to prescribe office-based buprenorphine for the purposes of treating opioid use disorder; no special waiver is necessary when prescribing buprenorphine for the treatment of pain. Office-based buprenorphine has helped to expand access to maintenance treatment to areas of the country that were previously underserved, as any physician may fulfill the requirements to obtain a waiver, whereas there are significant barriers to establishing an opioid treatment program. Office-based buprenorphine also does not need to be dispensed daily, so patients who are not able to travel daily to a clinic (due to distance, time, transportation, or mobility constraints) still are able to access maintenance treatment.

Smoking cessation is usually underaddressed by health care professionals, even in addiction treatment programs. However, tobacco (mostly used in the form of cigarettes) is the leading cause of preventable death in the United States and the world ("WHO Report on the Global Tobacco Epidemic 2008," n.d.), and the LGBT community is disproportionately affected, with some estimates placing rates of smoking at 50 to 200 percent that of the heterosexual population ("National LGBT Tobacco Control Network," n.d.). Seven medications are available for the treatment of nicotine use disorder, five of which are considered *nicotine replacement therapies* (NRT). NRTs provide a dose of nicotine (the addictive component of tobacco products) that can be gradually decreased over time until the patient is able to discontinue nicotine entirely. NRT is available as a patch, lozenge, inhaler, nasal spray, and gum; all have roughly equivalent efficacy, and some studies show these work best in combination—e.g., patch plus lozenge or patch plus gum (Piper et al., 2009). *Bupropion* is a medication that is used for the treatment of depression, but it also decreases cravings for nicotine by blocking the nicotinic acetylcholine receptor. This medication is taken daily and can also be used in combination with NRT with good effect. Finally, *varenicline* is a partial agonist at the nicotinic receptor. This medication, when take daily for a period of 12 to 24 weeks, can nearly triple the rates of smoking cessation (Gonzales et al., 2006). This medication should not be combined with NRTs, as it binds tightly to the nicotinic receptors, rendering NRTs ineffective.

Psychosocial Treatment of Substance Use Disorders

Given the limited number of medications, the majority of treatment for substance use disorders is psychosocial (individual, group, and family therapy, mutual help groups, sober companions, etc.). Many psychotherapy modalities exist to treat substance use disorders. While any therapy delivered by a competent, empathic clinician can be successful, there are some that have been specifically developed and/or studied for the treatment of substance use disorders.

Motivational interviewing (MI) is perhaps the best known of these therapies. MI was developed by two psychologists, Dr. William Miller and Dr. Stephen Rollnick, and evolved from their work treating problem drinkers. MI is a patient-centered approach to working with a client who is *ambivalent* about changing a behavior (e.g., whether to continue drinking vs. stop drinking) and serves to enhance a client's motivation to change. MI represented a shift away from the previously confrontational attitude that was frequently adopted by clinicians; it encourages a nonconfrontational, nonjudgmental, and nonadversarial style of interaction with patients. Despite that, it is not nondirective, and clinicians work to evoke motivation by highlighting change talk that ultimately leads patients to decisive action. It builds on the "transtheoretical model of change" proposed by Prochaska and DiClemente in 1983. This model views change as a fluid process that unfolds over time rather than an isolated event. A person moves through stages that include *pre-contemplation* (not ready to make a change), *contemplation* (considering change), *preparation* (getting ready for change), and *action* (making the change). After a change is made, a person can either *maintain* the change or *relapse*. The progress through the stages is not unidirectional, and a person may move back and forth through stages several times before ultimately making a change. MI is used to help a person process each step and facilitate movement through the stages. MI can be used in a long-term therapeutic relationship, but MI techniques have also shown efficacy when delivered in brief, one- or two-session interactions. When used in this way, it is called a *brief intervention*, and this modality has been shown to be effective in smoking cessation and moderating problematic drinking (Vasilaki, Hosier, & Cox, 2006; O'Donnell, Wallace, & Kaner, 2014; Fiore et al., 2008); efficacy has not been demonstrated for other substance use disorders.

Cognitive behavioral therapy (CBT) is a type of therapy used to treat a variety of psychiatric conditions. It is efficacious as a monotherapy for SUDs, and its principles also form the foundation for other types of therapies outlined below. One of the core principles of CBT is that cognitions (thoughts) and behaviors are learned over time; learning can be through *association* (classical conditioning) or *consequence* (operant conditioning). Most CBT approaches help a person manage the associations *antecedent* to use (commonly called "triggers") and focus on the consequences of use. *Reinforcement* of behavior is another key concept in CBT. A reinforcer is any stimulus that increases the chance that a behavior will be repeated in the future, and in the case of substance use, the substances themselves serve as powerful reinforcers. Reinforcement from substances can be *positive* or *negative*. In positive reinforcement, doing the behavior causes a pleasant stimulus to be added—e.g., a person snorts heroin, which causes her to feel euphoric. In negative reinforcement, doing the behavior causes a negative stimulus to be removed—e.g., a person with social anxiety has a drink, which causes his anxiety to resolve. In both cases, the person is more likely to remember this effect and repeat it in the future.

Relapse prevention (RP) focuses on the antecedents to substance use. The therapist and client work to identify situations, environments, and feeling states that contribute to relapse. Once these are identified, they work forward to see how these antecedents lead to relapse and also backward to see what factors led to exposure to these high-risk situations. Finally, the client works to build skills in order to cope with these triggers. Rather than managing triggers, *contingency management* instead uses positive consequences to reinforce behavior. In this model, patients are given tangible rewards for desired behaviors—for example, if a patient gives five drug-free urines, he earns a gift card for $10 to a local coffee shop. While studies show that this modality works very well, its use in the community is generally limited due to financial constraints. However, elements of contingency management often can be worked into a program's existing structure and budget, such as the "take-home" option in methadone maintenance (the more drug-free urines given over time, the more take-home bottles earned weekly).

Peer support groups can be an important part of recovery. The most well-known of the peer support groups is *Alcoholics Anonymous* (AA), which pioneered the *12-step model* of recovery. AA was originally founded in 1935 to help people recover from alcohol use disorder, but the model has now been expanded to include a variety of different addictive substances and behaviors (e.g., Narcotics Anonymous, Gamblers Anonymous, etc.). The core structure of the program is formed by groups consisting of recovering addicts meeting in order to aid one another in recovery; the program consists of 12 "steps" meant to guide the person through the recovery process. A text—*Alcoholics Anonymous: The Story of How More than One Hundred Men Have Recovered from Alcoholism*, known informally as the "Big Book"—outlines these steps. One particular benefit of AA for LGBT people is that there are a relatively large number of LGBT meetings in many areas of the country. Group therapy can pose some challenges in settings where LGBT and non-LGBT populations are mixed, as attitudes toward the LGBT population can be varied. Therefore, it is helpful to be able to access LGBT-identified peer support meetings. LGBT AA meetings also allow access to treatment for people who may not have options for other types of LGBT-affirming treatment. Some groups, such as Crystal Meth Anonymous and Sex Addicts Anonymous, are not specifically LGBT-identified but address issues that are more prevalent in certain LGBT communities. While LGBT-specific groups may be desirable for many people, there are also downsides for some. An LGBT person attempting to maintain sobriety may seek to avoid triggers, and seeing other community members at meetings can sometimes be a reminder of situations in which they use.

Though AA is the most widespread of the peer support groups, it is by no means the only option, and it is not an essential part of everyone's recovery. One aspect of AA that may be a barrier for some patients is its focus on a "higher power." AA originated from a religious perspective, with the original language referring to ceding control to God and asking God to remove defects of character. Though it has adapted over the years to remove overt religious references, it still has a spiritual focus. Critics also point to the lack of evidence for its success rates (because it is "anonymous," its claims of sobriety rates among its members are difficult to study or substantiate), its abstinence-only model, and its historically negative stance on use of psychotropic or maintenance medications as reasons that it may not be an appropriate treatment option for everyone. The largest alternative to AA is *Self-Management and Recovery Training* (SMART Recovery), a peer support group that uses a "4-Point Program" to teach participants skills and tools to manage urges to use and thoughts, feelings, and behaviors that lead to use. It employs principles drawn from MI, CBT, and rational emotive behavior therapy (REBT), and meetings are generally led by volunteer facilitators. Other alternatives, such as Moderation Management and Rational Recovery, exist but are much smaller in scale.

In conclusion, substance use disorders have a significant impact on the LGBT population, and certain characteristics (e.g., minority stress) may contribute to higher prevalence rates. Fortunately, resiliency in the community helps mitigate some of that impact, and for those who need more intensive intervention, effective treatments, both psychosocial and pharmacologic, are available. Though clearly, more research is needed in this area, there is enough to provide a foundation upon which to build further understanding of the development, diagnosis, and treatment of substance use disorders in the LGBT population.

REFERENCES

Anton, R. F., O'Malley, S. S., Ciraulo, D. A., Cisler, R. A., Couper, D., Donovan, D. M., . . . COMBINE Study Research Group. (2006). Combined pharmacotherapies and behavioral interventions for alcohol dependence: The COMBINE study: A randomized controlled trial. *JAMA, 295*(17), 2003–2017.

Brown, P. J., Recupero, P. R., & Stout, R. (1995). PTSD Substance abuse comorbidity and treatment utilization. *Addictive Behaviors, 20*(2), 251–254.

Cabaj, R. P. (1997). Gays, lesbians, and bisexuals. In J. H. Lowenson, P. Ruiz, & R. P. Millman (Eds.), *Substance abuse: A comprehensive textbook* (3rd ed., pp. 725–733). Baltimore: Williams and Wilkins.

Cabaj, R. P. (1998). Substance abuse and HIV Disease: Entwined and intimate entities. In E. F. McCanceKatz & T. R. Kosten (Eds.), *New treatments for chemical dependency* (pp. 113–149). Washington, DC: American Psychiatric Press.

Cabaj, R. P. (2014). Substance use issues among gay, lesbian, bisexual, and transgender people. In M. Galanter, H. Kleber, & K. Brady (Eds.), *The American Psychiatric Publishing textbook of substance abuse treatment* (pp. 702–722). Washington, DC: American Psychiatric Press.

CDC HIV/AIDS Fact Sheet: Methamphetamine Use and Risk for HIV/AIDS. (n.d.). Retrieved from http://www.cdc.gov/hiv/resources/factsheets/pdf /meth.pdf

Center for American Progress: How to Close the LGBT Health Disparities Gap. (n.d.). Retrieved from https://cdn.americanprogress.org/wp-content/uploads /issues/2009/12/pdf/lgbt_health_disparities.pdf

Center for Behavioral Health Statistics and Quality. (2015). Behavioral health trends in the United States: Results from the 2014 National Survey on Drug Use and Health (HHS Publication No. SMA 15-4927, NSDUH Series H-50). Retrieved from http://www.samhsa.gov/ data/

Choi, K. H., Operario, D., Gregorich, S. E., McFarland, W., MacKellar, D., & Valleroy, L. (2005). Substance use, substance choice, and unprotected anal intercourse among young Asian American and Pacific Islander men who have sex with men. *AIDS Education and Prevention, 17*(5), 418–429.

Clark, D. B., Kirisci, L., & Tatar, R. E. (1998). Adolescent versus adult onset and the development of substance use disorders in males. *Drug and Alcohol Dependence, 49*(2), 115–121.

Clements-Nolle, K., Marx, R., Guzman, R., et al. (2001). HIV prevalence, risk behaviors, health care use, and mental health status of transgender persons: Implications for public health intervention. *American Journal of Public Health, 91*(6), 915–921.

Cochran, B. N., & Cauce, A. M. (2006). Characteristics of lesbian, gay, bisexual, and transgender individuals entering substance abuse treatment. *Journal of Substance Abuse Treatment, 30*(2), 135–146.

Cochran, B. N., Peavy, K. M., & Robohm, J. S. (2007). Do specialized services exist for LGBT individuals seeking treatment for substance misuse? A study of available treatment programs. *Substance Use & Misuse, 42,* 161–176.

Cochran, S. D. (2001). Emerging issues in research on lesbians' and gay men's mental health: Does sexual orientation really matter? *American Psychologist, 56*(11), 931–947.

Cochran, S. D., Ackerman, D., Mays, V. M., & Ross, M. W. (2004). Prevalence of non-medical drug use and dependence among homosexually active men and women in the US population. *Addiction, 99*(8), 989–98.

Cochran, S. D., Sullivan, J. G., & Mays, V. M. (2003). Prevalence of mental disorders, psychological distress, and mental health services use among lesbian, gay, and bisexual adults in the United States. *Journal of Consulting and Clinical Psychology, 71,* 53–61.

D'Augelli, A. R. (2002). Mental health problems among lesbian, gay, and bisexual youths ages 14–21. *Clinical Child Psychology and Psychiatry, 7,* 439–462.

Eliason, M. J. (1996). An inclusive model of lesbian identity. *Journal of Gay, Lesbian, and Bisexual Identity, 1*(1), 3–9.

Fergusson, D. M., Horwood, L. J., & Beautrais, A. L. (1999). Is sexual orientation related to mental health problems and suicidality in young people? *Archives of General Psychiatry, 56,* 876–80.

Fiore, M. C., Jaen, C. R., Baker, T. B., Bailey, W. C., Benowitz, N. L., Curry, S. J., . . . Wewers, M. E. (2008). *Treating tobacco use and dependence: 2008 update.* Rockville, MD: U.S. Department of Health and Human Services Public Health Service.

Friedman, M. S., Marshal, M. P., Guadamuz, T. E., Wei, C., Wong, C. F., Saewyc, E., & Stall, R. (2011). A meta-analysis of disparities in childhood sexual abuse, parental physical abuse, and peer victimization among sexual minority and sexual nonminority individuals. *American Journal of Public Health, 101*(8), 1481–1494.

Garnets, L. D., Herek, G. M., & Levy, B. (1990). Violence and victimization of lesbians and gay men: Mental health consequences. *Journal of Interpersonal Violence, 5,* 366–383.

Gay and Lesbian Medical Association, United States. Department of Health and Human Services. (2001). *Healthy People 2010 companion document for lesbian, gay, bisexual, and transgender (LGBT) health.* San Francisco: Author.

Gillespie, W., & Blackwell, R. L. (2009). Substance use patterns and consequences among lesbian, gays, and bisexuals. *Journal of Gay and Lesbian Social Services, 21*(1), 90–108.

Gonzales, D., Rennard, S. I., Nides, M., Oncken, C., Azoulay, S., Billing, C., . . . Reeves, K. R. (2006). Varenicline, an α4β2 nicotinic acetylcholine receptor partial agonist vs. sustained-release bupropion and placebo for smoking cessation. *JAMA, 296*(1), 47–55.

Green, A. I., & Halkitis, P. N. (2006). Crystal methamphetamine and sexual sociality in an urban gay subculture: An elective affinity. *Culture Health and Sexuality, 8*(4), 317–333.

Green, K. E., & Feinstein, B. A. (2012). Substance use in lesbian, gay, and bisexual populations: an update on empirical research and implications for treatment. *Psychology of Addictive Behaviors, 26*(2), 265–278.

Greenwood, G. L., White, E. W., Page-Shafer, K., Bein, E., Osmond, D. H., Paul, J., . . . Stall, R. D. (2001). Correlates of heavy substance use among young gay and bisexual men: The San Francisco Young Men's Health Study. *Drug and Alcohol Dependence, 61*, 105–112.

Hellman, R. E., Stanton, M., Lee, J., Tytun, A., & Vachon, R. (1989). Treatment of homosexual alcoholics in government-funded agencies: Provider training and attitudes. *Hospital and Community Psychiatry, 40*, 1163–1168.

Hendricks, M., & Testa, R. J. (2012). Model for understanding risk and resiliency in transgender and gender nonconforming individuals. *Professional Psychology: Research and Practice, 43*(5), 460–467.

Herrick, A. L., Lim, S. H., Wei, C., Smith, H., Guadamuz, T., Friedman, M. S., & Stall, R. (2011). Resilience as an untapped resource in behavioral intervention design for gay men. *Journal of AIDS and Behavior, 15*(Suppl. 1), 25–30.

Hien, D. A., Cohen, L. R., Miele, G. M., Litt, L. C., & Capstick, C. (2004). Promising treatments for women with comorbid PTSD and substance use disorders. *American Journal of Psychiatry, 161*, 1426–1432.

Huebner, D. M., Rebchook, G. M., & Kegeles, S. M. (2004). Experiences of harassment, discrimination, and physical violence among young gay and bisexual men. *American Journal of Public Health, 94*(7), 1200–1203.

Hughes, T. L. (2003). Lesbians' drinking patterns: Beyond the data. *Substance Use and Misuse, 38*(11/13), 1739–1758.

Hughes, T. L., Wilsnack, S. C., Szalacha, L. A., Johnson, T., Bostwick, W. B., Seymour, R., . . . Kinnison, K. E. (2006). Age and racial/ethnic differences in drinking and drinking-related problems in a community sample of lesbians. *Journal of Studies on Alcohol and Drugs, 67*(4), 579–590.

Institute of Medicine Committee on Lesbian, Gay, Bisexual, and Transgender Health Issues and Research Gaps and Opportunities. (2011). *The health of lesbian, gay, bisexual, and transgender people: Building a foundation for better understanding.* Washington, DC: National Academies Press (US).

Kandel, D. B., Yamaguchi, K., & Chen, K. (1992). Stages of progression in drug involvement from adolescence to adulthood: Further evidence for the gateway theory. *Journal of Studies on Alcohol and Drugs, 53*, 447–457.

Kann, L., Kinchen, S. A., Williams, B. I., Ross, J. G., Lowry, R., Grunbaum, J. A., . . . State and Local YRBSS Coordinators. (1999). Youth risk behavior surveillance— United States. *MMWR CDC Surveillance Summary, 49*(5), 1–32, 60–68.

Kecojevic, A., Wong, C. F., Schrager, S. M., Silva, K., Bloom, J. J., Iverson, E., & Lankenau, S. E. (2012). Initiation into prescription drug misuse: Differences between lesbian, gay, bisexual, transgender (LGBT) and heterosexual high-risk young adults in Los Angeles and New York. *Addictive Behaviors, 37,* 1289–1293.

Kelly, B. C., Parsons, J. T., & Wells, B. E. (2006). Prevalence and predictors of club drug use among clubgoing young adults in New York City. *Journal Urban Health, 83*(5), 884–895.

Marshal, M. P., Friedman, M. S., Stall, R., King, K. M., Miles, J., Gold, M. A., . . . Morse, J. Q. (2008). Sexual orientation and adolescent substance use: A meta-analysis and methodological review. *Addiction, 103*(4), 546–556.

McGovern, M. P., Lambert-Harris, C., Alterman, A. I., Haiyi, X., & Meier, A. (2011). A randomized controlled trial comparing integrated cognitive behavioral therapy versus individual addiction counseling for co-occurring substance use and posttraumatic stress disorders. *Journal of Dual Diagnosis, 7*(4), 207–227.

Meyer, I. H. (2003). Prejudice, social stress, and mental health in lesbian, gay, and bisexual populations: Conceptual issues and research evidence. *Psychological Bulletin, 129*(5), 674–697.

Morgenstern, J., Irwin, T. W., Wainberg, M. L., Parsons, J. T., Muench, F., Bux, D. A., Jr., . . . Shulz-Heik, J. (2008). A randomized controlled trial of goal choice interventions for alcohol use disorders among men who have sex with men. *Journal of Consultative and Clinical Psychology, 75*(1), 72–84.

Najavits, L. M. (2002). *Seeking safety: A treatment Manual for PTSD and substance abuse.* New York: Guilford Press.

National LGBT Tobacco Control Network. (n.d.). Retrieved January 31, 2016, from http://lgbttobacco.org

Nuttbrock, L. A. (2012). Culturally competent substance abuse treatment with transgender persons. *Journal of Addictive Diseases, 31*(3), 236–241.

O'Donnell, A., Wallace, P., & Kaner, E. (2014). From efficacy to effectiveness and beyond: What next for brief interventions in primary care? *Frontiers in Psychiatry, 5,* 113.

Ostrow, D., & Shelby, D. (2000). Psychoanalytic and behavioral approaches to drug-related sexual risk taking. *Journal of Gay & Lesbian Psychotherapy, 3*(3–4), 123–139.

Piper, M. E., Smith, S. S., Schlam, T. R., Fiore, M. C., Jorenby, D. E., Fraser, D., & Baker, T. B. (2009). A randomized placebo-controlled clinical trial of 5 smoking cessation pharmacotherapies. *Archives of General Psychiatry, 66*(11), 1254–1262.

Polak, K., Haug, N., Drachenberg, H., & Svikis, D. (2015). Gender considerations in addiction: Implications for treatment. *Current Treatment Options Psychiatry, 2,* 326–338.

Rachlin, K., Green, J., & Lombardi, E. (2008). Utilization of health care among female-to-male transgender individuals in the United States. *Journal of Homosexuality, 54,* 243–258.

Roberts, S. J., Grindel, C. G., Patsdaughter, C. A., DeMarco, R., & Tarmina, M. S. (2004). Lesbian use and abuse of alcohol: Results of the Boston Lesbian Health Project II. *Substance Abuse, 25*(4), 1–9.

Rowe, C., Santos, G. M., McFarland, W., & Wilson, E. C. (2015). Prevalence and correlates of substance use among trans female youth ages 16–24 years in the San Francisco Bay Area. *Drug and Alcohol Dependence, 147,* 160–166.

Saewyc, E. M., Skay, C. L., Richens, K., Reis, E., Poon, C., & Murphy, A. (2006). Sexual orientation, sexual abuse, and HIV-risk behaviors among adolescents in the Pacific Northwest. *American Journal of Public Health, 96,* 1104–1110.

Santos, G. M., Rapues, J., Wilson, E. C., Macias, O., Packer, T., Colfax, G., & Raymond, H. F. (2014). Alcohol and substance use among transgender women in San Francisco: Prevalence and association with human immunodeficiency virus infection. *Drug and Alcohol Review, 33*(3), 287–295.

Semple, S. J., Strathdee, S. A., Zians, J., & Patterson, T. L. (2012). Factors associated with experiences of stigma in a sample of HIVpositive, methamphetamineusing men who have sex with men. *Drug and Alcohol Dependence, 125*(1–2), 154–159.

Sevelius, J. M., Reznick, O. G., Hart, S. L., & Schwarcz, S. (2009). Informing interventions: The importance of contextual factors in the prediction of sexual risk behaviors among transgender women. *AIDS Education and Prevention, 21,* 113–127.

Shoptaw, S., Reback, C. J., Larkins, S., Wang, P. C., Rotheram-Fuller, E., Dang, J., & Yang, X. (2008). Outcomes using two tailored behavioral treatments for substance abuse in urban gay and bisexual men. *Journal of Substance Abuse Treatment, 35,* 285–293.

Shoptaw, S., Reback, C. J., Peck, J. A., Yang, X., Rotheram-Fuller, E., Larkins, S., . . . Hucks-Ortiz, C. (2005). Behavioral treatment approaches for methamphetamine dependence and HIV-related sexual risk behaviors among urban gay and bisexual men. *Drug and Alcohol Dependence, 78,* 125–134.

Silvestre, A., Beatty, R., & Friedman, M. (2013). Substance use disorder in the context of LGBT health: A social work perspective. *Social Work in Public Health, 28,* 366–376.

Smith, A. M. A., Lindsay, J., & Rosenthal, D. A. (1999). Same sex attraction, drug injection and binge drinking among Australian adolescents. *Australian and New Zealand Journal of Public Health, 23,* 643–646.

Stall, R., Friedman, M., & Catania, J. (2008). Interacting epidemics and gay men's health: A theory of syndemic production among urban gay men. In R. J. Wolitski, R. Stall, & R. O. Valdiserri (Eds.), *Unequal opportunity: Health disparities affecting gay and bisexual men in the United States* (pp. 251–274). New York: Oxford University Press.

Stall, R., McKusick, L., Wiley, J., Coates, T. J., & Ostrow, D. G. (1986). Alcohol and drug use during sexual activity and compliance with safe sex guidelines for AIDS: The AIDS Behavioral Research Project. *Health Education Quarterly, 13,* 359–372.

Stall, R., Paul, J., Greenwood, G., Pollack, L., Bein, E., Crosby, G., . . . Catania, J. A. (2001). Alcohol use, drug use and alcohol-related problems among men who have sex with men: The Urban Men's Health Study. *Addiction, 96,* 1589–1601.

Stall, R., & Purcell, D. W. (2000). Intertwining epidemics: A review of research on substance use among men who have sex with men and its connection to the AIDS epidemic. *AIDS and Behavior, 4,* 181–192.

Stroumsa, D. (2014). The state of transgender health care: Policy, law, and medical frameworks. *American Journal of Public Health, 104*(3), e31–e38.

Substance Abuse and Mental Health Services Administration. (2010). *Results from the 2009 National Survey on Drug Use and Health: Volume I. Summary of national findings* (Office of Applied Studies, NSDUH Series H-38A, HHS Publication No. SMA 10-4586 Findings). Rockville, MD: Author.

Sullivan, P. S., Nakashima, A. K., Purcell, D. W., & Ward, J. W. (1998). Geographic differences in noninjection and injection substance use among HIV-seropositive men who have sex with men: Western United States versus other regions. *Journal of Acquired Immune Deficiency Syndromes & Human Retrovirology, 19*(3), 266–273.

Thiede, H., Valleroy, L. A., MacKellar, D. A., Celentano, D. D., Ford, W. L., Hagan, H., . . . Young Men's Survey Study Group. (2003). Regional patterns and correlates of substance use among young men who have sex with men in 7 US urban areas. *American Journal of Public Health, 93*(11), 1915–1921.

TolouShams, M., Tarantino, N., McKirnan, D. J., & Dyslin, K. J. (2013). Depressive symptoms, illicit drug use and HIV/STI risk among sexual minority young adults. *Journal of Gay and Lesbian Mental Health, 17*(1), 96–102.

Van Griensven, F., Kilmarx, P. H., Jeeyapant, S., Manopaiboon, C., Korattana, S., Jenkins, R. A., . . . Mastro, T. D. (2004). The prevalence of bisexual and homosexual orientation and related health risks among adolescents in northern Thailand. *Archives of Sexual Behavior, 33,* 137–47.

Vasilaki, E. I., Hosier, S. G., & Cox, W. M. (2006). The efficacy of motivational interviewing as a brief intervention for excessive drinking: A meta-analytic review. *Alcohol and Alcoholism, 41*(3), 328–335.

Wainberg, M. L., Kolodny, A. J., & Drescher, J. (2006). *Crystal meth and men who have sex with men: What mental health care professionals need to know.* Binghamton, NY: Haworth Medical.

Wang, P. S., Lane, M., Olfson, M., Pincus, H. A., Wells, K. B., & Kessler, R. C. (2005). Twelve month use of mental health services in the United States. *Archives of General Psychiatry, 62*(6), 629–640.

World Health Organization. (n.d.). WHO report on the global tobacco epidemic 2008. Retrieved from http://www.who.int/tobacco/mpower/2008/en/

4

Sexually Transmitted Infections and LGBT Populations

John A. Davis and Carl G. Streed Jr.

INTRODUCTION

Sexually transmitted infections (STIs) are a common source of morbidity and mortality in global and U.S. populations. It is estimated that 20 million new STIs occur in the United States annually, reflecting 110 million actual infections, and at a cost of $16 billion each year (Satterwhite et al., 2013; Owusu-Edusei et al., 2013). In some ways, it is inevitable that populations that are defined with respect to their sexual orientation would also be studied as a demographic for sex-associated outcomes, including "STIs." It is clear that marginalized groups may have differing sexual networks and that disease rates may differ between such networks. For example, rates of HIV (Centers for Disease Control and Prevention [CDC], 2017a) and syphilis (CDC, 2015b) are much higher in groups of men who have sex with men (MSM) when compared to their non-MSM counterparts, and rates of bacterial vaginosis (BV) and some STIs are higher in sexual minority women than in their sexual majority counterparts (Fethers, Fairley, Hocking, Gurrin, & Bradshaw, 2008; Marrazzo, 2010; Everett, 2013).

The purpose of this chapter is not to provide a comprehensive guide to the diagnosis and/or treatment of sexually transmitted infections. There are many good resources, including entire textbooks, on the subject—to which the authors kindly direct the reader who has further questions (Grimes, Fagerberg, & Smith, 2013; Handsfield, 1992; Holmes, 2007). Rather, the goal of this chapter is to provide an overview of the more common STIs in LGBT populations, and a context of these diseases as they pertain to LGBT populations.

Last, a caveat should be borne in mind when approaching data on LGBT populations, and with respect to STIs in LGBT populations in particular. There is a focus in much of the STI literature on behavior rather than identity, and thus, much of the statistical analysis focuses on "men who have sex with men" and "women who have sex with women"; so, much of the impact of identity and expression within data are lost. The terms "MSM" and "gay/bisexual men" are not synonymous; nor are "women who have sex with women" ("WSW") and "lesbian/bisexual women." Readers would do well to avoid conflation of such terms and to be aware of the limitations of research conclusions based on the selection of one set of terms over another.

HUMAN IMMUNODEFICIENCY VIRUS

Few conditions have affected the LGBT population as has the advent of the human immunodeficiency virus (HIV)/acquired immunodeficiency syndrome (AIDS) in the United States. From the time of its first recognition in the United States in 1981 (CDC, 1981), the HIV/AIDS epidemic was different. While other diseases disproportionately affect LGBT populations, the deadly nature of HIV infection, with greater than 80 percent mortality through 1988 (CDC, 1989), combined with our lack of knowledge about the disease and its management, and its rise in particularly marginalized populations in U.S. society (such as MSM), led to the loss of significant numbers, and even greater percentages, of gay/bisexual men, other MSM, and trans women. While the history and impact of HIV/AIDS on the LGBT population cannot be summarized adequately here, the reader is encouraged to review any of the excellent resources that currently exist on the subject (Shilts, 1988, Engel, 2006), as the epidemic has had a profound effect on many aspects of society, including health care and, apropos of this chapter and book, LGBT health care in particular.

It is also worth noting that much research is being conducted on the nature of the disproportionate burden of HIV among gay men and other MSM. In particular, there is now a body of literature on the framework of syndemics—two or more afflictions interacting synergistically, contributing to excess burden of disease in a population (Milstein, 2002). Research has shown that conditions such as depression, substance use, intimate partner violence, and high-risk sex, all of which are found disproportionately in LGBT populations, can combine in a way that is more than additive to increase risk of other conditions, such as acquisition of HIV (Stall et al., 2003).

Currently, HIV is a global pandemic affecting (and infecting) over 30 million people worldwide, growing at a rate of approximately 2 million people per year and killing approximately 1.2 million people a year (WHO, 2014). The United States contributes approximately 50,000 new HIV diagnoses annually and about 1 million persons living with HIV to the overall prevalence (CDC, 2017a). Unfortunately, statistics continue to bear out the significant impact that HIV has on MSM (and gay/bisexual-identified men). In 2010, the most recent year for which the CDC has published data at the time of this writing, men who have sex with men (MSM) made up 63 percent of all new HIV diagnoses, and the rate of HIV infection was approximately an order of magnitude greater (or more) for white, black, and Latino MSM when compared to their male, non-MSM counterparts (CDC, 2017a). Additionally, while rates of HIV infection have decreased overall in the United States, rates among certain communities, notably young MSM of color, have actually been increasing.

HIV infection has three main clinical manifestations. In the very early stages of infection, or acute HIV, infected individuals may experience a mononucleosis-like syndrome (fever, lymphadenopathy), occasionally with rash (Braun et al., 2015). More severe, end-organ-specific manifestations of acute HIV have been reported (e.g., meningitis/encephalitis, psychiatric disturbance, hepatitis, etc.) (Braun, 2015). Some 50 to 60 percent of those infected with HIV may not experience any symptoms in the acute phase, and symptoms may only be encountered later in the course of disease after a variable latent period, when immunosuppression is severe enough to permit opportunistic infection or other symptoms of immune dysfunction. Symptoms are thus dependent upon the end organ affected and the infectious etiology.

Diagnosis of HIV infection is primarily by detection of HIV-specific antibodies in the serum or in some other bodily fluids (such as saliva). In some instances, detection of viral components (such as HIV p24 antigen, or HIV nucleic acids) is performed, and this approach is particularly important for diagnosis of infection in the "window period"—the time between infection and formation of measurable antibody response (seroconversion), sometime in the first two to six weeks. Current CDC recommendations regarding HIV testing are summarized in Figure 4.1 (CDC & Association of Public Health Laboratories [APHL], 2014). The importance of diagnosis cannot be overstated. The CDC estimates that approximately 25 percent of those in the United States with HIV are unaware of their status (Branson et al., 2006).

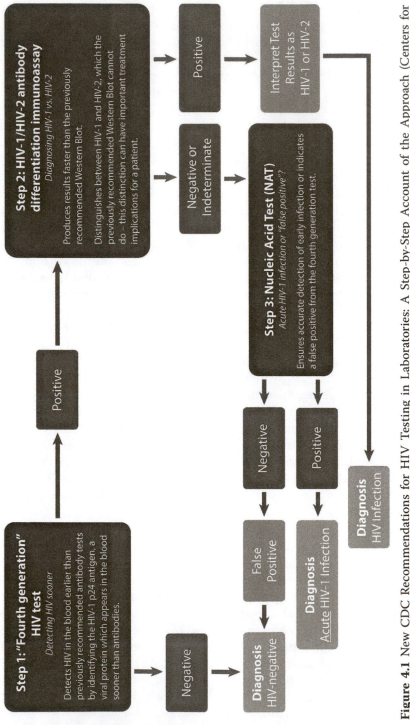

Figure 4.1 New CDC Recommendations for HIV Testing in Laboratories: A Step-by-Step Account of the Approach (Centers for Disease Control and Prevention)

It is important to note that the U.S. Department of Health and Human Services (HHS) recommends antiretroviral treatment for all persons infected with HIV (HHS, 2018). The treatment of HIV has been, since the discovery of effective regimens in the mid-1990s, focused on continuous virologic suppression, thus halting further destruction of CD4+ T cells and permitting immune reconstitution. Pharmacologic advances have permitted development of multiple single-pill, once-daily regimens for the effective treatment of HIV. Regimens that are recommended by the HHS are summarized in the current version of the treatment guidelines from 2018. Treatment of HIV continues to evolve at a rapid pace, and review of treatment regimens is beyond the scope of this chapter. However, guidelines are updated regularly, and the reader is referred to those sources for further information (HHS, 2018). In general, goals of treatment are, as above, to halt human immunodeficiency viral replication, thus permitting immune reconstitution. Antimicrobial prophylaxis can be lifesaving for those who are severely immunocompromised. Goals of treatment are also to monitor for side effects of treatment and prevent/manage possible complications of both HIV infection and its treatment (HHS, 2018; Aberg et al., 2014).

HIV, as with many other STIs, is preventable. Condoms and other barrier methods have proven effective in prevention of transmission of HIV. For those in serodiscordant relationships, effective treatment of the positive partner has also been shown to be effective in prevention of transmission of HIV (Cohen et al., 2011).

More recently, biomedical methods (particularly pre-exposure prophylaxis, or PrEP) have proven quite effective at HIV prevention (Partners PrEP, TDF2), including in LGBT populations (namely MSM and transwomen) (Grant et al., 2010). In addition, PrEP has been demonstrated to be effective in a variety of settings, including the prevention of nonsexual transmission of HIV (Choopanya et al., 2013). These studies, and others, led the CDC to recommend PrEP for HIV prevention (HHS & CDC, 2014), and also led the FDA to approve the main study agent, a combination pill of tenofovir disoproxil fumarate and emtricitabine (TDF/FTC, or Truvada), for the PrEP indication. As approved, the PrEP regimen consists of a single pill taken once daily for the duration of significant risk.

In the time since the initial studies were done, others have demonstrated the efficacy of PrEP in real-world settings (Volk et al., 2015). The availability and efficacy of PrEP have significantly altered the HIV prevention landscape and discussions about approaches to prevention in the United States and abroad. It is important to note that currently, PrEP is not without side effects (of highest concern are renal and bone) and is only approved for HIV prevention as part of a more comprehensive approach. As with the medical management of HIV, the medical prevention of HIV is an area of active research and is evolving rapidly. There are studies currently underway to determine alternate dosing frequencies (e.g., event-triggered dosing) and alternate regimens. These and other studies will undoubtedly lead to optimization of PrEP over time. It is safe to say that, in the absence of an effective vaccine, PrEP has proven to be a tolerable and effective means of HIV prevention, achieving the goal of reducing new diagnoses to a degree that other prevention efforts have been unable to achieve.

HEPATITIS

Hepatitis broadly involves any inflammation of the liver. For the purposes of this text, we will discuss viral hepatitis, the most common cause of hepatitis. There are five hepatitis viruses (A, B, C D, E), of which we will be discussing those that cause a majority of disease: hepatitis A (HAV), hepatitis B (HBV), and hepatitis C (HCV). According to the CDC, viral hepatitis is the leading cause of liver cancer and the most common reason for liver transplantation (although transplantation due to alcoholic cirrhosis is fast rising). It is estimated that 4.4 million individuals in the United States and hundreds of millions worldwide are living with chronic hepatitis, and most do not know they are infected (CDC, 2013).

Men who have sex with men (MSM) are at elevated risk for HAV and HBV. Yet, despite the availability of safe and effective vaccines, many MSM have not been adequately vaccinated against viral hepatitis. Approximately 15 to 25 percent of all new HBV infections in the United States are among MSM. The Advisory Committee on Immunization Practices recommends HAV and HBV vaccination for MSM. Because of higher rates of infection among this population, CDC also recommends testing MSM for chronic HBV infection. As of publication, there remains no effective vaccination against HCV. However, recent developments in treatment have made it possible to cure individuals of persistent HCV infection.

What follows is a more in-depth discussion of HAV, HBV, and HCV.

Hepatitis A (HAV)

Hepatitis A (HAV) is a self-limited viral infection of the liver transmitted through virus shed in the host's feces. Initial presentation is characterized by mild flu-like symptoms, including anorexia, nausea/vomiting, fatigue, malaise, myalgias, and low-grade fevers. Following these symptoms, urine becomes dark (bilirubinuria), stool becomes pale, and jaundice can occur in a majority of adults (70 to 85 percent). Acute liver failure is a rare complication of infection, and HAV thankfully does not result in chronic infection. In addition to contact with contaminated foods, person-to-person sexual contact can cause transmission through a fecal-oral route (e.g., rimming, felching, ass play, et cetera) (CDC, 2009). Approximately 10 percent of all new HAV cases are MSM, and therefore it is recommended that all MSM receive the HAV vaccine (CDC, 1996).

Hepatitis B (HBV)

Like HAV, HBV infection can present as mild flu-like symptoms, including anorexia, nausea/vomiting, fatigue, malaise, myalgias, and low-grade fevers. Similarly, those infected may experience elevated bilirubin, pale stool, and jaundice. Unlike HAV, HBV is spread through bodily fluids such as blood and semen; it is most often transmitted sexually, and incidence is noted to be high among MSM (Gorgos, 2013). HBV causes approximately 1 to 2 million deaths a year. In the United States alone, 700,000 to 1.4 million persons are estimated to be infected (Ioannou, 2011; Wasley et al., 2010), many of whom are unaware they are infected (Spradling, 2012). It is important to note that HBV is not spread through sharing eating utensils or casual contact such as hugging and kissing.

HBV can either be acute or chronic; likelihood of chronic HBV infection decreases with age at time of infection. During acute infection, HBV surface antigen (HBsAg) and HBVe antigen (HBeAg) become detectable within four weeks of infection. Immunity and resolution of the infection develop following development of antibodies to HBsAg (anti-HBsAg Ab) and HBeAg (anti-HBeAg Ab); detection of anti-HBsAg antibodies indicates immunity. Lack of antibodies to HBsAg indicates chronic HBV infection.

Chronic HBV infection increases the risk for hepatocellular carcinoma. As MSM are at increased risk for HBV infection, making up 20 percent of new cases, vaccination is strongly encouraged (CDC, 2005). Vaccination against HBV has been an effective method of reducing infections but also essentially preventing hepatocellular carcinoma; the HBV vaccine is considered the first vaccine against a cancer (Chang, 2009). In addition to vaccination, public health efforts have been made to improve access to care and treatment for persons living with HBV. CDC guidelines addressing chronic HBV infection stress the importance of testing, conducting contact management, educating patients, and administering FDA-approved therapies for treating HBV, including new antiviral medications (CDC, 2008).

Hepatitis C (HCV)

Similar to HAV and HBV, HCV has higher rates among MSM, but unlike the other two hepatitis strains, an effective vaccine has yet to be developed for it (Bradshaw, Matthews, & Danta, 2013). As the most common chronic blood-borne infection in the United States, HCV is not classically categorized as an STI; however, reports of sexual transmission continue, particularly among MSM and HIV-infected MSM (CDC, 2011; van de Laar et al., 2009). In light of this and reported high rates of reinfection after treatment, HIV-infected individuals should undergo HCV screening and have their liver function monitored (Lambers et al., 2011). Like HBV, untreated HCV can lead to liver cirrhosis, liver failure, and hepatocellular carcinoma; approximately 75 to 85 percent of individuals infected with HCV develop chronic infection.

HCV is transmitted primarily through percutaneous exposure that can result from injection drug use, needle-stick injuries, and inadequate infection control in health care settings. Much less often, HCV transmission occurs among persons living with HIV, especially MSM, as a result of sexual contact with an HCV-infected partner (CDC, 2011).

As there is no effective vaccine available against HCV infection, and burden of disease remains significant, prevention focuses on behavior modification and screening (CDC, 1998).

Given limited prevention options, providing access to care and treatment is critical to improving health outcomes for individuals infected with HCV. Connecting patients to care is especially important given the significant advancements in HCV therapies; treatment previously consisted of PEGylated interferon combined with oral doses of ribavirin, a regimen that has improved health outcomes for many infected persons but had limited efficacy and significant side effects (e.g., flu-like symptoms and occasional exacerbation of mental illness due to interferon-containing agents, and dose-limiting anemia with ribavirin). Novel agents that have direct action against HCV have recently been approved with higher cure rates and lower side effect profiles (Asselah & Marcellin, 2011; Poordad et al., 2013). Current attention has been focused on affordability of oral regimens, which are still currently cost prohibitive for many people living with HCV.

OTHER SEXUALLY TRANSMITTED INFECTIONS

Syphilis

Syphilis, the disease caused by infection with *Treponema pallidum*, is a disease known from antiquity ("the great pox"). It is well known for its protean manifestations ("the great imitator"), and, as with many other STIs, persons may be infected with—and transmit—the disease with few or no symptoms at all. Rates of syphilis are currently increasing in the United States, particularly in gay and bisexual men, and are presently at incidence/prevalence levels not seen since the 1970s.

According to the most recent CDC estimates, MSM accounted for approximately 75 percent of all syphilis cases (CDC, 2015). Furthermore, MSM continue to make up a large percentage of syphilis prevalence, and cases are often associated with HIV coinfection (Foggia et al., 2014). Black, Hispanic, and young MSM are at increased risk for primary and secondary syphilis (Su, Beltrami, Zaidi, & Weinstock, 2011).

Spread of syphilis is a result of direct contact with sores that can be found on the penis, vagina, anus, lips, or in the rectum or mouth. Even MSM who do not practice anal sex may have similar risk of urethral primary syphilis (PS) to MSM who do (Nash et al., 2014), specifically, receptive unprotected oral sex as well as use of anal sex toys have been positively correlated with syphilis despite low risk of HIV transmission (Champenois et al., 2013; Thurnheer et al., 2010).

Syphilis has three major stages: primary, secondary, and tertiary. The natural history of the disease also includes a latent stage, most often between secondary and tertiary syphilis. Primary syphilis is characterized by a local infection with *T. pallidum*, during which patients may have a genital ulcer, classically painless, that occurs at the site of initial exposure/ inoculation. Occasionally, the site of inoculation may be on a mucous membrane that is not easily visible (e.g., rectal mucosa), and thus may go unnoticed. Diagnosis requires a high index of suspicion, as testing of the lesion for presence of *T. pallidum* is the primary means of diagnosis. Secondary syphilis represents dissemination of the organism and is often associated with systemic symptoms (fevers, chills, malaise), a generalized rash that classically involves the palms and soles, lesions of the mucous membranes (mucous patches), and lesions of the genitals (condyloma lata). If left untreated, most symptoms resolve within a few weeks, giving rise to latent syphilis. Diagnosis during secondary and early latent syphilis is usually made with serologic testing, including a combination of treponemal (specific) and nontreponemal (nonspecific) tests; e.g., fluorescent treponemal antibody absorptiometry (FTA-ABS) and rapid plasma reagin (RPR), respectively. Tertiary syphilis is marked by inflammatory complications of sites of infection (gummas) that may occur in any organ, other complications such as aortitis, and neurologic disease such as tabes dorsalis and general paresis. During late latent and tertiary syphilis, the total organism burden in a host may be small, and nontreponemal tests typically lose sensitivity in these settings. Again, diagnosis relies on a high index of suspicion, and definitive diagnosis may require biopsy of affected tissue. Some treponemal tests (e.g., syphilis IgG) will typically remain positive but are unable to distinguish latent from previously treated infection and thus must be interpreted carefully. Long-term consequences can occur as a result of untreated syphilis.

Treatment relies on penicillin or, in some cases, particularly in early syphilis and when a patient may have a penicillin allergy, doxycycline. Current guideline recommendations are publicly available with the CDC (CDC, 2015). Management is complex and requires knowledge of both the stage of syphilis as well as whether there is central nervous system involvement, as intramuscular penicillin and oral therapies have been associated with treatment failure in the presence of CNS infection.

Prevention is key but is made more challenging by the fact that only traditional safer sex methods (barrier methods) are associated with meaningful prevention efficacy. Some have expressed concern that the possible discrepant message between prevention of HIV (biomedical/PrEP) and other STIs (barrier/condom), along with the possible perception of syphilis as a "lesser" STI due to its curable nature, may lead to a more permissive attitude and thus contribute to the rising rates of STIs in general and syphilis in particular, especially in those populations at highest risk (e.g., MSM).

Gonorrhea and Chlamydia

Gonorrhea, infection with *Neisseria gonorrhea* (NG), and chlamydia, infection with *Chlamydia trachomatis* (CT), are two of the most common of the classically nonulcerative STI. Infection with these agents typically presents with inflammation of the inoculated site: this usually manifests as inflammation of the urinary tract (urethritis) and cervix (cervicitis) but may also manifest as inflammation of the rectum (proctitis) or throat (pharyngitis). Of note, infection with certain types of *Chlamydia trachomatis* (serovars L1–L3) may cause a particularly aggressive form of proctitis and superinfected inguinal lymph node enlargement known as lymphogranuloma venereum (LGV). Additionally, a significant minority of infections—and depending on the site, a majority of infections—are asymptomatic, though they still may be transmissible. Last, it is worth noting that individuals may suffer a variety of complications of GC/CT, both infectious (e.g., disseminated gonococcal infection, Fitz-Hugh-Curtis syndrome, pelvic inflammatory disease) and noninfectious (e.g., reactive arthritis [formerly Reiter syndrome], keratoderma blenorrhagicum).

Diagnosis is usually made by nucleic acid amplification testing (NAAT) of the affected site. Culture is possible for gonorrhea, and this may be particularly important for susceptibility testing (see below). It is important to remember that testing should not only be triggered by compatible symptoms but also by discovery of other STI, contact exposure (though some areas practice expedited partner treatment, EPT, see below), and routine screening for sexually active adults.

CDC screening guidelines recommend annual screening for gonorrhea and chlamydia for sexually active gay, bisexual, and other MSM. MSM with more than one partner, anonymous partners, and those who use or are sexually active with those who use illicit drugs should increase the frequency of screening (CDC, 2017b). MSM must be screened for both CT in addition to gonorrhea, or more than 70 percent of cases may be missed (Kent et al., 2005). Clinicians have cited various barriers to maintaining these screening standards, such as time restraints, lack of staff, cultural/language barriers and, as a result, self-testing, self-collected rectal/pharyngeal swabs, and Internet-based testing may be better alternatives (van der Helm et al., 2009). Condom use with anal sex has been shown to be protective against infection (Nash et al., 2014).

Distressingly, drug-resistant strains of gonorrhea are on the rise, particularly among MSM (Kirkcaldy et al., 2015; Kirkcaldy et al., 2013). Therefore, patients should be instructed to return for follow-up if symptoms do not improve after a few days of treatment.

Treatment is often performed presumptively, based on symptoms, exam findings, and pending test results. Treatment may also be initiated in sexual partners of diagnosed patients (EPT); the optimal mode of initiating treatment (from the partner, versus from a health care provider) is currently debated. Treatment of CT infection is usually with doxycycline or azithromycin, with a duration dictated by site and type of infection. Treatment of GC is made more complex by evolving resistance patterns. Because of increased resistance of GC to fluoroquinolones and, more recently, to oral cefixime, current guidelines are for dual therapy with IM ceftriaxone (or cefotaxime or cefoxitin) with oral azithromycin. This dual therapy has the added advantage of built-in treatment for CT coinfection, as is often present in those who test positive for GC.

Among MSM, sexual partners who do not come into clinic to be tested and treated may benefit from patient-delivered partner therapy (PDPT) (Kerani, Fleming, DeYoung, & Golden, 2011). Treatment failures should be expected, since MSM are particularly susceptible to antimicrobial-resistant strains (Kirkcaldy et al., 2013).

Prevention of infection is best achieved by traditional safer-sex methods, most notably with barrier protection/condoms. Concerns raised about the public perception of STI (see syphilis above) apply to GC/CT infection as well, and such perceptions have been hypothesized as at least part of the reason for the observed rise in cases in the United States over the last few years.

Human Papillomavirus

Human papillomavirus (HPV) is the most common STI worldwide (Brown et al., 2012). While many HPV infections are asymptomatic (~50 percent of sexually active persons) certain strains are associated with genital warts (e.g., HPV-6, -11) or cancers of the cervix, anal canal, and throat (e.g., HPV-16, -18) (CDC & APHL, 2014). Of note, HIV-infected MSM populations have higher incidences of anal cancer that exceed those of cervical cancer in women.

One method of prevention of HPV-associated cancer is screening for precancerous lesions. Cytologic screening of the cervix (by Papanicolau smear) has proven effective at reducing both incidence of—and deaths due to—cervical cancer, and cervical cytologic screening is recommended by the USPSTF (Moyer & U.S. Preventive Services Task Force, 2012). At this time, evidence is limited, but some studies have called for an increase in HPV vaccine coverage and cancer surveillance in MSM (CDC & APHL, 2014), in part driven by the higher incidence of HPV-associated anal cancer noted in the paragraph above. The cost-effectiveness of anal cytologic screening is an area of debate and is dependent upon multiple factors: provider experience/comfort with obtaining anal cytology specimens, expertise in interpreting smears, availability of appropriate follow-up diagnostic testing (such as high-resolution anoscopy), and availability of appropriate therapeutic referrals (such as therapeutic high-resolution anoscopy and colorectal surgical expertise). While most factors weigh in favor of screening for those with immunosuppressive conditions such as HIV, conclusions are not as clear-cut for HIV-uninfected MSM, women, and other men (Long et al., 2016). Additionally, WSW are less likely to undergo regular cervical screening. However, HPV can be transmitted from woman to woman via finger-to-genital contact (Sonnex, Strauss, & Gray, 1999). While more studies are needed to determine rates of HPV among WSW, this population should be encouraged to undergo regular screening (Henderson, 2009). If left untreated, infection with high-risk HPV can result in cervical, anal, and pharyngeal cancer.

The epidemiology and impact of HPV infection and disease burden are in flux due to the relatively recent availability of several effective vaccines against many strains of HPV, including some of the strains most commonly associated with cancer (Pahud & Ault, 2015). The efficacy of these vaccines, particularly in prevention of cervical infection and precancerous lesions (FDA, 2014), have led to their incorporation into the recommended pediatric vaccine schedule by the ACIP (Markowitz et al., 2014).

CONCLUSIONS

This chapter has provided a brief overview of the importance of STIs to LGBT populations and illustrates how STIs represent another aspect of health and health care disparities suffered by minority sexual orientation/gender identity populations. Addressing this disparity will require increased efforts in research to better identify magnitudes and etiologies of these disparities, and in education to generate providers who are competent in the knowledge, skills, and behaviors needed for LGBT health care. We hope that this overview contributes to those mission areas.

REFERENCES

Aberg, J. A., Gallant, J. E., Ghanem, K. G., Emmanuel, P., Zingman, B. S., Horberg, M. A., & Infectious Diseases Society of America. (2014). Primary care guidelines for the management of persons infected with HIV: 2013 update by the HIV Medicine Association of the Infectious Diseases Society of America. *Clinical Infectious Diseases : An Official Publication of the Infectious Diseases Society of America, 58*(1), 1–10. doi:10.1093/cid/cit757

Asselah, T., & Marcellin, P. (2011). New direct-acting antivirals' combination for the treatment of chronic hepatitis C. *Liver International : Official Journal of the International Association for the Study of the Liver, 31*(Suppl 1), 68–77. doi:10.1111/j.1478-3231.2010.02411.x

Bradshaw, D., Matthews, G., & Danta, M. (2013). Sexually transmitted hepatitis C infection: The new epidemic in MSM? *Current Opinion in Infectious Diseases, 26*(1), 66–72. doi:10.1097/QCO.0b013e32835c2120

Branson, B. M., Handsfield, H. H., Lampe, M. A., Janssen, R. S., Taylor, A. W., Lyss, S. B., . . . Centers for Disease Control and Prevention (CDC). (2006). Revised recommendations for HIV testing of adults, adolescents, and pregnant women in health-care settings. *Morbidity and Mortality Weekly Report, 55*(RR-14), 4 (rr5514a1 [pii]).

Braun, D. L., Kouyos, R. D., Balmer, B., Grube, C., Weber, R., & Gunthard, H. F. (2015). Frequency and spectrum of unexpected clinical manifestations of primary HIV-1 infection. *Clinical Infectious Diseases : An Official Publication of the Infectious Diseases Society of America, 61*(6), 1013–1021. doi:10.1093/cid/civ398

Brown, B., Davtyan, M., Galea, J., Chow, E., Leon, S., & Klausner, J. D. (2012). The role of human papillomavirus in human immunodeficiency virus acquisition in men who have sex with men: A review of the literature. *Viruses, 4*(12), 3851–3858. doi:10.3390/v4123851

Centers for Disease Control and Prevention (CDC). (1981). Pneumocystis pneumonia—Los Angeles. *Morbidity and Mortality Weekly Report, 30*(21), 1-3.

Centers for Disease Control and Prevention (CDC). (1989). AIDS and human immunodeficiency virus infection in the United States: 1988 update. *MMWR Supplements, 38*(4), 1–38.

Centers for Disease Control and Prevention (CDC). (1996). Prevention of hepatitis A through active or passive immunization: recommendations of the Advisory Committee on Immunization Practices. *Morbidity and Mortality Weekly Report, 45*(RR-15), 1–30.

Centers for Disease Control and Prevention (CDC). (1998). Recommendations for prevention and control of hepatitis C virus (HCV) infection and

HCV-related chronic disease. *Morbidity and Mortality Weekly Report, 47*(RR-19), 1–54.

Centers for Disease Control and Prevention (CDC). (2005). A comprehensive immunization strategy to eliminate transmission of hepatitis B virus infection in the United States. Part 1: Immunization of infants, children, and adolescents. *Morbidity and Mortality Weekly Report, 54*(RR-16), 1–31.

Centers for Disease Control and Prevention (CDC). (2008). Recommendations for identification and public health management of persons with chronic hepatitis B virus infection. *Morbidity and Mortality Weekly Report, 57*(RR-08), 1–18.

Centers for Disease Control and Prevention (CDC). (2009). *Epidemiology and prevention of vaccine-preventable diseases* (11th ed.). Atkinson, W., Wolfe, S., Hamborsky, J., McIntyre, L. (Eds.). Washington, DC: Public Health Foundation.

Centers for Disease Control and Prevention (CDC). (2011). Sexual transmission of hepatitis C virus among HIV-infected men who have sex with men—New York City, 2005–2010. *Morbidity and Mortality Weekly Report, 60*, 945–950.

Centers for Disease Control and Prevention (CDC). (2013). *Surveillance for viral hepatitis—United States, 2012.* Atlanta: U.S. Department of Health and Human Services.

Centers for Disease Control and Prevention (CDC). (2015a). *Sexually transmitted disease surveillance 2014.* Atlanta: U.S. Department of Health and Human Services.

Centers for Disease Control and Prevention (CDC). (2015b). Sexually transmitted diseases treatment guidelines: Syphilis. Retrieved from https://www.cdc.gov/std/tg2015/syphilis.htm

Centers for Disease Control and Prevention (CDC). (2017a). HIV surveillance report, 2016; vol. 28. Retrieved from http://www.cdc.gov/hiv/library/reports/hiv-surveillance.html

Centers for Disease Control and Prevention (CDC). (2017b). Special populations, 2015 sexually transmitted diseases treatment guidelines. Retrieved from https://www.cdc.gov/std/tg2015/specialpops.htm.

Centers for Disease Control and Prevention (CDC) & Association of Public Health Laboratories. (2014). Laboratory testing for the diagnosis of HIV infection: Updated recommendations. Retrieved from http://stacks.cdc.gov/view/cdc/23447

Champenois, K., Cousien, A., Ndiaye, B., Soukouna, Y., Baclet, V., Alcaraz, I., . . . Yazdanpanah, Y. (2013). Risk factors for syphilis infection in men who have sex with men: Results of a case-control study in Lille, France. *Sexually Transmitted Infections, 89*(2), 128–132. doi:10.1136/sextrans-2012-050523

Chang, M. H. (2009). Cancer prevention by vaccination against hepatitis B. *Recent Results in Cancer Research. Fortschritte der Krebsforschung. Progrès dans les recherches sur le cancer, 181*, 85–94.

Choopanya, K., Martin, M., Suntharasamai, P., Sangkum, U., Mock, P. A., Leethochawalit, M., . . . Bangkok Tenofovir Study Group. (2013).

Antiretroviral prophylaxis for HIV infection in injecting drug users in Bangkok, Thailand (the Bangkok tenofovir study): A randomised, double-blind, placebo-controlled phase 3 trial. *Lancet, 381*(9883), 2083–2090. doi:10.1016/S0140-6736(13)61127-7

Cohen, M. S., Chen, Y. Q., McCauley, M., Gamble, T., Hosseinipour, M. C., Kumarasamy, N., . . . HPTN 052 Study Team. (2011). Prevention of HIV-1 infection with early antiretroviral therapy. *The New England Journal of Medicine, 365*(6), 493–505. doi:10.1056/NEJMoa1105243

Engel, J. (2006). *The epidemic: A global history of AIDS*. New York: Smithsonian Books/Collins. Retrieved from http://www.loc.gov/catdir/toc/fy0705/2006044285.html; http://www.loc.gov/catdir/enhancements/fy0911/2006044285-b.html; http://www.loc.gov/catdir/enhancements/fy0911/2006044285-d.html

Everett, B. G. (2013). Sexual orientation disparities in sexually transmitted infections: Examining the intersection between sexual identity and sexual behavior. *Archives of Sexual Behavior, 42*(2), 225–236. doi:10.1007/s10508-012-9902-1

Fethers, K. A., Fairley, C. K., Hocking, J. S., Gurrin, L. C., & Bradshaw, C. S. (2008). Sexual risk factors and bacterial vaginosis: A systematic review and meta-analysis. *Clinical Infectious Diseases: An Official Publication of the Infectious Diseases Society of America, 47*(11), 1426–1435. doi:10.1086/592974

Foggia, M., Gentile, I., Bonadies, G., Buonomo, A. R., Minei, G., Borrelli, F., . . . Borgia, G. (2014). A retrospective study on HIV and syphilis. *Le infezioni in medicina: Rivista periodica di eziologia, epidemiologia, diagnostica, clinica e terapia delle patologie infettive, 22*(1), 26–30.

Food and Drug Administration (FDA). (2014). Product approval-prescribing information [Package insert, online]. Gardasil [human papillomavirus quadrivalent (types 6, 11, 16, and 18) vaccine, recombinant], Merck & Co, Inc. Silver Spring, MD. Retrieved from http://www.fda.gov/downloads/BiologicsBloodVaccines/Vaccines/ApprovedProducts/UCM111263.pdf

Gorgos, L. (2013). Sexual transmission of viral hepatitis. *Infectious Disease Clinics of North America, 27*(4), 811–836. doi:10.1016/j.idc.2013.08.002

Gottlieb, M. S. (2006). Pneumocystis pneumonia—Los Angeles. 1981. *American Journal of Public Health, 96*(6), 3 (96/6/980 [pii]).

Grant, R. M., Lama, J. R., Anderson, P. L., McMahan, V., Liu, A. Y., Vargas, L., . . . iPrEx Study Team. (2010). Preexposure chemoprophylaxis for HIV prevention in men who have sex with men. *The New England Journal of Medicine, 363*(27), 2587–2599. doi:10.1056/NEJMoa1011205

Grimes, J., Fagerberg, K., & Smith, L. (2013). *Sexually transmitted disease: An encyclopedia of diseases, prevention, treatment, and issues*. Santa Barbara, CA: Greenwood.

Handsfield, H. H. (1992). *Color atlas and synopsis of sexually transmitted diseases*. New York: McGraw-Hill, Health Professions Division.

Henderson, H. J. (2009). Why lesbians should be encouraged to have regular cervical screening. *The Journal of Family Planning and Reproductive Health Care, 35*(1), 49–52. doi:10.1783/147118909787072315

Holmes, K. K. (2007). *Sexually transmitted diseases* (4th ed.). New York: McGraw-Hill Medical. Retrieved from http://www.loc.gov/catdir/toc/ecip 0714/2007013008.html; http://www.loc.gov/catdir/enhancements/fy0726 /2007013008-b.html; http://www.loc.gov/catdir/enhancements/fy0726/20070 13008-d.html

Ioannou, G. N. (2011). Hepatitis B virus in the United States: Infection, exposure, and immunity rates in a nationally representative survey. *Annals of Internal Medicine, 154*(5), 319–328. doi:10.7326/0003-4819-154-5-201103010-00006

Kent, C. K., Chaw, J. K., Wong, W., Liska, S., Gibson, S., Hubbard, G., & Klausner, J. D. (2005). Prevalence of rectal, urethral, and pharyngeal chlamydia and gonorrhea detected in 2 clinical settings among men who have sex with men: San Francisco, California, 2003. *Clinical Infectious Diseases: An Official Publication of the Infectious Diseases Society of America, 41*(1), 67–74 (CID35177 [pii]).

Kerani, R. P., Fleming, M., DeYoung, B., & Golden, M. R. (2011). A randomized, controlled trial of inSPOT and patient-delivered partner therapy for gonorrhea and chlamydial infection among men who have sex with men. *Sexually Transmitted Diseases, 38*(10), 941–946. doi:10.1097/OLQ.0b013e 318223fcbc

Kirkcaldy, R. D., Hook, E. W., Soge, O. O., del Rio, C., Kubin, G., Zenilman, J. M., & Papp, J. R. (2015). Trends in *Neisseria gonorrhoeae* susceptibility to cephalosporins in the United States, 2006–2014. *JAMA, 314*(17), 1869–1871. doi:10.1001/jama.2015.10347

Kirkcaldy, R. D., Zaidi, A., Hook, E. W., Holmes, K. K., Soge, O., del Rio, C., . . . Weinstock, H. S. (2013). *Neisseria gonorrhoeae* antimicrobial resistance among men who have sex with men and men who have sex exclusively with women: The Gonococcal Isolate Surveillance Project, 2005–2010. *Annals of Internal Medicine, 158*(5, Part 1), 321–328. doi:10.7326/0003-4819 -158-5-201303050-00004

Lambers, F. A., Prins, M., Thomas, X., Molenkamp, R., Kwa, D., Brinkman, K., . . . MOSAIC (MSM Observational Study of Acute Infection with hepatitis C) study group. (2011). Alarming incidence of hepatitis C virus re-infection after treatment of sexually acquired acute hepatitis C virus infection in HIV-infected MSM. *AIDS (London, England), 25*(17), 21. doi:10.1097 /QAD.0b013e32834bac44

Long, K. C., Menon, R., Bastawrous, A., & Billingham, R. (2016). Screening, surveillance, and treatment of anal intraepithelial neoplasia. *Clinics in Colon and Rectal Surgery, 29*(1), 57–64. doi:10.1055/s-0035-1570394

Markowitz, L. E., Dunne, E. F., Saraiya, M., Chesson, H. W., Curtis, C. R., Gee, J., . . . Centers for Disease Control and Prevention (CDC). (2014). Human papillomavirus vaccination: Recommendations of the advisory committee on immunization practices (ACIP). *Morbidity and Mortality Weekly Report, 63*(RR-05), 1–30 (rr6305a1 [pii]).

Marrazzo, J. M., Thomas, K. K., Agnew, K., & Ringwood, K. (2010). Prevalence and risks for bacterial vaginosis in women who have sex with women. *Sexually Transmitted Diseases, 37*(5), 335–339.

Milstein, B. (2002). Introduction to the Syndemics Prevention Network. Retrieved from http://www.cdc.gov/syndemics/

Moyer, V. A., & U.S. Preventive Services Task Force. (2012). Screening for cervical cancer: U.S. preventive services task force recommendation statement. *Annals of Internal Medicine, 156*(12), 91, W312. doi:10.7326/0003-4819 -156-12-201206190-00424

Nash, J. L., Hocking, J. S., Read, T. R., Chen, M. Y., Bradshaw, C. S., Forcey, D. S., & Fairley, C. K. (2014). Contribution of sexual practices (other than anal sex) to bacterial sexually transmitted infection transmission in men who have sex with men: A cross-sectional analysis using electronic health records. *Sexually Transmitted Infections, 90*(1), 55–57. doi:10.1136/sextrans -2013-051103

Owusu-Edusei, K., Chesson, H. W., Gift, T. L., Tao, G., Mahajan, R., Ocfemia, M. C., & Kent, C. K. (2013). The estimated direct medical cost of selected sexually transmitted infections in the United States, 2008. *Sexually Transmitted Diseases, 40*(3), 197–201. doi:10.1097/OLQ.0b013e318285c6d2

Pahud, B. A., & Ault, K. A. (2015). The expanded impact of human papillomavirus vaccine. *Infectious Disease Clinics of North America, 29*(4), 715–724. doi:10.1016/j.idc.2015.07.007

Poordad, F., Lawitz, E., Kowdley, K. V., Cohen, D. E., Podsadecki, T., Siggelkow, S., . . . Bernstein, B. (2013). Exploratory study of oral combination antiviral therapy for hepatitis C. *The New England Journal of Medicine, 368*(1), 45–53. doi:10.1056/NEJMoa1208809

Satterwhite, C. L., Torrone, E., Meites, E., Dunne, E. F., Mahajan, R., Ocfemia, M. C., . . . Weinstock, H. (2013). Sexually transmitted infections among US women and men: Prevalence and incidence estimates, 2008. *Sexually Transmitted Diseases, 40*(3), 187–193. doi:10.1097/OLQ.0b013e318286bb53

Shilts, R. (1988). *And the band played on: Politics, people, and the AIDS epidemic.* New York: Penguin Books.

Sonnex, C., Strauss, S., & Gray, J. J. (1999). Detection of human papillomavirus DNA on the fingers of patients with genital warts. *Sexually Transmitted Infections, 75*(5), 317–319.

Spradling, P. R., Rupp, L., Moorman, A. C., Lu, M., Teshale, E. H., Gordon, S. C., . . . Chronic Hepatitis Cohort Study Investigators. (2012). Hepatitis B and C virus infection among 1.2 million persons with access to care: Factors associated with testing and infection prevalence. *Clinical Infectious Diseases: An Official Publication of the Infectious Diseases Society of America, 55*(8), 1047–1055 (cis616 [pii]).

Stall, R., Mills, T. C., Williamson, J., Hart, T., Greenwood, G., Paul, J., . . . Catania, J. A. (2003). Association of co-occurring psychosocial health problems and increased vulnerability to HIV/AIDS among urban men who have sex with men. *American Journal of Public Health, 93*(6), 939–942.

Su, J. R., Beltrami, J. F., Zaidi, A. A., & Weinstock, H. S. (2011). Primary and secondary syphilis among black and Hispanic men who have sex with men: Case report data from 27 states. *Annals of Internal Medicine, 155*(3), 145–151. doi:10.7326/0003-4819-155-3-201108020-00004

Thurnheer, M. C., Weber, R., Toutous-Trellu, L., Cavassini, M., Elzi, L., Schmid, P., . . . Swiss HIV Cohort Study. (2010). Occurrence, risk factors, diagnosis and treatment of syphilis in the prospective observational Swiss HIV Cohort Study. *AIDS (London, England), 24*(12), 1907–1916. doi:10.1097/QAD.0b013e32833bfe21

U.S. Department of Health and Human Services (HHS). (2018). Guidelines for the use of antiretroviral agents in HIV-1-infected adults and adolescents. Retrieved from https://aidsinfo.nih.gov/contentfiles/lvguidelines/adultand adolescentgl.pdf

U.S. Department of Health and Human Services (HHS) & Centers for Disease Control and Prevention (CDC). (2014). United States public health services: Preexposure prophylaxis for the prevention of HIV Infection in the United States—2014 clinical practice guideline. Retrieved from http://www.cdc.gov/hiv/pdf/prepguidelines2014.pdf

van de Laar, T., Pybus, O., Bruisten, S., Brown, D., Nelson, M., Bhagani, S., . . . Danta, M. (2009). Evidence of a large, international network of HCV transmission in HIV-positive men who have sex with men. *Gastroenterology, 136*(5), 1609–1617 (S0016-5085(09)00184-X [pii]).

van der Helm, J. J., Hoebe, C. J., van Rooijen, M. S., Brouwers, E. E., Fennema, H. S., Thiesbrummel, H. F., & Dukers-Muijrers, N. H. (2009). High performance and acceptability of self-collected rectal swabs for diagnosis of Chlamydia trachomatis and Neisseria gonorrhoeae in men who have sex with men and women. *Sexually Transmitted Diseases, 36*(8), 493–497. doi:10.1097/OLQ.0b013e3181a44b8c

Volk, J. E., Marcus, J. L., Phengrasamy, T., Blechinger, D., Nguyen, D. P., Follansbee, S., & Hare, C. B. (2015). No new HIV infections with increasing use of HIV preexposure prophylaxis in a clinical practice setting. *Clinical Infectious Diseases: An Official Publication of the Infectious Diseases Society of America, 61*(10), 1601–1603. doi:10.1093/cid/civ778

Wasley, A., Kruszon-Moran, D., Kuhnert, W., Simard, E. P., Finelli, L., McQuillan, G., & Bell, B. (2010). The prevalence of hepatitis B virus infection in the United States in the era of vaccination. *The Journal of Infectious Diseases, 202*(2), 192–201. doi:10.1086/653622

Workowski, K. A., Berman, S., & Centers for Disease Control and Prevention (CDC). (2010). Sexually transmitted diseases treatment guidelines, 2010. *Morbidity and Mortality Weekly Report, 59*(RR-12), 1–110 (rr5912a1 [pii]).

World Health Organization (WHO). (2014). *Global update on the health sector response to HIV, 2014.* Geneva, Switzerland: World Health Organization. Retrieved from https://www.who.int/hiv/pub/progressreports/update2014/en/

5

Cancer in Sexual Minority Women

Deborah Bowen and Jennifer Jabson

Cancer is a cluster of diseases that occur all through life, although cancer occurs much more frequently in older years (American Cancer Society [ACS], 2010). Cancer, at its simplest, comes from groups of cells growing and multiplying in ways that interfere with functioning and, in many cases, cause mortality and morbidity (ACS, 2010). Cancer occurs in all races and in both women and men. Remarkably little is known about specific issues of cancer in sexual minority women. This chapter will briefly review the patterns of cancer in women, noting where possible any information specific to sexual minority women. We will end with a call for more research into areas that particularly need addressing.

DEFINING CANCER SURVIVORSHIP

Cancer survivorship is defined by the National Institute of Cancer (2008) as the "physical, psychosocial and economic issues of cancer, from diagnosis until the end of life. It includes issues related to the ability to get health care and follow-up treatment, late effects of treatment, second cancers, and quality of life." Mullan (1990) suggests three distinct phases of cancer survival, each characterized by different behavioral, physical, and emotional disruptions. According to Mullan (1990), the first phase, acute survival, accompanies diagnosis and continues through the first year, which is often highlighted by cancer treatments. For example, Bloom (2002) reports that individuals in the acute survival phase report emotional distress and depression related to diagnosis and treatments but that these symptoms abate near the end of the first year. The second phase of survivorship is defined as extended survival and begins at the end of the first year after diagnosis and lasts until three years after diagnosis. Extended survival is characterized by physical disruptions similar to the first phase, including low levels of physical energy and compromises in physical functioning. Additionally, during the second stage of survivorship or extended survival, some individuals experience difficulty returning to employment and engaging previously rewarding interpersonal relationships. These disturbances are expected during the second phase, given that it is also the period when most survivors have the highest probability of cancer recurrence—a stressful reality for many survivors.

A survivor is said to enter the third phase of survivorship, permanent survival, after the first three years since diagnosis pass without a recurrence of cancer. The third and final phase, or permanent survival, is characterized by a return to precancer levels of functioning for some, but in other cases by permanent loss of physical energy and problems with interpersonal relationships. Although some survivors experience this phase of cancer survival with minimal negative outcomes, many other survivors in this phase of survival report continuing problems with social reintegration, including close friendships, employment, and leisure activities.

The complexity of quantifying the multifactorial qualities and characteristics of cancer survivorship is enormous. Very generally, and based on the current definition of survivorship, measuring the quality of one's survivorship results in two broadly defined categories of cancer survivorship: physical health and psychosocial health (Rowland, 2004; Fobair, 2007). Physical health includes factors such as physiologic reactions to treatments, health consequences of cancer treatment, physical functioning, and physical health outcomes. Psychosocial health includes factors such as stress, social support, affect/mood, and quality of life—composed of four types of well-being, including social, physical, spiritual, and psychological well-being. Both physical health and psychosocial health are vulnerable in the experiences of cancer diagnosis, treatment, and survivorship.

The research that supports our understanding of the stages and experiences of women's cancer survivorship is largely based on the experiences of heterosexual, or assumed heterosexual, cancer survivors. Despite the growing interest in understanding cancer survivorship of diverse groups, there exists a dearth of information pertaining to the experiences of cancer survivors who are also sexual minority women (SMW). In what follows, we discuss what is known about women's cancer survivorship and, where data is available, SMW's cancer survivorship. Notably, there is limited information regarding cancer survivorship among SMW. The notable lack of information about cancer survivorship among SMW reflects, among other factors, an absence of population-based demographic questions in cancer surveillance and registries and therefore an inability to analyze for differences in SMW's cancer survivorship experiences, physical health, and psychological health outcomes.

PHASE 1: ACUTE CANCER SURVIVORSHIP

According to Mullan (1990), the first phase of cancer survivorship, acute cancer survival, occurs from the moment of one's cancer diagnosis through treatments and to the first year after diagnosis. Most commonly diagnosed cancers among women include breast cancer, lung cancer, and colorectal cancers (ACS, 2010). Other cancers of importance for women include gynecologic cancer, including ovarian cancer and cervical cancer.

Breast Cancer

An estimated 268,670 new cases of invasive breast cancer were expected to be diagnosed as of 2018 (ACS, 2018). Breast cancer led to an estimated 41,400 deaths among women in 2018.

Lung Cancer

Lung cancer is the second most commonly diagnosed cancer in women in the United States (ACS, 2018). Women's rates of lung cancer have recently begun to plateau after a long period of increased rates over two decades. Estimated cancer incidence among women is 112,350 in 2018 (ACS, 2018). In 2018, it was estimated that 70,500 women would die from lung cancer.

Colorectal Cancer

Colorectal cancer is the third most common form of cancer to affect women. It was expected that in 2018, there would be 64,640 new cases of colon cancer among women (ACS, 2018). A steady decline in colorectal cancer cases among women has been attributed to increases in the use of colorectal cancer screening. In 2018, it was estimated that 23,240 women would die from colorectal cancer (ACS, 2018).

Gynecological Cancers

The American Cancer Society (2018) estimated that there would be 22,240 new cases of ovarian cancer diagnosed in 2018. Ovarian cancer rates have declined gradually over the past two decades. It was expected that 14,070 deaths would occur from ovarian cancer in 2018. The fourth most commonly occurring new cancer cases among women in 2018 was estimated to be uterine cancer, with 63,230 new uterine corpus cancer cases and 11,350 cancer-related deaths expected to occur among women.

Other Cancers

Other cancers occur in women, although their incidence is less than the four previously mentioned sites. In 2018, there was an estimate of 22,660 new cases of kidney and renal cancer cases diagnosed among women. Incidence of pancreatic cancer has been steadily increasing annually among women since 2000. It was estimated that 26,240 new cases of pancreatic cancer would be diagnosed among women in 2018. In 2018, it was estimated that 21,310 female deaths would be attributed to pancreatic cancer. The American Cancer Society estimated that in 2018, 36,120 cases of melanoma of the skin would occur among women. Among women in 2018, an estimated 40,900 new cases of thyroid cancer would occur.

Incidence of Cancer in Sexual Minority Women

Little definitive data has existed on potential disparities the incidence of cancer for sexual minority women. The major problem has been that sexual orientation is not routinely collected in population-based cancer surveillance efforts, including cancer registries, the gold-standard system in the United States for understanding cancer patterns by demographic groups (Bowen & Boehmer, 2007). Studies with limited or poor sampling have found potentially higher incidence of breast cancer among sexual minority women, but these cannot be considered definitive (Dibble & Roberts, 2002; Valanis et al., 2000). Recent research has identified a method of matching registry data sets with other large data sets that do contain sexual orientation, among other health variables, and using this method, the investigators did find disparities in breast and lung cancer among sexual minority women compared to heterosexual women (Boehmer, Ozonoff, & Timm, 2011; Boehmer, Miao, & Ozonoff, in press). Therefore, we finally have data to indicate that there are disparities among sexual minority women, but the mechanisms of these disparities are not known.

Diagnosis and Follow-Up

The diagnosis of cancer, from initial testing through definitive diagnosis, is a multistep process, different for each type of cancer and often involving multiple providers, multiple visits to health care facilities, many scans and tests, and complex feedback. A diagnosis of cancer often begins with one of two events: a routine screening test that identifies a possible cancer, or the experience of symptoms that leads the woman or her provider to request further testing. Both of these types of events often occur in the context of primary care, and the connection is made to oncology and further testing at that point. Zapka and colleagues have articulated models of care that involve several steps with different tests and providers, painting the picture of complexity and technical innovation required to accurately diagnose and label cancer in the current medical system (Zapka et al., 2004).

There are no known or published differences between sexual minority women and heterosexual women in the diagnosis or follow-up process of cancer.

Treatment of Cancer

Treatment of cancers is usually based on the stage (extent of growth and invasion) of cancer at diagnosis and is different for each cancer site. Treatment activities often involve chemotherapy, targeted radiation, surgery, or an increasingly complex combination of some or all of these treatments. For example, in order to down-stage cancerous tumors and to test for chemosensitivity, a Cochrane Review recommends that women diagnosed with operable breast cancer undergo preoperative chemotherapy (van der Hage, van der Velde, & Mieog, 2007) followed by surgery and a combination of other targeted treatments. Several policy-setting medical organizations, such as the National Cancer Institute and the American Cancer Society, identify state-of-the-science treatment options and targeted therapies for cancer type specific to stage and tumor characteristics, and these guidelines provide standards for appropriate therapy of cancers across the country and internationally.

There are no known differences in cancer treatment between sexual minority women and heterosexual women.

Palliative Care During and After Cancer Treatment

Palliative care in the treatment of cancer patients is defined as assisting patients with the side effects, long-term effects, and late effects of cancer diagnosis and treatment (National Consensus Project for Quality Palliative

Care, 2009; Frager, 1996). Palliative care can address the physical side effects of specific chemotherapeutic agents, mental health needs of patient and family due to the stress of diagnosis and/or treatment, or any changes in functioning as a result of treatment. Surviving treatment of the diagnosis of cancer often comes with a price for the survivors, who frequently experience harsh, life-altering side effects during and after treatment. The principal methods of managing the side effects of cancer treatment and cancer are pharmacologic. Over the last three decades, however, substantial research has shown that behavioral techniques are beneficial in controlling cancer treatment–related side effects and the pain and emotional effects of cancer (Kirsch, 1997). Behavioral treatments have several assets that contribute to their usefulness. They are cost-effective, noninvasive, and accepted by the patient; they require little training and can be implemented by psychologists, nurses, physicians, social workers, and others (Redd, 1994). These interventions also have few side effects, which is not the case with anti-nausea medication or other drugs (Morrow & Hickok, 1993). Furthermore, behavioral techniques empower patients to assume control over an aspect of their care, thereby enhancing patient feelings of self-efficacy and control (Molassiotis, Yung, Yam, Chan, & Mok, 2002). Indeed, at a time when people may feel that their lives and bodies are out of their own control regarding what and when substances are put into them, interventions that are not based on chemicals and/or drugs have a great deal to offer the patient.

There are no known differences between sexual minority women and heterosexual women in palliative care needs or responses.

Interactions with the Health Care System and Sexual Minority Status

Access to quality health care is a critical part of many of the actions needed to diagnose and treat cancer. LGBT patients face considerable barriers when seeking care or engaging in care (Institute of Medicine, 2011). These barriers can limit the quality or amount of care that is provided in any single clinical encounter and, when summed across a cancer experience, could lead to lower-quality care for patient and family. Little support and training is provided to health care professionals to help them engage in quality care with LGBT patients and families, so the problem rests with the system as well as the provider and patient. Little is known about the care experiences of subpopulations of sexual minority women, such as older SMW or SMW of color. This area is ripe for improvements in practice, including training, and needs critical attention during this time of current major changes in health care provision in the United States.

PHASE 2: EXTENDED SURVIVAL

Physical Health and Functioning

Complex treatment regimens with surgery, chemotherapy, radiation therapy, and supportive care procedures have improved in recent years, resulting in better survival rates for individuals with a diagnosis of cancer. As the number of cancer survivors continues to grow from the advances in therapy, we are able to identify the consequences of cure since the impact can be far-reaching. Both pediatric and adult cancer diagnosis and treatment produce effects that can have profound impact on the survivor's and the family's life and quality of life. Chronic effects are outcomes that occur as a result of cancer treatment, either during or after treatment and persist for longer than three months after the time of initial presentation. A late effect is an outcome that occurs greater than five years from time of diagnosis of cancer as a result of the previous cancer treatment and may be physical, psychological, or social in nature.

There are no known differences between sexual minority women and heterosexual women in long-term or late effects of cancer during survivorship.

Psychosocial Health and Functioning

In the field of cancer survivorship research, quality of life has become a highly regarded measure of women's survivorship characteristics. The extraordinary gains in cancer screening and treatment technology have resulted in steady improvements in quality of life among many survivors in recent decades. Quality of life measurement is of particular utility in assessing cancer survivorship because it quantifies one's well-being in the multiple domains of life, including psychological well-being, physical well-being, social well-being, and spiritual well-being (Bloom, Petersen, & Kang, 2007).

Several studies of breast cancer survivorship have used quality of life to assess breast cancer survivors' survivorship and adjustment (Ganz, et al., 1996; Tomich & Helgeson, 2002; Cimprich, Ronis, & Martinez-Ramos, 2002; Ganz et al., 2002). Quality of life indicators have been used to determine differences among older versus younger women (Cimprich et al., 2002), women who have opted for surgery or not (Rowland, et al., 2000), who are going through menopause (Durna, Crowe, Leader, & Eden, 2002; Biglia et al., 2003), and who are experiencing cognitive dysfunction (Lemieux, Bordeleau, & Goodwin, 2007). For example, in Cimprich and colleagues' 2002 study, quality of life indicators are used to determine the differences in breast cancer survivorship by age. In their study of 105 long-term breast cancer survivors, Cimprich, Ronis, and Martinez-Ramos (2002) determined that women diagnosed with breast cancer at an older age (greater than 65) had worse physical quality-of-life scores than women diagnosed at younger ages (27 to 44 years). However, the younger age group showed worse social quality-of-life scores than the older survivors. Women diagnosed at midlife were the most likely to have positive physical quality-of-life scores as well as a positive overall quality of life compared to the younger and older survivors.

The majority of studies pertaining to quality of life either assumes women's heterosexuality or does not consider the role of sexual orientation in quality of life as an outcome of survivorship. The minimal focus on sexual minority women (SMW) in studies pertaining to quality of life restricts our knowledge about sexual minority breast cancer survivorship as measured by quality of life. The few published quality-of-life breast cancer survivorship studies that expressly focused on sexual minorities (Matthews, Peterman, Delaney, Menard, & Brandenburg, 2002; Boehmer, Linde, & Freund, 2005) indicate that there are few or no differences in survivorship between heterosexual and sexual minority breast cancer survivors. Matthews and colleagues (2002) conducted a qualitative study using quality of life as a primary outcome for heterosexual and sexual minority women coping with breast cancer. Interviews with 13 sexual minority women and 28 heterosexual women revealed similarities in quality of life. However, sexual minority women reported significantly more stress and greater dissatisfaction with provider care than did heterosexual breast cancer survivors. In a quantitative online study conducted by Jabson and colleagues (Jabson, Donatelle, & Bowen, 2011) 68 sexual minority and 143 heterosexual breast cancer survivors reported similar quality of life scores. Like Matthews et al. (2002), Jabson also found elevated perceived stress scores among sexual minority breast cancer survivors. Comparing population-based methodologies, including cancer registries and online convenience sampling, Boehmer and colleagues (2005) also determined that there were no discernable differences in measures of quality of life between heterosexual and sexual minority breast cancer survivors.

Social Support and Survivorship

The importance of social support among cancer survivors in alleviating negative cancer experiences has been documented (Kneier, 2003). Breast cancer survivors, in particular, are known for their established and well-promoted social support systems and supportive survivor activities (Nausheen, Gidron, Peveler, & Moss-Morris, 2009). These are important for cancer survivors because women who perceive that they have adequate social support resources also report more positive physical and psychological outcomes, including better symptom management and better quality of life than socially isolated cancer survivors. Social support may come in the form of close friends, family members, or other sources such as support group members. Heterosexual cancer survivors are more likely to report that social support is received from "traditional" family members than sexual minority cancer survivors (Barnoff, Sinding, & Grassau, 2005; Fobair et al., 2002; Boehmer et al., 2005) who are much more likely to report receiving support from partners and close friends (Arena et al., 2006; Fobair et al., 2002). Few studies have been published regarding the social support of sexual minority breast cancer survivors, but those that have been produced indicate that sexual minority women may have unique needs and desires pertaining to social support compared to heterosexual cancer survivors (Barnoff et al., 2005). In a qualitative research study Barnoff, Sinding, and Grassau (2005) highlight the voices of 26 breast cancer survivors. Three distinct themes emerged from their interviews: (1) a need for treatment and breast cancer information that includes and reflects the reality of SMW diagnosed with breast cancer; (2) a need for breast cancer support services and activities designed and tailored for SMW and their families, and (3) a need for medical service providers who are conscious of, and sensitive to, the reality and experiences of SMW diagnosed with breast cancer.

In terms of support groups and support group activities, SMW appear to be less likely to participate than heterosexual cancer survivors. Barbara, Quandt, and Anderson (2001) determined that SMW were less likely to participate in breast cancer support groups for fear of marginalization and stigma related to their sexual orientation. This suggests that the perceived and anticipated stigma and marginalization experienced by SMW may significantly impact their perceptions of social support. This could have meaningful effects on their ability to engage positive aspects and outcomes associated with high-quality breast cancer survivorship.

Few interventions have been conducted to enhance and tailor social support resources and support group participation for sexual minority breast cancer survivors. Fobair and colleagues (2002) designed one such intervention that provided a support group for SMW diagnosed with breast cancer. A convenience sample of 20 women consented to participate in a 12-week group support intervention program. The women were assessed at baseline, 3, 6, and 12 months after the group intervention to detect changes in coping, adjustment to disease, and social support. Results revealed an unexpected finding: group participants demonstrated reduced levels of support. However, family conflict also declined, and trends toward increased cohesiveness and expressiveness were evident. The increases in cohesiveness and expressiveness, paired with a decline in family conflict, lead one to think that the reports of instrumental and informational support declined because of the reduced need for these forms of support. Consequently, it appears that a SMW-specific breast cancer support group may be beneficial to SMW who are surviving breast cancer.

Affect/Mood and Survivorship

Cancer diagnosis, treatment, and survivorship have all been shown to stimulate distress and mood disturbance in the form of depression, anger, apathy, and other emotions (Mullan, 1990; National Cancer Institute [NCI], 2008) among cancer survivors. Mood and affect are indicators for the quality of a woman's cancer survivorship. For example, a woman who reports low levels of distress, depression, anger and anxiety, and high levels of friendliness, activity, and vigor would be demonstrating a positive degree of survivorship and might be characterized as "thriving." Another woman who reports high levels of stress, distress, anger, and low levels of friendliness and vigor would be demonstrating a compromised survivorship experience.

There is a preponderance of studies of mood disturbance and affect among heterosexual breast cancer survivors and a paucity of studies that address the experiences of sexual minority cancer survivorship. One of the few available studies revealed that despite elevated mood disturbances (measured by the Profile of Mood States [POMS]) among SMW, there were no statistically significant differences between SMW and heterosexual women on mood disturbance and distress (Fobair et al., 2001). The ability to generalize the findings resulting from these studies is limited due to methodological constraints, qualitative approaches, and small sample sizes. Due to the dearth of research concerning sexual minority breast cancer survivors' affect/mood, the field is left with an incomplete understanding of the characteristics and quality of affect/mood among sexual minority breast cancer survivors.

Perceived Stress and Survivorship

The negative influence of perceived stress on health is well documented among both cancer-free and cancer populations (Kasl, 1984; Arnetz & Ekman, 2006; Seyle, 1976). Those who perceive a high level of stress report poorer mental and physical health. Perceived stress is important to cancer survivorship research for several reasons. The cancer experience is stressful. Stress is stimulated by experiences with cancer diagnosis, cancer treatment, and some aspects of cancer survivorship (Mullan, 1990; IOM, 2006; NCI, 2008).

Growing evidence from multiple studies suggests that SMW surviving breast cancer report higher levels of stress than heterosexual breast cancer survivors (Matthews et al., 2002; Boehmer et al., 2005; Fobair et al., 2002). Minority stress and heterosexism may contribute to SMW's cancer experience and elevate their levels of perceived stress above and beyond the stress caused by a breast cancer diagnosis, treatment, and survivorship compared to those of heterosexual breast cancer survivors.

Minority Stress, Sexual Minority Women, and Survivorship

Sexuality-based minority stress is an important and negative consequence of heterosexism. Ilan Meyer and colleagues (2003, 2007, 1995) have developed a conceptual model of sexuality-based minority stress that explains the unique forces and characteristics of sexuality-based discrimination and heterosexism on the health of sexual minority individuals.

According to Meyer and Northridge (2007), minority stress is distinct from "regular" stress experienced in everyday living and is distinguished by three specific characteristics. First, minority stress is additive. The sexuality-based stressors experienced by sexual minority people occur in addition to the "regular" daily-living and life stressors experienced by all people. In the case of cancer survivors, the overlay of minority stress occurs on top of the stressors experienced in daily living and dealing with cancer. This requires sexual minorities to develop and utilize additional coping strategies or resources above and beyond those required for successfully coping with everyday life and cancer. Second, minority stress is chronic. This means that minority stress is constant. The constancy or chronicity occurs because sexuality-based minority stress is supported by well-established sociocultural frameworks and traditions that undergird institutions and society, including the health care system. Consequently, sexual minority cancer survivors may be exposed to additional stress via their exposure to the health care system while undergoing cancer diagnoses and treatments. The third characteristic that sets minority stress apart from "regular" stress is that it is socially based. This means that minority stress stems from sources beyond individual control, such as institutions and social processes. When we apply the conceptual model of sexuality-based minority stress to sexual minority women, we have a clearer picture of how heterosexism, sexuality-based prejudice, and discrimination can influence cancer survivors' health adversely.

Discrimination and Survivorship

Limited research exists regarding the experiences of sexual minority breast cancer survivors and discrimination in the health care setting. However, one possible channel of influence in SMW's cancer survivorship may involve the experience of perceived discrimination in the health care setting during cancer treatments and care. In a cross-sectional examination of SMW's breast cancer survivorship, Jabson and colleagues (2011) found that most women reported low perceptions of discrimination but that this measure was significantly associated with quality of life. Additionally, most women in this study indicated that providers assumed that they were heterosexual. This finding is important because it indicates a heterosexist norm that could have negative implications for SMW cancer survivors who do not pass as heterosexual in the health care setting. Such norms may adversely influence cancer survivors by restricting discussions between providers and SMW about the intimacies of their experiences with breast cancer treatments and symptom management for fear of the risk of negative consequences associated with revealing their concealed minority identity (Jabson et al., 2011).

Coming Out and Survivorship

Heterosexual female cancer survivors do not "come out" to health care providers, because our heterocentric cultural orientation facilitates provider assumptions of women's heterosexuality. Consequently, SMW face the unique reality of having to choose whether or not to reveal their sexual orientation to providers. For some SMW surviving cancer, the risk of discrimination in the health care setting is a barrier that keeps them from disclosing their sexual orientation to providers (Boehmer & Case, 2004). The risk-of-discrimination barrier can have a negative impact on survivor experiences. Dibble and Roberts (2002) report that the fear of discrimination acts as a barrier to symptom management among SMW undergoing cancer treatments, where sexual minority women experienced worse cancer treatment side effects than those experienced by heterosexual cancer survivors. Coming out to providers could allow for more thorough discussions of symptom management and other cancer-related experiences between SMW cancer survivors and their providers.

PHASE 3: PERMANENT SURVIVORSHIP

Years since Diagnosis and Survivorship

The factors reviewed up to this point are all important in discussions related to breast cancer survivorship. There is some disagreement in the literature pertaining to the influence of the years since diagnosis on women's cancer survivorship. Some research has found that quality of life and life satisfaction improve with a longer post-diagnosis period (Kessler, 2002). In a study of breast cancer survivors, Kessler (2002) found that both

the greater the time since diagnosis and the severity of disease were associated with improvements in quality of life and health-related quality of
life. Kessler's work also found that treatment-related issues and concerns
persisted long term among breast cancer survivors. Others have found that
health and quality of life diminish over time (Ganz et al., 1996, 2002).
Ganz and colleagues (1996) found that women's health, mood, quality of
life, and functional status improved the most between one month and one
year post diagnosis, without subsequent improvements in later years. In a
later study of women one to five years post diagnosis, Ganz and colleagues
(2002) found that women's quality of life and functional status had diminished since diagnosis rather than improved.

Although it remains unclear how the duration of time since breast cancer diagnosis influences survivorship outcomes such as quality of life and
affect, it is clear that time since diagnosis does influence survivorship.
Additionally, studies concerning breast cancer survivorship and the role of
years since diagnosis have historically not analyzed data as they pertain to
SMW's cancer survivorship experiences.

There were no published studies available at the time of this writing that
specified the influence of years since diagnosis in sexual minority women
cancer survivors.

End-of-Life Care for Women Dying of Cancer

End-of-life care and issues for women dying of cancer is complex for
practitioners and for cancer patients. For practitioners, end-of-life care signals a significant shift in the approach to patient care, from treatment and
curative strategies to palliative care strategies (Baile, Aaron, & Parker,
2009). Palliative care strategies involve communication and coordination
of patient comfort and quality of life through the relief of the patient's suffering, as well as symptom management through the end of life. This may
include, but is not limited to, pain management and relief from symptoms
such as nausea, shortness of breath, and even fatigue. Emotional and spiritual support is also a key component in palliative care for cancer patients
dying of cancer.

End-of-life issues for women dying of cancer are numerous and vary
from woman to woman. End-of-life-related concerns can be psychosocial,
physical, spiritual, and/or emotional. Some women will experience concerns in one domain, and others experience concerns across all domains.
Some women may struggle with changes in their inability to fulfill "normal" social roles, while yet others may experience difficulty with the loss of
control and concern about the burdening of loved ones for care (Singer,
Martin, & Kelner, 1999). Some women also report concerns about physical
issues such as deteriorating mental awareness and fear of pain. Others also

report concerns about having a "good" death, fears of abandonment, separation from loved ones, and quality of life and dignity (Chochinov et al., 2002). Research pertaining to end-of-life issues among women dying of cancer suggests that many individuals benefit from the opportunity to discuss and talk about their concerns about death and end-of-life topics (Adelbratt & Strang, 2000). Cancer patients who do not have the opportunity to discuss these concerns report feelings of isolation and separation.

At the time of this writing, there have been no published studies of sexual minority women and end-of-life issues unique to them. In a single, conveniently sampled study of gay and lesbian individuals, gay and lesbian participants reported perspectives consistent with the general population about end-of-life care topics (Stein & Bonuck, 2001). However, this study did not involve an investigation of sexual minorities at the end of life. It yet remains unknown if there are unique concerns and end-of-life issues to be considered among sexual minority women dying of cancer. Certainly, the complexity of LGBT families suggests that end-of-life issues must be clearly identified for this population and that these issues could be very different for these special populations.

KEY AREAS OF FUTURE RESEARCH

As can be seen from this overview, many areas of potential relevance to sexual minority women and cancer have been left un- or underresearched. The most critical areas of research are proposed here.

- *Studies of cancer incidence in sexual minority women.* This area of study is sadly underresearched and in some ways drives much of the rest of this field. The efforts to match databases and therefore identify sexual orientation as a potential disparity marker for cancer incidence is well underway, but it needs more money and research attention.

- *Research into the effects of health care difficulties on screening, diagnosis, and care for sexual minority women.* Currently there is preliminary evidence suggesting difficulties in health care access and care among sexual minority women (Boehmer & Case, 2004; Dibble & Roberts, 2002). Population-based study designs that include questions about sexual orientation could significantly contribute to our understanding about the presence and effects of health care difficulties experienced by sexual minority women when dealing with cancer screening, diagnosis, care, and surveillance. The extant literature is largely based on small, conveniently sampled groups, which results in threats to scientific constructs—including limitations to external validity, bias (including phenomena such as the healthy volunteer effect), and an inability to fully describe the difficulties in access to care, treatment, and screening among this population of interest. Practically speaking, the existing data and study methodology keep us from fully realizing the effects of any difficulties experienced by SMW in accessing cancer screenings, diagnosis, and care and therefore, we are unable to develop successful interventions to improve access and care for sexual minorities dealing with cancer.

• *Studies into the palliative care and long-term survivorship experiences for sexual minority women and their families.* Few studies that involve palliative care and long-term survivorship among sexual minorities and their families currently exist. This significantly hampers our ability to identify recommendations for improving palliative care and long-term survivorship among SMW and their families. Future research must be committed to investigating the experiences of sexual minority long-term cancer survivors and identifying their palliative care needs. This should overtly include the role of family—and the unique family composition among long-term cancer survivors who are also sexual minorities. This type of research would contribute richly to long-term survivorship among sexual minorities and allow for the development of efficacious interventions for unmet palliative care needs. Family is increasingly understood as a fertile social context for health and intervention implementation. By including family in research pertaining to sexual minority long-term cancer survivors, there is a rich potential for improving the health of family members while improving our understanding of the role of family among the lives of sexual minority long-term cancer survivors.

• *Research into the health behaviors of sexual minority cancer survivors.* Growing research involving cancer survivors highlights the importance of modifying health behaviors, including tobacco control, participation in regular physical activity and cancer surveillance, and screenings for second primaries in an effort to reduce risk for recurrence, second primaries, and comorbid chronic disease, and to improve quality of life (Mariotto, Rowland, Reis, Scoppa, & Feuer, 2007; Demark-Wahnefried, Pinto, & Gritz, et al. 2006). However, none of this research has intentionally focused on the health behaviors of sexual minority cancer survivors. Despite the strong line of evidence regarding sexual minority women's cancer risk behaviors, including tobacco use and higher rates of obesity, there has been next to no research published on the health behaviors of sexual minority cancer survivors. Survivorship research indicates that as much as 15 percent of cancer survivors continue to use tobacco products after cancer diagnosis and treatment (Gritz et al., 2006), and many cancer survivors deal with the adverse effects of obesity and overweight (Rock and Demark-Wahnfried, 2002). However, research specific to the health behaviors of sexual minority cancer survivors is decidedly absent. Such research would help us to develop an evidence base from which to design and implement interventions to improve quality of life and reduce the risk for second primaries, cancer recurrence, and the development of additional chronic conditions such as heart disease and diabetes among sexual minority cancer survivors.

CONCLUDING STATEMENTS

Despite the overwhelming focus on sexual majorities in the cancer survivorship literature, there are a growing number of publications that reflect an also growing scholarly and clinical interest in the unique issues and experiences of sexual minority cancer survivors. The studies reviewed here showcase what the field is beginning to understand as important and distinct differences in women's cancer survivorship experiences according to sexual orientation. The literature indicates that SMW experience and respond to breast cancer differently from heterosexual women. SMW's social support is qualitatively different from heterosexual female cancer survivors (Fobair et al., 2001, 2002), SMW experience more stress than heterosexual cancer survivors and yet appear to have very similar quality of life as heterosexual cancer survivors (Matthews et al., 2002). Unfortunately, this literature is plagued by issues with convenience sampling and the difficulty that comes with locating an "invisible" population, self-selection bias, the healthy volunteer effect, and small sample sizes inherent to studying a minority population (Brogan et al., 2001; Bowen & Boehmer, 2007). For example, when registries are used to study cancer, the prevalence of minority sexual orientation was 6.3 percent in women, suggesting that sexual minority women are entered in higher prevalence in a registry than in the general population (Boehmer et al., 2010) These initial works are showcased here as first steps toward understanding some of the important and influential differences between women who survive cancer and how these differences may impact cancer survivorship and the growing numbers of female cancer survivors.

REFERENCES

Adelbratt, S., & Strang, P. (2000). Death anxiety in brain tumor patients and their spouses. *Palliative Medicine, 14,* 499–507.

American Cancer Society. (2018). Cancer statistics center. Retrieved December 6, 2018, from https://cancerstatisticscenter.cancer.org/#!/

Arnetz, B., & Ekman, R. (2006). *Stress in health and disease.* Wernheim: Wiley-VCH.

Baile, W. F., Aaron, J., & Parker, P.A. (2009). Practitioner-patient communication in cancer diagnosis and treatment. In S. M. Miller, D. J. Bowen, R. T. Croyle, & J. H. Rowland (Eds.), *Handbook of cancer control and behavioral science* (pp. 327–346). Ann Arbor, MI: McNaughton and Gunn.

Barbara, A. M., Quandt, S. A., & Anderson, R. T. (2001). Experiences of lesbians in the health care environment. *Women & Health, 34*(1), 45–62.

Barnoff, L., Sinding, C., & Grassau, P. (2005). Listening to the voices of lesbians diagnosed with cancer: Recommendations for change in cancer support services. *Journal of Gay & Lesbian Social Services, 18*(1), 17–35. doi:10.1300/J041v18n0103

Biglia, N., Cozzarella, M., Cacciari, F., Ponzone, R., Roagna, R., Maggirotto, F., & Sismondi, P. (2003). Menopause after breast cancer: A survey on breast cancer survivors. *Maturitas, 45*(1), 29–38.

Bloom, J. R. (2002). Surviving and thriving? *Psycho-Oncology, 11,* 89–92.

Bloom, J. R., Petersen, D. M., & Kang, S. H. (2007). Multi-dimensional quality of life among long-term (5+ years) adult cancer survivors. *Psycho-Oncology, 16*(8), 691–706.

Boehmer, U., & Case, P. (2004). Sexual minority women's interactions with breast cancer providers. *Women & Health, 44*(2), 41–58.

Boehmer, U., Clark, M., Glickman, M., Timm, A., Sullivan, M., Bradford, J., & Bowen, D. J. (2010). Using cancer registry data for recruitment of sexual minority women: Successes and limitations. *Journal of Women's Health, 19*(7), 1289–1297.

Boehmer, U., Linde, R., & Freund, K. M. (2005). Sexual minority women's coping and psychological adjustment after a diagnosis of breast cancer. *Journal of Women's Health, 14*(3), 214–224.

Boehmer, U., Miao, X., & Ozonoff, A. (2011). Cancer survivorship and sexual orientation. *Cancer, 117*(16), 3796–3804.

Boehmer, U., Ozonoff, A., & Timm, A. (2011). County-level association of sexual minority density with breast cancer incidence: results from an ecological study. *Sexuality Research and Social Policy, 8*(2), 139–145.

Bowen, D. J., & Boehmer, U. (2007). The lack of cancer surveillance data on sexual minorities and strategies for change. *Cancer Causes and Control, 18,* 343–349.

Brogan, D. J., Denniston, M. M., Liff, J. M., Flagg, E. W., Coates, R. J., & Brinton, L. A. (2001). Comparison of telephone sampling and area sampling: Response rates and within-household coverage. *American Journal of Epidemiology, 153*(11), 1119–1127.

Chochinov, H. M., Hack, T., Hassard, T., Kristjanson, L. J., McLement, S., & Harlos, M. (2002). Dignity in the terminally ill: A cross-sectional cohort study. *Lancet, 360,* 2026–2030.

Cimprich, B., Ronis, D. L., & Martinez-Ramos, G. (2002). Age at diagnosis and quality of life in breast cancer survivors. *Cancer Practice, 10*(2), 85–93.

Demark-Wahnefried, W., Pinto, B. M., & Gritz, E. R. (2006). Promoting health and physical function among cancer survivors: Potential for prevention and questions that remain. *Journal of Clinical Oncology, 24*(32), 5125–5131.

Dibble, S., & Roberts, S. (2002). A comparison of breast cancer diagnosis and treatment between lesbian and heterosexual women. *Journal of the Gay and Lesbian Medical Association, 6*(2), 9–17.

Durna, E. M., Crowe, S. M., Leader, L. R., & Eden, J. A. (2002). Quality of life of breast cancer survivors: The impact of hormone replacement therapy. *Climacteric, 5*(3), 266–276.

Fobair, P. (2007). Oncology social work for survivorship. In P. A. Ganz (Ed.), *Cancer survivorship* (pp. 14–27). New York: Springer.

Fobair, P., Koopman, C., DiMiceli, S., O'Hanlan, K., Butler, L. D., Classen, C., . . . Spiegel, D. (2002). Psychosocial intervention for lesbians with primary breast cancer. *Psycho-Oncology, 11*(5), 427.

Fobair, P., O'Hanlan, K., Koopman, C., Classen, C., Dimiceli, S., Drooker, N., . . . Spiegel, D. (2001). Comparison of lesbian and heterosexual women's response to newly diagnosed breast cancer. *Psycho-Oncology, 10*(1), 40.

Frager, G. (1996). Pediatric palliative care: Building the model, bridging the gaps. *Journal of Palliative Care, 12*(3), 9–15.

Ganz, P. A., Coscarelli, A., Fred, C., Kahn, B., Polinsky, M. L., & Peterson, L. (1996). Breast cancer survivors: Psychosocial concerns and quality of life. *Breast Cancer Research and Treatment, 38*, 183–199.

Ganz, P. A., Desmond, K. A, Leedham, B., Rowland, J. H. Meyerowitz, B. E., & Belin, T. R. (2002). Quality of life in long-term, disease-free survivors of breast cancer: A follow up study. *Journal of the National Cancer Institute, 94*, 39–49.

Gritz, E. R., Cororve Fingeret, M., Vidrine, D. J., Lazev, A. B., Mehta, N. V., & Reece, G. P. (2006). Successes and failures of the teachable moment. *Cancer, 106*(1), 17–27.

Hewitt, M., Greenfield, S., & Stovall, E. (Eds.). (2006). *From cancer patient to cancer survivor: Lost in transition* (Institute of Medicine Report). Washington, DC: National Academies Press.

Institute of Medicine (IOM). (2011). *The health of lesbian, gay, bisexual and transgender people: Building a foundation for better understanding.* Washington, DC: National Academies Press.

Jabson, J. M., Donatelle, R. J., & Bowen, D. J. (2011). Relationship between sexual orientation and quality of life in female breast cancer survivors. *Journal of Women's Health, 20*(12), 1819-1824.

Kasl, V. S. (1984). Stress and health. *Annual Review of Public Health, 5*, 319–341.

Kessler, T. A. (2002). Contextual variables, emotional state and current and expected quality of life in breast cancer survivors. *Oncology Nursing Forum, 29*, 1109–1116.

Kirsch, I. (1997). Response expectancy theory and application: A decennial review. *Applied Preventive Psychology, 6*(2), 69–79.

Kneier, A. W. (2003). Coping with melanoma—Ten strategies that promote psychological adjustment. *Surgical Clinics of North America, 83*(2), 417–430.

Lemieux, J., Bordeleau, L. J., & Goodwin, P. J. (2007). Medical, psychosocial, and health-related quality of life issues among cancer survivors. In P. A. Ganz (Ed.), *Cancer survivorship* (pp. 28–42). New York: Springer.

Mariotto, A. B., Rowland, J. H., Reis, L. A. G., Scoppa, S., & Feuer, E. J. (2007). Multiple cancer prevalence: A growing challenge in long term survivorship. *Cancer Epidemiology, Biomarkers and Prevention, 16*, 566–571.

Matthews, A. K., Peterman, A. H., Delaney, P., Menard, L., & Brandenburg, D. (2002). A qualitative exploration of the experiences of lesbian and heterosexual patients with breast cancer. *Oncology Nursing Forum, 29*(10), 1455–1462.

Meyer, I. H. (1995). Minority stress and mental health in gay men. *Journal of Health and Social Behavior, 36*(1), 38.

Meyer, I. H. (2001). Why lesbian, gay, bisexual and transgender public health? *American Journal of Public Health, 91*(6), 856–859.

Meyer, I. H. (2003). Prejudice, social stress, and mental health in lesbian, gay, and bisexual populations: Conceptual issues and research evidence. *Psychological Bulletin, 129*(5), 674.

Meyer, I. H., & Northridge, M. (2007). *The health of sexual minorities.* New York: Springer.

Meyer, I. H., Rossano, L., Ellis, J. M., & Bradford, J. (2002). A brief telephone interview to identify lesbian and bisexual women in random digit dialing sampling. *The Journal of Sex Research, 39*(2), 139–144.

Molassiotis, A., Yam, B., Yung, H., Chan, F., & Mok, T. (2002). Pretreatment factors predicting the development of postchemotherapy nausea and vomiting in Chinese breast cancer patients. *Supportive Care in Cancer, 10*(2), 139–145.

Morrow, G. R., & Hickok, J. T. (1993). Behavioral treatment of chemotherapy-induced nausea and vomiting. *Oncology, 7*(12), 83–89.

Mullan, F., & Hoffman, B. (1990). *Charting the journey: Almanac of practical resources for cancer survivors.* Mount Vernon, NY: Consumers Union.

National Cancer Institute. (2008). NCI dictionary of cancer terms. Retrieved November 2008 from http://www.cancer.gov/dictionary/?CdrID=445089

National Consensus Project for Quality Palliative Care. (2009). *Clinical practice guidelines for quality palliative care* (2nd ed.). Retrieved from http://www.nationalconsensusproject.org

Nausheen, B., Gidron, Y., Peveler, R., & Moss-Morris, R. (2009). Social support and cancer progression: A systematic review. *Journal of Psychosomatic Research, 67*(5), 403–415.

Redd, W. H. (1994). Advances in behavioral intervention in comprehensive cancer treatment. *Supportive Care in Cancer, 2*(2), 111–115.

Rock, C. L., & Demark-Wahnefried, W. (2002). Can lifestyle modification increase survival in women diagnosed with breast cancer? *The Journal of Nutrition, 132*, 3504S–3509S.

Rowland, J. H. (2004). Survivorship research: Past, present and future. In P. A. Ganz (Ed.), *Cancer survivorship* (pp. 28–42). New York: Springer.

Rowland, J. H., Desmond, K. A., Meyerowitz, B. E., Belin, T. R., Wyatt, G. E., & Ganz, P. A. (2000). Role of breast reconstructive surgery in physical and emotional outcomes among breast cancer survivors. *Journal of the National Cancer Institute, 92*(17), 1422–1429.

Selye, H. (1976). Forty years of stress research: principle remaining problems and misconceptions. *Canadian Medical Association Journal, 115*(1), 53–56.

Singer, P. A., Martin, D. K., & Kelner, M. (1999). Quality end of life care: Patients' perspectives. *Journal of the American Medical Association, 271,* 163–168.

Solarz, A. L. (Ed.). (1999). *Lesbian health: Current assessment and directions for the future.* Washington, DC: National Academy Press.

Stein, G. L., & Bonuck, K. A. (2001). Attitudes on end of life care and advance care planning in the lesbian and gay community. *Journal of Palliative Medicine, 4*(2), 173–191.

Tomich, P. L., & Helgeson, V. S. (2002). Five years later: A cross sectional comparison of breast cancer survivors with healthy women. *Psycho-Oncology, 11*(2), 154–169.

Valanis, B. G., Bowen, D. J., Bassford, T., Whitlock, E., Charney, P., & Carter, R. A. (2000). Sexual orientation and health. *Archives of Family Medicine, 9,* 843–853.

van der Hage, J. H., van de Velde, C. C. J. H., & Mieog, S J. S. D. (2007). Preoperative chemotherapy for women with operable breast cancer. *Cochrane Database of Systematic Reviews, Issue 2,* Article CD005002. doi:10.1002/14651858.CD005002.pub2

Weitzner, M. A., Meyers, C. A., Stuebing, K. K., & Saleeba, A. K. (1997). Relationship between quality of life and mood in long term survivors of breast cancer treated with mastectomy. *Supportive Care in Cancer, 5,* 241–248.

Zapka, J. G., Puleo, E., Taplin, S. H., Valentine Goins, K., Ulcickas Yood, M., Mouchawar, J., . . . Manos, M. M. (2004). Process of care in cervical and breast cancer screening and follow-up—The importance of communication. *Preventive Medicine, 39,* 81–90.

6

Cancer in Men and Transgender Women

Darryl Mitteldorf, Gerald Perlman, and David M. Latini

Cancer patients live two lives: one lived before diagnosis and one to be lived after diagnosis.

Men who have been diagnosed with cancer inhabit a small community of peers who share unique experiences of cancer survivorship. Gay and bisexual men and transgender women diagnosed with cancer are part of an even smaller community of survivors who navigate both the minority-status challenges of self-identity, stigmatization, and disclosure—and the barriers and issues regarding their cancer treatment.

This chapter covers how being a man who has sex with men, or being a transgender woman, is relevant to cancer diagnosis, treatment, and survivorship. It also discusses how coming out as a gay, bisexual, or transgender female is parallel to coming out as a cancer survivor. It looks at the ways that being a gay or bisexual man or transgender woman diagnosed with cancer are different from being a heterosexual diagnosed with cancer during each of the three stages of cancer survivorship: diagnosis, treatment, and post-treatment survivorship. It explores the ways that being gay impact the choices one makes about professional and personal caregivers as well as cancer treatments. It also touches on issues relevant to bisexual men and transgender women. A variety of helpful strategies for patients and clinicians are offered. Finally, some cancer-specific coping devices, as well as ways in which gay and bisexual men and transgender women patients can become cancer advocates and health care navigators, are provided.

For ease of reading, the term "gay" is used here as inclusive of all iterations of men who have sex with men; those who identify as gay, whether sexually active or not; and transgender women who may or may not have sex with men. The inclusion of transgender women here is relevant because, although self-identified as female, they are at risk for the same diseases common to all people assigned male at birth. Distinctions are made where relevant to the discussion.

"Cancer" is a frightening word. Cancer reminds us that we are mortal and that our lives are replete with unknowns. There are no certainties about which physician is the best health care professional, which hospital is the best, which treatment is most likely to work, or what pains or side effects might result from treatments. Cancer is a realm of many unknowns and potentially grave consequences that a diagnosis forces a person to inhabit. Being diagnosed with cancer creates a new form of identity that joins with, and usually trumps, all other self-identities: that of cancer survivor.

SPECIFIC CONCERNS

Significant issues around being a cancer survivor who is a gay man or transgender woman revolve around causes of cancer, disclosure of cancer status, and working with health care professionals. A primary question is: How is cancer different for these populations?

Cancer impacts one's sexual and social identities and returns one to a time when understanding these identity issues, and how one presents himself to others, was paramount. Most cancer clinics, clinicians, and informational materials present discussions about cancer based on the assumption that the patient is heterosexual. When most of the discussion is focused on heterosexual men, important discussions around gay experiences—such as sexual identity, sexual behaviors and desires, and some physical issues that only men who have sex with men may experience as a consequence of some cancer treatments (including concerns about anal and oral sex, about one's sperm being banked if there might be a desire to father a child, and about the appropriateness of bringing a partner to a consultation)—often do not occur.

Gay men may notice that intake forms and brochures are beginning to use words like "partner" or "life-friend," and many people, including gay men, think that is enough—or they may feel that this is all they are going to get in terms of gay-relevant discussions about their cancer. But there is much more about being gay and having cancer that needs expression, research, and understanding.

DIAGNOSIS

People assigned male at birth can be diagnosed with cancer in several ways. Some may find themselves diagnosed as a consequence of a test at a community health fair or during an annual physical or health care professional's visit. Some may have noticed aches or pains, or changes in their physical behavior or appearance, such as having to urinate more frequently or noticing a lump below their skin or an odd-shaped mole. Some may even be diagnosed while receiving treatment for another disease. Others may age into a set of tests that health care professionals routinely begin at a specific age.

Hearing a health care provider say, "Your test results came back . . . you have cancer," affects most people with a unique and powerful thrust. This is a solitary experience for most; there is usually a period of time, from minutes to months, before a person tells anyone else that he has been diagnosed with cancer. Cancer is a life-threatening illness, and most people need time to absorb the truth that they are mortal and that they may die sooner than they had thought or hoped. There are moments of denial, bargaining, and begging for a return to the past, but ultimately, most individuals adapt to the negative news and get to work understanding what needs to be done to stay alive.

The question of cause is somewhat different for gay than for heterosexual men. Everyone diagnosed with cancer asks, "Was it diet, on-the-job stress, exposure to chemicals or weapons, or sexual behavior? Did I spend too much time in the sun? Or was it because I smoked?" Everyone diagnosed with cancer asks all sorts of variations of "How did my cancer happen?" However, individuals often have questions that are specific to their sexual activities. For example, "Was prostate or anal cancer caused by anal- receptive sex, or did my throat cancer occur from swallowing during oral sex?" For many, there is some degree of concern that being gay is somehow causal.

Trying to understand cause is a way of regaining a sense of control after hearing the diagnosis. Understanding cause creates an emotional implication that maybe, if he has caused it, he can also fix it.

Some LGBT people feel that others are going to blame them for causing the onset of their own disease. This may cause them to feel even more concern that being gay or transgender caused their cancer or that their cancer is somehow a punishment for being gay or transgender. Uncertainty about the future can cause individuals to internalize their fears and doubts, causing them to blame themselves, and this may perhaps be more common in individuals who have had to cope with the stigma of redefining their sexual orientation or gender identity.

There are prominent authors who believe that the stress of "being in the closet" caused their cancer (Murphy, 2010). Although a recent research study (Boehmer, Miao, & Ozonoff, 2011) suggests that gay men are 1.9 times as likely to be diagnosed with cancer, there is currently no evidence-based study in the literature that suggests why men who have sex with men report a higher burden of cancer diagnosis.

Being part of a sexual or gender minority group does not cause cancer. But emerging research suggests that oral and anal sex may, indeed, lead to increased incidence of throat and rectal cancer among gay men (Kreimer et al., 2004).

In addition, sexually transmitted infections may create opportunity for cancer. For example, there is growing evidence that human papillomavirus (HPV), which can be transmitted orally or anally, is related to high-grade anal intraepithelial neoplasia, which often precedes the onset of cancers specific to the anus, rectum, and throat (Palefskey, 2011). Cancers of the mouth and oropharynx (the top of the throat) used to be mainly diagnosed in older men who drink or smoke. But increasingly, they are being seen in younger gay men.

The relationship of HPV to anal and oral cancer does not mean that gay men, any more than heterosexual men, are responsible for their cancer. Transmission is not cause. Prudence and use of dental dams, condoms, and common sense may prove helpful for men who would like to reduce the possibility of cancer in their lives. And a new vaccine against HPV may prove useful in reducing anal and oral cancer incidence.

COMING OUT WITH CANCER

Soon after cancer diagnosis, people are referred to health care professionals who specialize in treating specific types of cancers. Almost always, this will be someone the patient has never seen before. They may not have known that such a specialist even existed. There is usually a period of time, days to weeks, between scheduling an appointment and seeing the health care provider. It is during this time that people begin to wonder what they will tell their provider about themselves and whom else they are going to tell about their cancer. This is the coming-out period of being an LGBT person living with cancer.

For LGBT people, coming out is familiar and replete with memories of experiences and emotions ranging along a positive-to-negative continuum. Common to both coming out with cancer and coming out as a gay man or transgender person is a sense of not knowing what might be next and being riddled with degrees of anxiety, depression, and, often, paranoia. Feeling some degree of fear during the coming-out process is common to all men, no matter where and at what age they decide to be open about being gay or transgender. Most people will likely agree that some degree of fear is a natural, healthy emotional response to the unknown and is usually mitigated by the quality of the experience the man meets over time. The reality of harm that might occur as a result of coming out as a gay man or transgender person varies from community to community worldwide. Most gay men and transgender people develop an authentic sense of self and cultivate a positive minority identity after coming out within supportive peer communities, but this is significantly less the case within communities hostile to gender or sexual minorities (Legate, Ryann, & Weinstein, 2011).

It is rare to identify social communities that are entirely accepting of LGBT people in all situations and circumstances. Most LGBT people are rarely out in all settings in their communities. Feelings of safety and of the social utility or danger of being out usually determine in which settings a person is out. For many people, selectivity in disclosure is a common way of protecting oneself from harm. Disclosing in some situations, but not in others, in total, may be neither helpful nor harmful. But being gay or transgender and also having a diagnosis of cancer provokes concerns that most people have not considered in relation to self-disclosure.

There is no easy formula for understanding when, where, and to whom being out with cancer is helpful or benign. Nor is it possible to say that disclosing a cancer diagnosis gets easier with experience over time. The passage of time and the building of close social relationships may ease fears about being out as a gay man or transgender person; with cancer, time presents new challenges and milestones but rarely eliminates fear. A graph comparing fear experienced from coming out versus coming out as an LGBT person living with cancer might look like a parabola versus a series of waves with varying amplitudes.

Experiences reported to the authors (who have led gay men's prostate cancer support groups) in gay cancer-survivor support groups show that being out as a gay man to one's cancer health care professional is helpful for increasing the chances of satisfactory treatment and minimizing long-term feelings of regret. There are two main reasons for this. First, a person needs to understand that some types of cancer may present them with a variety of treatment choices, many with consequences that impact heterosexual people differently than they do LGBT people.

As has been suggested, many health care professionals assume that their male patients are heterosexual or that their patients with female identities have natal female reproductive organs. Population-wise, there are, indeed, more heterosexual cancer survivors than gay or transgender cancer survivors in most communities. Gay men and transgender women almost always find themselves in the minority when presenting outside LGBT community-specific realms. Cancer units within hospitals are no exception. Even rarer is the cancer health care provider who is out as an LGBT person.

People rarely ask questions regarding subjects about which they are reluctant to know the answers. It is to be expected that health care professionals with limited knowledge or desire to know more about gay life are less likely to ask a patient whether he is gay or heterosexual. It is far easier to generalize about a patient's sexual orientation than it is to spend time learning about what, specifically, might impact his quality of life. Most cancer specialists focus on removing the threat of cancer as a primary goal and are less inclined to consider the relevance of LGBT-appropriate treatment choices, even when there are choices that are equivocal. Because it is unlikely that a health care professional will directly ask questions related to sexual orientation and gender identity, the newly diagnosed cancer patient is burdened with the challenge of deciding whether to be open and honest and ask the questions he or she needs to ask.

It is difficult for most LGBT people to know whether to come out to their health care professional and, if so, how and when. Feeling safe with the person whom a patient is trusting to save their life is, quite understandably, a primary concern for all cancer patients. Nothing in this chapter should be construed as saying that one must or even should come out to one's health care professional or that a health care professional should press one into coming out. There is no right or wrong solution to this issue, but there are good and less-than-optimal consequences from either decision.

Remaining quiet about being gay or trans limits the conversation about treatment choices regarding sexual and physical appearance and identity issues that an individual might feel are important. On the other hand, not fully disclosing one's sexual orientation or gender identity to one's health care professional reduces any concerns and delusions that he or she might treat one differently and perhaps with less quality then he or she might treat a heterosexual patient. Not being out reduces the patient's possibility of worry that nurses and allied health staff will treat one with less care and dignity than they would treat heterosexual patients. Last, less stress based on less worry about homophobia or transphobia is a valuable and valid context on which to base one's choice not to disclose.

When an individual feels that they understands the protocol and treatments, there is usually less perceived emotional stress. Men who avoid asking many questions, or simply are afraid to anger or upset their health care professionals with many questions, usually feel more stress than men who understand their cancer treatments (Degner & Davison, 1997). Gay men typically feel less stress when they understand the impact of cancer treatments relative to their sexual and emotional lives. Mutual consent and understanding between health care professional and patient enhance treatment decision making and play a positive role in post-treatment quality of life (MacDonagh & Cliff, 2000). Being out to one's health care professional allows an open and free-flowing conversation about how treatment impacts quality of life. Many people choose to be out to their health care professionals and do so in a variety of ways.

DIFFERENTIAL EFFECTS OF AND ATTITUDES TOWARD TREATMENT CHOICES FOR GAY MEN

Cancer treatments can alter a man's libido and ability to perform sexually. For example, the primary treatments for prostate cancer are surgery and/or radiation. These either eliminate or reduce, respectively, a man's ability to produce seminal fluid, thus decreasing the possibility of ejaculation (differentiated from the ability to have an orgasm). The physical and psychological implications of that for a gay man can be overwhelming because of the eroticization of the ejaculate that may be greater for men who have sex with men (Schilder et al., 2008). Impotence, urinary incontinence, and reduced enjoyment of anal-receptive sex may also follow primary prostate cancer treatments. Anal penetration requires a greater degree of rigidity than vaginal intercourse (Goldstone, 2005), yet treatments for erectile dysfunction focus on creating an erection sufficient for vaginal penetration. Oral sex enjoyment may also be reduced because of urinary incontinence. While the research remains limited, early work suggests that gay men may have worse quality of life after prostate cancer treatment than other men (Hart, Coon, Kowalkowski, & Latini, 2011). Those suffering from anal cancer and throat cancer, among others, have similar obstacles to face.

Later-stage prostate cancer treatments include androgen deprivation therapy, which reduces testosterone levels, impacting a man's feelings and sexual desires. Hormonal treatments create difficulties in feeling attraction beyond sexual desire and can have an impact on developing or maintaining emotional connections with others. Body changes, such as flabbiness and breast enlargement, often also occur, along with hot flashes. Radiation treatments for several types of cancer may lead to anal and bowel irritation sufficient to reduce sexual pleasure in that region.

Male breast cancer treatment often involves surgery, which may leave a concave depression where the breast was removed. Orchiectomy, the removal of testicles, impacts sperm production and physical appearance. More advanced skin cancers require removal of some tissue surrounding the cancer site to ensure that all cancer cells are excised. Many other types of cancer have similar side effects from various treatments. And gay men often have very different post-treatment quality-of-life goals than do heterosexual men. For example, gay men diagnosed with prostate cancer may choose surgery over radiation, with the goal of minimizing risk of radiation-induced rectal irritation, while heterosexual men may choose radiation without any regard to concerns of post-treatment anal-receptive sex.

Gay male partners and heterosexual female partners seem to present an equally dissimilar set of concerns. Treatment-related worries and concerns among heterosexual partners are typically more about pain and physical limitation, while the male partners who have been treated may worry more about urinary incontinence. Among gay men, however, there seems to be equal concern about urinary symptoms in the patient and his partner; sexual concerns are the least prevalent for partners and the most for the men treated (Roesch, 2005). From support groups for the partners of gay cancer survivors, there is anecdotal evidence suggesting that the healthy partner is often envious about the ejaculate play and penile erectile functioning that the gay patient still gets to enjoy with him, while he may no longer be able to get the same satisfaction and opportunity from his partner that he had prior to treatment. Cancer treatment also excites concerns about partner infidelity. More research of gay partners of cancer survivors' emotional and sexual concerns is needed to fully understand the responses of gay partners to cancer diagnosis and treatment.

It is usually the nondiagnosed partner that becomes a filter and manager of care and treatment adherence. In his state of anxiety, the diagnosed partner may want either to rush into or delay treatment, and it is the nondiagnosed partner who often presents a more reasoned view about the timing of treatment and other decisions that need to be made about treatment choices. Research suggests that in heterosexual couples, the female spouse becomes the conduit for information between professionals and her husband. Couples view the wife as the primary partner who manages the cancer, and she may even act on behalf of her husband (Rosner & Heyman, 1996). Gay men's partner support groups suggest that this dynamic also occurs in gay couples.

TOWARD A BETTER OUTCOME AND QUALITY OF LIFE

Understanding how the variety of treatments affects future quality-of-life issues will minimize regret and anger later. If one feels that they have taken appropriate steps from the beginning, it is less likely that years later, they will regret earlier missed opportunities. Based on what the authors have noticed in both gay and mixed gay and heterosexual prostate cancer support groups, it seems reasonable to say that a well-informed patient with a good relationship with their health care professional is less likely to experience anger, regret, and depression later on in his life.

It appears to be helpful for patients to be out to health care professionals so that the treatment experience feels honest and safe; coming out this way also feels empowering. While it is not entirely clear what specific effects stress has on cancer, many articles have been written suggesting the benefits of stress reduction during cancer treatment. A gay man or transgender person may find themselves feeling less stress by choosing not to be out to his health care professional and nurses, but the authors have seen many men relating that they received more supportive care when they early on presented themselves as gay to their health care staff. Each individual needs to understand the sexual and gender-friendly temperature of the environment in which they are being treated.

Research suggests that men who learn about their disease and participate in discussions with their health care professionals are able to make treatment choices sooner and with more confidence than men who do not (Degner & Davison, 1997). Many people find that it is beneficial to learn as much as they can about their proposed cancer treatment and then to question their care providers about why a particular treatment protocol is being suggested, what side effects may be expected, and how success and failure will be measured.

MEETING THE PROFESSIONAL CARE PROVIDERS

Most people diagnosed with cancer are consulting with health care professionals with whom they have had no prior relationship. Cancer health care professionals are specialists and rarely participate in any part of a patient's life prior to their diagnosis. Thus, in the beginning, a health care provider knows little more about a person beyond the results of the tests and scans that he or she reads in his chart. Rarely do intake forms ask about orientation or identity. Many health care professionals feel that technical information is all that they need to provide to their patients regarding the type of treatment required. Treatment suggestions are usually made from a heterosexual perspective and a presumption that the patient is hoping to continue to enjoy a happy and healthy heterosexual lifestyle after treatment. For most cancer health care providers, their priority is saving life; other concerns regarding quality of life may not be a top priority. On the contrary, a patient's priorities may be quite at odds with those of the health care professional. This needs to be openly discussed.

All people who have decided to be out to their health care professional have to specifically ask how treatment will affect their lives. They cannot assume that their health care professional knows that they enjoy particular activities and are concerned about effects of specific types of treatment—such as, for example, radiation irritating the anus. A health care professional is unlikely to volunteer information regarding when it is safe to begin or revisit anal or oral sex after treatment. Counseling on sexual activity may come from a hetero-normative perspective. Because a cisgender man may present himself as gay, his health care professional may assume that he is not interested in having children and may not discuss oncofertility options.

It is important to discuss pretreatment sperm banking. Even if one feels confident that biological children are unlikely, sperm banking can bring a degree of emotional solace during the first year or two after treatment. If the gay man or transgender woman remains clear about his or her fertility needs, later on, he or she can choose to cancel or continue his sperm-banking agreement.

The patient needs to be clear with his health care professional about to whom she/he can or cannot reveal medical information. This, of course, is the duty of every health care professional: to provide confidentiality and written document authorizing the person of his choice as a partner in his care is very useful. This continues to be important even now that same-sex marriage is legal. A simple statement on paper, early on, reduces stress and problems that may occur later.

It is always advisable to bring another person along to all medical consultations. The second person becomes a note taker, sounding board, advocate, and emotional support. Some people show up at their consultations with another person, introducing them clearly as their partner. It is worth noting that one should never assume that their health care professional understands what being a partner is. Just because the patient understands what they mean does not mean others do. Simply showing up with another person is not sufficient for conveying a sexual or gender minority status. It is helpful for the patient to actually say what the relationship is between themselves and the person accompanying them. Even if the other is not a partner, one can say that he or she is a friend and that currently there is no partner, or that the partner is unable to be at that particular consultation.

LGBT people who are not out to their health care professionals and other professional care providers are less likely to take their partners to their consultations, missing out on their partner's help and support and denying their partners the voice in treatment decisions and the support provided to partners in heterosexual relationships. Collaborative treatment decision making between health care professional and patient may be impaired when the couple's partnership is not understood or is denied or trivialized by the health care professional. As Santillo and Lowe (2005) have noted, the value of a partner's input is limited by the extent and quality of his involvement in the process. The partner's interpretation of information gathered helps the patient formulate a final decision, but if the partner is excluded due to homophobic or transphobic reasons emanating from the health care professional, the partner's input is less likely to be of value. The partners of cancer patients often experience significant psychological and social turmoil and benefit from mutual support offered in the context of partnerships and in close friendships (Rosner & Heyman, 1996).

WHAT HEALTH CARE PROFESSIONALS NEED TO KNOW

Health care professionals need to be aware of the effect of real or imagined issues between themselves and patients around sexual orientation and gender identity. Just because an individual believes that he/she is not homophobic or transphobic does not mean that his/her patient knows or expects that about him/her. For example, a health care professional may think that a cancer patient with advanced disease may benefit from being in a clinical trial or being placed on a newly developed protocol. LGBT people, like most stigmatized/minority patients, may be more suspicious than others that their health care professional may be inclined to suggest something new or experimental for them because they are from a minority population and more socially acceptable "test patients." Health care professionals need to comprehensively state the reasons that novel treatment options are being offered.

Health care professionals need to be aware of the ethnic and economic diversity of the LGBT community and to actively build a rapport with their LGBT patients across a range demographic groups. Empathy can be communicated through simple gestures such as including copies of LGBT publications and newspapers in waiting rooms and including inclusive questions on their intake forms. It is just as true that health care professionals are afraid to ask patients about their sexual orientation and gender identity as patients might be to disclose it. Health care professionals may fear not knowing what to do with the answer. And patients fear what the health care professional might do after hearing the answer. Health care professionals need to ask about a patient's lifestyle and identity just as he/she would ask about all the aspects of a patient's life that cancer may directly affect.

Health care professionals often miss the opportunity to explore dual diagnosed cancers in couples. For example, a health care professional may be called to consult with a testicular cancer patient but may not be aware that the patient's partner may also have been diagnosed with testicular cancer. Heterosexual couples have a one-in-six chance of dealing with prostate cancer during their lifetime. When both partners in a couple have prostates, there is close to a one-in-three chance that one of the partners will be diagnosed with prostate cancer. For example, more and more gay men are presenting as couples, each sharing similar male cancer–type diagnoses.

Health care professionals need also to be aware that gay men may use anabolic steroids more than the general population; steroids are being prescribed to gay men with AIDS as part of their treatment. The drugs replenish testosterone levels and help to fight fatigue (Santillo & Lowe, 2005). Many gay men also strive for an "ideal" body, often involving being trim and muscular, and may use steroids to achieve that goal (Tiggemann & Yeland, 2003). Accordingly, gay men and their health care professionals need to be aware of the use of testosterone and other anabolic steroids, whether prescribed for AIDS or as a performance enhancer. They also need to be aware of the use of finasteride (Propecia) for hair loss and HIV status and its influence on treatment options, as well as the use of alcohol and anal sex, as they affect prostate-specific antigen (PSA) tests.

ISSUES CONCERNING BISEXUAL AND TRANSGENDER WOMEN CANCER SURVIVORS

Bisexual men have specific difficulties engaging their health care professionals in understanding their quality-of-life issues. Many men, of many different cultures and races, are enjoying same-sex relationships, but they are not necessarily self-identifying as bisexual or gay. Some men, particularly in the African American community, may participate in sex with other men but do so without disclosure and without necessarily identifying as gay. Health care professionals should always offer one-on-one private time with their patients, gay and heterosexual, and offer the opportunity to discuss any sexual or cultural practices that they engage in but are reticent to discuss with others. Health care professionals need to offer confidential time, apart from any present partner, for the patient to discuss concerns that he might otherwise keep cloistered. They should never assume that a man who comes with a female spouse is not interested in sex with other men. Nor should health care professionals assume that a man presenting with a gay partner or husband is solely interested in sex with other men.

Trans female or feminine cancer survivors also have unique issues that rarely fit into any one particular category. Cancer survivorship for this group ought to be studied more and is likely to earn its own set of psychosocial and treatment protocols. The following covers some concerns that are clearly present for trans feminine people. They often find themselves diagnosed with later-stage cancer because they are less likely than others to get appropriate medical care. Transgender people are 30 to 40 percent less likely to regularly visit a primary care health care professional and are often less inclined to seek out cancer screening out of concern that disclosing their transgender status will cause more harm to them than good (Hibbs, 2008).

Transgender people are often reluctant to describe parts of their anatomy that correlate with their gender identity, a gender that they feel has no relationship to who they really are. For example, transgender men are often loath to perform breast self-examinations, and transgender women are less likely than heterosexual men to request prostate cancer testing, even though breast tissue remains in the former and prostate tissue remains in the latter. Thurston (1994) suggests that those who use hormone therapy but decide not to undergo surgery continue to be at risk for endometrial cancer (transgender men) and prostate cancer (transgender women). For transgender men, androgen therapy carries an increased risk for heart disease, endometrial hyperplasia, and subsequent endometrial carcinoma (Futterweit, 1998). Gynecologic health care needs assessment of transgender men characterizes the barriers they face when seeking health care (Dutton, Koenig, & Fennie, 2008).

Health care professionals treating transgender individuals may not be aware that their patients have transitioned. A health care professional who is not aware of a patient's biological sex might not consider sex-specific disorders, even if the patient presents with classic symptoms, e.g., prostate cancer in a transgender woman or cervical cancer in a transgender man. This lack of awareness could lead to a life-threatening delay in diagnosis and treatment (Molokwu, Appelbaum, & Miksad, 2008).

THE LGBT COMMUNITY, FAMILY AND FRIENDS

Telling friends of a cancer diagnosis in the context of a community historically focused on HIV and AIDS is another challenge. The LGBT community continues to rise to meet the health care challenge that HIV and AIDS have wrought since the early 1980s. In light of the latter, it is not always easy for LGBT cancer survivors to feel fully supported by the LGBT community that is now just beginning to understand the importance of advocating for LGBT cancer survivorship research and appropriate treatment. Indeed, the first lesbian-, gay-, bisexual- and transgender-inclusive national nonprofit cancer survivor organization, the National LGBT Cancer Project (lgbtcancer.org), came on the scene only in 2005. Coming out about cancer means coming out to a generation of people already decimated by HIV.

Disclosing one's cancer diagnosis to one's family becomes an occasion for many more people besides the patient revisiting the coming-out process. Family members usually share the patient's initial concerns about what caused the cancer and often will consider whether or not being from a sexual or gender minority group was causal.

From gay cancer-survivor support groups, it has been noted that men report how their families were able to handle disclosure about a diagnosis of cancer with greater ease than they did when the family member came out as a gay man. Family members may have more experience or knowledge about cancer than they might have had about being gay, so it is not surprising that they are better navigators of cancer than of disclosure of a family member's being gay. Nor does cancer carry the stigma it once did, whereas being gay in many parts of the world is still something of which to be ashamed. Nevertheless, for the diagnosed man, the ease with which a family can cope with his cancer versus the way it may have managed his coming out as a gay man can be unsettling. Many men also wonder if their lives will become burdensome on their family and friends; often they wonder if their friends and family will avoid them and if loneliness will be their fate (Schaffner, 2005).

Coming out as a cancer survivor will almost certainly be influenced by the patient's previous experience in coming out. Revisiting that experience may be painful or of no consequence, but the methods that a person developed in coming out will certainly be helpful in coming out as a cancer survivor. Theoretically, LGBT people may be better at coming out as cancer survivors than heterosexual or cisgender counterparts for the very reason that they are already experienced at coming out. Clearly, there is room for research here.

There are also cases reported in support groups facilitated by one of the authors, where a cancer diagnosis created an avenue for coming out as a gay man. For example, one man who was living a heterosexual life, with wife and children, found himself diagnosed with an advanced-stage prostate cancer in his mid-forties. He spent several months discussing treatment choices, when it was clear that time for treatment was critical. He later revealed that the time that appeared as a delaying tactic toward treatment was actually the time he needed to come out as someone who had fantasized about sex with other men most of his life. His cancer diagnosis created a now-or-never moment, a time for him to come out and actively create relationships with other men. Remarkably, his family was understanding and remained supportive, even with his change in identity.

Survivorship is the period of time after initial treatment. Between diagnosis and treatment, there are many opportunities for action: choosing, carrying out, and monitoring the treatment (which entails seeing whether it is working or needs to be altered), and then monitoring and coping with the side effects. After treatment, the patient is told to take regularly scheduled tests, scans, and examinations until a period of time passes when the treatment may be considered a success or failure. Health vigilance for all cancer survivors is on order for the rest of their lives. Cancer survivors often quip that they want to live long enough to die from something other than their cancer.

PARTICIPATING IN ADVOCACY

LGBT people, young and old, have grown up in an atmosphere of activism and advocacy around HIV and AIDS. LGBT cancer survivors should be aware that there is a small but growing world of cancer-related advocacy organizations that they are encouraged to support and participate in.

There is both empowerment and honor in helping newly diagnosed LGBT people navigate cancer treatment. Being part of finding a cure for cancer is life affirming, and it validates a person's purpose and survivorship (Clarke & Stovall, 1996). Active rather than avoidant activities are correlated with positive psychological and physical outcomes and are associated with a better return to precancer activities (Roesch, 2005). People who actively participate in support groups after their treatment find gratification and renewed purpose by helping and mentoring newly diagnosed persons. LGBT people who are cancer survivors are indeed role models for others, who often hear nothing more about health care advocacy beyond that around HIV and AIDS. Participating in advocacy also helps build the LGBT community's presence in the heterosexually dominant health care world.

Founded in 1998, Malecare (www.malecare.org) is the national nonprofit support and advocacy organization for gay, bisexual, and transgender men diagnosed with cancer. Malecare facilitates peer-to-peer support groups, many led by social workers and psychologists diagnosed with cancer, for prostate, testicular, anal and/or male breast cancer. The ability to speak of sexuality and identity, without fear and without having to explain, is a critical benefit of cancer-survivor support groups for gay, bisexual, and transgender people. LGBT people are best served by support groups that feature peer-to-peer conversations rather than podium speakers. Peer-to-peer support groups have been shown to be more helpful in dealing with sexual problems and issues associated with maintaining employment than lecture-style groups (Lepore & Helgeson, 2003).

Malecare wants all sexual and gender minority people to feel encouraged to participate in its work. As demand for services from Malecare grew, discussions developed around the idea that there might be commonly held LGBT issues regarding cancer survivorship. In 2005, members of Malecare and its lesbian allies worked together to create the National LGBT Cancer Project, America's first national advocacy and support organization focused on supporting the advocacy and psychosocial issues of all gay, lesbian, bisexual, and transgender cancer survivors. The National LGBT Cancer Project provides opportunities for LGBT people to participate in advocacy issues such as reversing a law that prohibits men who have sex with men from donating bone marrow to people with leukemia, lymphoma, and other diseases. It also promotes research in our community in collaboration with universities around the world. The National LGBT Cancer Project now includes the LGBT cancer-survivor support-group network Out With Cancer (www.outwithcancer.org), creating opportunities for cancer survivors to benefit from inclusion within the broader LGBT cancer-survivor support community.

FINAL THOUGHTS

It is clear that a cancer diagnosis alters people's lives, but it does not change their identities. It is possible to navigate cancer and live a happy, purposeful, and love-filled life. The cancer may or may not be fatal. The side effects of treatment may or may not impede one from fully enjoying life. It is the unknowns that affect most people—that live in their hearts and minds and persist. Learning to enjoy life with cancer as an LGBT person helps the cancer survivor beat cancer at its own game.

REFERENCES

Boehmer, U., Miao, X., & Ozonoff, A. (2011). Cancer survivorship and sexual orientation. *Cancer, 117*(16), 3796–3804.

Clarke, E. J., & Stovall, E. L. (1996). Advocacy: The cornerstone of cancer survivorship. *Cancer Practice, 4*(5), 239–244.

Degner, D., & Davison, B. J. (1997). Empowerment of men newly diagnosed with prostate cancer. *Cancer Nursing, 20*, 187–196.

Dutton, L., Koenig, K., & Fennie, K. (2008). Gynecologic care of the female to male transgender man. *Journal of Midwifery and Women's Health, 53*(4), 331–337.

Futterweit, W. (1998). Endocrine therapy of transsexualism and potential complications of long-term treatment. *Archives of Sexual Behavior, 27*(2), 209–226.

Goldstone, S. E. (2005). The ups and downs of gay sex after prostate cancer treatment. In G. Perlman & J. Drescher (Eds.), *A gay man's guide to prostate cancer* (pp. 43–55). Binghamton, NY: Haworth Medical Press.

Hart, S. L., Coon, D. W., Kowalkowski, M. A., & Latini, D. M. (2011). Gay men with prostate cancer report significantly worse HRQOL than heterosexual men. *The Journal of Urology, 185*(4S), e68–e69.

Hibbs, D. (2008). Hormone replacement and the transgender patient. In M. Chesnay & B. A. Anderson (Eds.), *Caring for the vulnerable: Perspectives in nursing theory, practice and research* (pp. 351–353). Sudbury, MA: Jones and Bartlett.

Hoffman, B., & Stovall, E. (2006). Survivorship perspectives and advocacy. *Journal of Clinical Oncology, 24*(32), 5154–5159.

Kreimer, A. R., Alberg, A. J., Daniel, R., Gravitt, P. E., Viscidi, R., Garrett, E. S., . . . Gillison, M. L. (2004). Oral human papillomavirus infection in adults is associated with sexual behavior and HIV serostatus. *Journal of Infectious Diseases, 189*, 686–698.

Legate, N., Ryan, R. M., & Weinstein, N. (2011). Is coming out always a good thing? Disclosing sexual orientation makes people happier than thought, but mainly in supportive settings. *Social Psychological and Personality Science, 3*(2), 145–152..

Lepore, S. J., & Helgeson, V. S. (2003). Improving quality of life in men with prostate cancer: A randomized controlled trial of group education interventions. *Health Psychology, 22*, 443–452.

MacDonagh, R. P., & Cliff, A. M. (2000). Psychosocial morbidity in prostate cancer: A comparison of patients and partners. *British Journal of Urology, 86*, 834–839.

Miksad, R. A., & Bubley, G. (2006). Prostate cancer in a transgender woman 41 years after initiation of feminization. *Journal of the American Medical Association, 296*(19), 2316–2317.

Mitteldorf, D. (2013). What I have learned from working with gay men who have prostate cancer. In G. Perlman (Ed.), *What every gay man needs to know about prostate cancer* (pp. 128–135). New York: Magnus Books.

Molokwu, C., Appelbaum, J., & Miksad, R. (2008). Detection of prostate cancer following gender reassignment. *British Journal of Urology International, 101*, 259.

Murphy, M. (2010). *At five in the afternoon: My battle with male cancer.* Kerry, Ireland: Brandon Books.

Palefskey, J. M. (2011). HPV vaccine against anal HPV infection and anal intrapithelial neoplasia. *The New England Journal of Medicine, 365*(17), 1576–1585.

Pirl, W., & Siegel, G. (2002). Depression in men receiving androgen deprivation therapy for prostate cancer: A pilot study. *Psycho-Oncology, 11*, 518–523.

Roesch, S. C. (2005). Coping with prostate cancer: A meta-analytic review. *Journal of Behavioral Medicine, 28*(3), 281–293.

Rosner, E. N., & Heyman, T. T. (1996). Prostate cancer: An intimate view from patients and wives. *Urologic Nursing, 6*(2), 37–44.

Santillo, V., & Lowe, F. (2005). Prostate cancer and the gay male. In G. Perlman & J. Drescher (Eds.), *A gay man's guide to prostate cancer* (pp. 9–29). New York: Haworth Press.

Schaffner, B. (2005). Prostate cancer at age 84. In J. Drescher & G. Perlman (Eds.), *A gay man's guide to prostate cancer* (pp. 131–137). New York: Haworth Press.

Schilder, A. J., Orchard, T. R., Buchner, C. S., Miller, M. L., Fernandes, K. A., Hogg, R. S., & Strathdee, S. A. (2008). "It's like the treasure": Beliefs associated with semen among young HIV-positive and HIV-negative gay men. *Culture, Health & Sexuality, 10,* 667–679.

Thurston, A. (1994). Carcinoma of the prostate in a transsexual. *British Journal of Urology International, 73*(2), 217.

Tiggemann, C., & Yeland, M. (2003). Muscularity and the gay ideal: Body dissatisfaction and disordered eating in homosexual men. *Eating Behaviors, 4*(2), 107–116.

7

Tobacco Use in LGBT Populations

NFN Scout

Tobacco use is the leading global cause of preventable death. The World Health Organization reports it currently kills 6 million people each year, and if current trends continue, that will grow to 8 million by 2030 (World Health Organization, 2011). People who use tobacco will lose an average of 10 years of their lives as a result (Jha et al., 2013).

In the United States, cigarette smoking prevalence has dropped from 42.4 percent in 1965 to its current full population rate of 15.5 percent (Jamal et al., 2018). A series of tobacco control actions have helped drive this rate down. Notable among them was the 1999 Master Settlement Agreement, a result of a lawsuit by state attorneys general against the tobacco industry. This settlement funded a surge in tobacco control programs at the state level and established many new regulations prohibiting some tobacco industry tactics, notably those that attempted to market directly to youth (Jones & Silvestri, 2010). Still, smoking kills an estimated 480,000 people each year and costs an estimated $156 billion in productivity losses and $170 billion in direct health costs (Warren, Alberg, Kraft, & Cummings, 2014; Xu, Bishop, Kennedy, Simpson, & Pechacek, 2015). Reviews of data and modeling of future health costs have highlighted the key role that changing smoking behavior will play in any efforts to reduce spiraling health care costs (Institute of Medicine, 2009) Several other milestones have enhanced tobacco control in recent years. In 2009, Congress passed the Family Tobacco Control and Prevention Act, giving the Food and Drug Administration (FDA) authority to regulate many tobacco products. In 2010, lawmakers passed the Affordable Care Act, including provisions to set up several new funding streams and coordination mechanisms to further push down the rates of tobacco use. In 2011, the Centers for Disease Control considered reducing the smoking rate to be one of their six "winnable battles" ("CDC Winnable Battles," 2011).

Today the spotlight on reducing health care costs has brought more focus to successful tobacco control strategies than ever before. Full-population smoking rates have largely slowed their decline over recent years (Jamal et al., 2018). The CDC has called for greater funding to state tobacco programs to keep the progress on track. Community leaders posit another reason for the plateau: that we only have limited focus on countering tobacco use in populations with the highest smoking rates—such as certain racial/ethnic groups, those of lower socioeconomic status, people with mental illness, veterans, and LGBT communities (Drope et al., 2018). Community advocates argue that in order to move the needle on overall prevalence, tobacco control leaders must adopt the strategies of the tobacco industry, which has for years tailored its outreach to vulnerable communities such as LGBT people.

LGBT TOBACCO PREVALENCE

The first organization to fight against the harms of tobacco in the LGBT community, the Coalition of Lavender-Americans on Smoking and Health (CLASH), was founded in 1991 by Naphtali Offen, then the director of the Medical Expertise Retention Program of the Gay and Lesbian Medical Association (GLMA); Gloria Soliz, the originator of The Last Drag, the first smoking-cessation program for LGBT and HIV-positive smokers; and Len Casey and Kevin Goebel, advocates at the pioneer tobacco control organization, Americans for Nonsmokers Rights. They were joined shortly thereafter by Galen Ellis and Bob Gordon. CLASH suspected that LGBT people smoked more than the mainstream, but it had no reliable studies. It successfully lobbied UCSF to study smoking prevalence rates of gay and bisexual men in its landmark late 1990s Urban Men's Health Study, producing some of the earliest results corroborating high smoking rates in this population (Stall, Greenwood, Acree, Paul, & Coates, 1999).

As with many rare populations, data for determining prevalence of smoking among the LGBT communities are scarce. Most of the national full-population surveillance surveys used to gauge these numbers do not include LGB or T (transgender) measures. Even of the available studies, most collect LGB but not T status. Nonetheless, there is a consistent pattern among available LGBT smoking data, demonstrating that the population has a profound smoking disparity.

The most recent systematic review of the literature focused on sexual minority data (L, G, B) was published in 2009. After reviewing the 42 studies that met their criteria, the authors found that the data generally showed a positive correlation between being a sexual minority and smoking, with reported odds ratios between 1.5 to 2.5 (Lee, Griffin, & Melvin, 2009).

Full-probability surveys that report LGBT smoking are especially valuable. In the several years that the National Adult Tobacco Survey (NATS) was used as a prevalence marker, only the first wave (2009–2010) collected trans data. From that, we see that LGBT smoking rates were 68 percent higher than in the general population (King, Dube, & Tynan, 2012). This echoes an earlier full-probability study from California, where LGBT men's prevalence rate was almost 50 percent higher than that of the other men, and disturbingly, LGBT women's prevalence rate was almost 200 percent higher than for other women. The next wave of NATS (trans exclusive) showed LGB people smoking at rates 58 percent higher than others (Agaku et al., 2014). After that, the full-population marker for smoking switches to the National Health Interview Survey (NHIS). In the NHIS, information about gender identity is not collected, and there is evidence that because of methodological artifact, bisexual respondents are undercounted. Waves of NHIS data show that LGB persons use tobacco products at rates 33 to 36.3 percent higher than others (Jamal et al., 2016, 2018). Because of changes in the question wording and scope of the measure (all tobacco products), evidence about any reduction of disparity would need to be corroborated through other sources.

One set of researchers sought to examine sexual minority youth data to clarify if that gap was staying steady, increasing, or decreasing over time. They found that while smoking rates were dropping for all groups, the disparity was not decreasing between LGB youth and others; in some cases, it was even increasing (Watson, Lewis, Fish, & Goodenow, 2018).

Other Tobacco Products

Likely in direct relation to the FDA's new authority to regulate tobacco, the number of tobacco products available to consumers has increased substantively in recent years. When data are available on LGBT use of these products, the profile follows that of cigarette smoking; in most cases, there is an increased risk to use other tobacco products.

Researchers found LGBT people to be 1.66 times more likely to have tried disposable tobacco products than others (Cabrera-Nguyen, Cavazos-Rehg, Krauss, Kim, & Emery, 2016). In a review of the National Adult Tobacco Survey, LGB people showed greater water pipe tobacco smoking than non LGB people (Ortiz, Mamkherzi, Salloum, Matthews, & Maziak, 2017).

Likewise, LGBT people smoked flavored cigars at higher rates than non-LGBT people (King, Dube, & Tynan, 2013).

Flavorings deserve special note because of how changes in their regulation have affected the market. After the Family Tobacco Control and Prevention Act prohibited certain types of flavored cigarettes in an effort to deter youth smoking, the tobacco industry unveiled flavored cigarillos—small "cigars" that looked very much like cigarettes but were brown in color. Eventually, the FDA sent warning letters to several tobacco manufacturers about this practice, but that was seven years after it had started to enforce the ban on flavored cigarettes (FDA, 2016). In that time, many new tobacco users were lured into smoking via cigars or cigarillos with wild cherry, grape, and strawberry flavorings.

In an odd twist, the most prominent tobacco flavoring, menthol (mint), was not banned in the original legislation. Advocates have asked for action on this point, because menthol cigarettes are disproportionately used by some of the most vulnerable people—those with low income, who are black, or who are Hispanic. It is not widely known that LGBT people also fall into this subgroup. Researchers found that 36.3 percent of LGBT smokers reported using menthol cigarettes versus 29.3 percent of other smokers (Fallin, Goodin, & King, 2015).

Another area where flavorings are prominent is in e-cigarette use. Many of the vape stores combine the appeal of a trendy coffeehouse with a wide range of youth-friendly flavors—for example, banana nut bread, Gummi Bear, and Blue Razz Cotton Candy. While using an e-cigarette may help established smokers reduce the harm from cigarettes, new evidence shows that they do not actually facilitate cessation—and the biggest impact is in luring new smokers into the market, tipping the balance of their impact away from harm reduction. A large-scale full-probability sample showed significant elevations in LGBT electronic cigarette use: ever use was 25.1 percent versus 14.3 percent for non-LGBT; current use was 9.4 percent versus 4.9 percent for non-LGBT (Huang, Kim, Vera, & Emery, 2016).

NATS data show that overall, use of other tobacco products is significantly higher for sexual minority people: prevalence of women's e-cigarette (12.4 percent), hookah (10.3 percent), and cigar use (7.2 percent) was more than triple that of other women (3.4 percent, 2.5 percent, and 1.3 percent, respectively); prevalence of men's e-cigarette (7.9 percent) and hookah (12.8 percent) use exceeded that of other men (4.7 percent and 4.5 percent, respectively) (Johnson et al., 2016).

LGBT People of Color

Extremely limited data on subpopulations within LGBT communities continue to provide cause for concern. From the very earliest reported

LGBT data, we see disparities experienced by LGBT people of color. In an early full-probability phone survey, black gay or bisexual men had almost double the smoking rates of heterosexual black men (62 percent versus 34 percent) (Stall et al., 1999). In a longitudinal study of adolescent health (ADD Health), 58.4 percent of LGB Asian American/Pacific Islander women smoked versus 38.3 percent of other AA/PI women (S. B. Austin et al., 2004; Easton & Sell, 2004). While prevalence rates reported for LGBT of color in one survey had sample sizes too small to achieve significance, the raw frequencies showed each of the LGBT black, AA/PI, and Latino subgroups had prevalence rates *at least* 100 percent higher than their non-LGBT referent ethnic groups (Bye, Gruskin, Greenwood, Albright, & Krotski, 2004; Greenwood & Gruskin, 2007). Researchers who are able to explore this subpopulation continue to find these disparities through to today. Researchers looking at NHANES found that LGBT Latino people were 1.93 times more likely to be smokers than their non-LGB Latino counterparts (Martinez et al., 2017). Likewise, other researchers found that racial discrimination is a significant factor influencing tobacco smoking and health behaviors within two-spirit populations. (Johnson-Jennings, Belcourt, Town, Walls, & Walters, 2014).

There has been notable government attention on the tobacco-related disparities experienced by racial and ethnic minority communities, but LGBT overlap is often omitted. In 1998, the surgeon general published *Tobacco Use Among U.S Racial/Ethnic Minority Groups: A Report of the Surgeon General.* There was no mention of the LGBT communities in this report. In general, it has been found that prevalence rates for communities of color vary widely by subpopulation and are plagued by similar data gaps as for LGBT data. Tobacco disparities for LGBT of color are not always about prevalence. For example, African Americans smoke at rates not dissimilar to the full population, but they experience notably higher mortality from tobacco-related illnesses (Fagan, Moolchan, Lawrence, Fernander, & Ponder, 2007). The authors urged people to consider a continuum of tobacco effects when considering the burden of tobacco on a vulnerable population, including differences in tobacco use, exposure, initiation, treatment, and subsequent health outcomes. Similarly, an analysis of a national college data set demonstrated that all LGB racial groups smoked more than their referent heterosexual racial groups, including significantly more hookah use among white and Hispanic LGB people (J. R. Blosnich, Jarrett, & Horn, 2011).

In 2006, the National Cancer Institute worked with other tobacco leaders to address the data gaps in LGBT of color and smoking. They identified a primary obstacle as lack of sampling methodologies for such a relatively rare population as LGBT of color. As a result, they convened a meeting of experts and prepared the report *Lesbians, Gays, Bisexuals, and Transgenders of*

Color Sampling Methodology: Strategies for Collecting Data in Small, Hidden, or Hard-to-Reach Groups to Reduce Tobacco-Related Health Disparities (Buchting & Fagan, 2008). The experts reviewed published and unpublished data before concurring that available data supported the hypothesis that the effect of dual discrimination is additive: LGBT people of color, as expected, smoke more than their referent racial/ethnic categories. Blosnich et al. have confirmed this hypothesis with their analysis of a large youth sample, finding that every racial/ethnic minority had an increased level of smoking when compared with their non–sexual minority referent groups (J. R. Blosnich et al., 2011).

The supreme challenge in analyzing this subgroup of a subgroup is in obtaining a sample large enough to provide statistical power. The 2012–2013 NATS sample size was over 60,000 respondents. In both of the subgroups, researchers were able to report that racial minority people experienced elevated smoking rates, but the biggest takeaway is that they were unable to achieve enough power to report data from most racial and ethnic subgroups (Johnson et al., 2016). Currently, the Behavioral Risk Factor Surveillance System (BRFSS) has the largest sample size of any surveillance instrument, with 400,000 surveys completed annually. While more states are adding sexual and/or gender minority measures to that survey, the final measures are decided at the state, not the federal, level, making it a challenge to get uniformity in LGBT data collection across the full sample.

Gay/Bisexual Men versus Lesbian/Bisexual Women

Many available studies report gay and bisexual categories together for both men and women (G/B and L/B). The evidence of distinctions in the smoking disparities between these two populations is mixed. The 2007 Lee review of research found that among existing studies, G/B men had a slightly higher odds ratio for smoking than L/B women: 1.5 to 2.5 for gay men (compared to heterosexual) versus 1.5 to 2.0 for lesbians (Lee et al., 2009). On the other hand, the large 2003 California LGBT Tobacco Use Survey, not included in that review, found that gay men smoke at rates 35 percent higher than their referent groups, and lesbians almost 200 percent higher (Bye et al., 2004). A later study combining those data with the California Health Interview Survey data upheld the slightly greater gap for lesbians (Gruskin, Greenwood, Matevia, Pollack, & Bye, 2007). Researchers were finally able to report on a full-probability, large-scale sample from the 2012–2013 NATS wave: gay men 26.1 percent; bi men 20.7 percent; straight men 20.5 percent; lesbian/gay women 22.2 percent; bi women 36 percent, straight women 14.3 percent. Gay men's and lesbian/gay women's smoking rates are not appreciably different; the most prominent issue is the elevated rates of smoking for bi women, which would push L/B women's smoking rates above that of G/B men's. The further breakout shows the power of disaggregating information, since the anomaly of bi women's smoking rates would be masked in the earlier reporting (Johnson et al., 2016).

Bisexuals

As stated above, LG and B data are too rarely disaggregated. When they are, there is evidence that bisexuals experience increased health challenges compared to L and G populations. The NATS data were not the only ones pointing to a pronounced disparity for bi people and especially women. In one full-population study, the odds of bi women using some form of tobacco were 2.6 that of non-LB women (lesbians were 1.7 times as likely to use tobacco). Bi women also had 2.9 times the odds of using regular cigars and 2.4 times the odds of using small cigars (Emory et al., 2016). Identifying as a female bisexual has also been associated with fewer past quit attempts, lower age at first cigarette, and higher nicotine dependence when compared to straight women (Fallin, Goodin, Lee, & Bennett, 2015). In another study, bisexual females were most likely to report concurrent tobacco use, binge drinking, and marijuana use in the past 30 days (Schauer, Berg, & Bryant, 2013).

In an analysis of the National Health Interview Survey data, bi men were 2.1 times more likely to report heavy smoking than non-GB men, and bi women were 1.6 times as likely to report moderate smoking than non-LG women (Gonzales, Przedworski, & Henning-Smith, 2016). Likewise, an analysis of a large surveillance instrument found that the range of people who were attracted to both sexes, acted on that attraction, and identified as bisexual were all at greatest risk for tobacco use (compared to LG and non-LGB) (McCabe et al., 2017). This study illuminates one of the factors that may contribute to this disparity. It is well documented that bi people experience discrimination both from LG and non-LGB populations; in the study, people who experienced greater sexual orientation discrimination had significantly greater change of past-year smoking. Another study explored not just identity but behavior and attraction as well; it found that bi-attracted people have the highest rates of smoking (Dai, 2017; McCabe et al., 2017).

The experience of stigma and discrimination is likely heightened among the bi population, since bi identified people get less than average support from the LG communities. These tobacco data support the connection between increased stigma and smoking.

Men Who Have Sex with Men and HIV

Data from the Multicenter AIDS Cohort Study were used to assess smoking patterns for men who have sex with men (MSM) over the 30-year window since the study started. Researchers found baseline smoking rates to be high among both HIV-positive (44.1 percent) and HIV-negative (37.9 percent) men. Over time, both declined; multivariate analyses showed no significant connection to HIV status but a positive correlation with measurable viral load. Demographic and health variables that positively correlated with current smoking included: black, non-Hispanic, lower education, enrollment wave, alcohol use, and marijuana use (Akhtar-Khaleel, Cook, Shoptaw, Surkan, Stall, et al., 2016). Interestingly, a related study illuminated smoking patterns among all enrolled men; it found 55.9 percent to be persistent nonsmokers, 11 percent to be persistent light smokers, 10 percent to be intermittent smokers, and 23.1 percent to be persistent heavy smokers. Being a persistent heavy smoker was positively correlated with low education and being HIV positive (Akhtar-Khaleel, Cook, Shoptaw, Surkan, Teplin, et al., 2016). This smoking disparity among HIV-positive men is persisting into the young population: a study of HIV-positive MSM enrollees in the Adolescent Trials network found 32.9 percent of them reported at least weekly tobacco use (Gamarel, Brown, et al., 2016).

Transgender People

Data on transgender smoking is even rarer than for communities of color. Many studies initiated by sexual minority researchers do not also collect gender identity data, thus echoing the gap in the governmental surveillance instruments. The current best evidence is from a recent full probability study (Buchting et al., 2017). From that panel of over 17,000 people, researchers report that transgender adults had higher 30-day use of any tobacco product, 39.7 percent trans versus 25.1 percent of others. Current use of all products was also notably elevated: cigarettes 35.5 percent trans versus 20.7 percent of others; cigars 26.8 percent trans versus 9.3 percent of others; e-cigarettes 21.3 percent trans versus 5.0 percent of others.

More information about the nexus between trans people and smoking can be found in the first of two large-scale but convenience samples of national transgender people. The first such survey engaged 6,450 respondents; data from that survey echo many of the themes in larger LGB data (Grant, Mottet, & Tanis, 2010).

Transgender respondents report smoking at rates 50 percent higher than the general population (30 percent versus 20 percent). Race, age, educational attainment, citizenship status, region, and income all affected smoking rates. Black respondents reported current daily or occasional smoking at a rate of 50 percent; Latino and multiracial respondents were at 37 percent; respondents with high school degrees (only) were at 46 percent; respondents earning incomes of $10,000 annually or less report 43 percent; undocumented noncitizens were at 40 percent; respondents in the 18 to 24 year-old cohort were at 37 percent; and respondents in the South were at 34 percent. Those who have been involved in the street economies at any level appear to be at the highest risk of smoking, reporting a rate of 51 percent (Grant, Mottet, & Tanis, 2010).

Respondents on the female-to-male (FTM) spectrum smoke at higher rates than those on the male-to-female spectrum (MTF), with FTMs at 34 percent and MTFs at 29 percent. There was no significant difference between smoking rates of those who identify as transgender and those who identify as gender nonconforming/genderqueer (Grant, 2010).

In a San Francisco study of smoking patterns among trans women, 83 percent reported smoking in the last month and 62.3 percent reported daily smoking (Gamarel, Mereish, et al., 2016). For transgender people, "passing" as gender conforming can minimize their internal stress as well as reduce their experience of stigma. Researchers showed that transgender people whose identity documents matched their true gender had only 0.84 times the odds of smoking versus those with incongruent identity documents. In a similar vein, transgender people who experienced structural discrimination were 1.65 times as likely to smoke as those who had not (Shires & Jaffee, 2016).

Later researchers found that people who experienced transphobic discrimination in health care were most likely to experience multiple negative health indicators: depression, alcohol use, smoking, physical inactivity, and overweight status (Reisner, Gamarel, Dunham, Hopwood, & Hwahng, 2013).

Contradicting most literature, the later iteration of the National Trans Health Survey, with an even larger convenience sample, reported that trans people did not smoke at appreciably different rates than the general population—21 percent general versus 22 percent trans (James et al., 2016). A relative level of detail about these numbers has not yet been published. This anomaly in the trend of data for this population could be related to the reference data set: the National Survey on Drug Use and Health. CDC publishes smoking surveillance data based on the National Health Interview Survey, which reported a 15.1 percent smoking rate for the same year, thus yielding a 45 percent excess smoking rate for trans survey respondents (Jamal et al., 2016).

INITIATION AND PREVENTION

Smoking is a pediatric epidemic. Most people start smoking in their teens; very few adults initiate tobacco use. There is evidence that LGBT people do not vary from this pattern. In the largest LGBT study to date, average age of initiation was 12 (Bye et al., 2004). Thus, the discussion of initiation and prevention is one about LGBT youth.

There has been growing attention to the stressors that LGBT youth experience. Publicity about LGBT teen suicides has shed light on the difficult circumstances that LGBT youth are often asked to navigate. Lack of parental acceptance is common, as is lack of acceptance at school. Reports of even more extreme responses, including bullying, are frequent. LGBT youth experience particular stressors based on their LGBT status, particularly internalized homophobia and reactions to disclosures of sexual orientation or gender minority status. They also experience increased rates of other factors, including stress, depression, alcohol use, and victimization (J. Blosnich, Lee, & Horn, 2013).

In what is perhaps the single most illustrative research study on LGB youth and smoking, researchers studied adverse childhood experiences (ACEs). They found that LGB youth (data were pulled from a surveillance system that did not collect T data) had 1.4 to 3.1 times the odds of experiencing ACEs versus other youth. Importantly, once adjusted for ACEs, sexual orientation was no longer correlated with poor physical health, current smoking, or binge drinking (A. Austin, Herrick, & Proescholdbell, 2016). This points to the impact that negative events have on the health trajectory of LGBTQ youth.

Stress

The inordinate level of stress experienced by LGBT youth is identified by many researchers as a leading contributor to disproportionate smoking initiation. In a study by Remafedi, stress was identified by LGBT youth themselves as the most frequent experience contributing to tobacco use (2017). In the words of one 19-year-old African American youth from that study,

> You're at higher risk if you are gay. We go through SO MUCH. It is STRONG . . . only thing that can calm our nerves now is cigarettes, weed, alcohol. I mean they have been through so much. . . . If you hear the stories, you can cry. . . . They are escaping a lot of stuff in their lives. You know, some of them were molested, raped, beaten on, abandoned.

Stress continues to be cited as a factor among youth. A 2015 study of sexual minority women found that youth thought smoking was a way to overcome general life stressors and sexuality-related stressors and that it was ingrained into LGBTQ culture (Youatt, Johns, Pingel, Soler, & Bauermeister, 2015). Tobacco is not the only substance used to mediate this stress; one study found that sexual minority girls were nearly seven times as likely to be using tobacco, marijuana, and alcohol (Dermody et al., 2016). Researchers attributed part of this disparity to participants' experiences of discrimination, victimization, and social isolation.

Researchers found that, even controlling for other demographic factors, negative reactions to disclosure of LGBT status were directly correlated with youth smoking, as well as with using marijuana and alcohol (Rosario, Schrimshaw, & Hunter, 2009). In another study, higher rates of experienced violence among LGB people were directly associated with higher smoking rates (J. R. Blosnich & Horn, 2011). In others, higher levels of anti-gay prejudice were correlated with higher current smoking rates (J. R. Blosnich, Gordon, & Fine, 2015; Coulter, Bersamin, Russell, & Mair, 2017; D'Avanzo, Halkitis, Yu, & Kapadia, 2016). The harassment does not have to be pronounced to have an effect on smoking; researchers studying micro-aggressions found frequent experience with them increased odds of recent smoking by 72 percent (Ylioja, Cochran, Woodford, & Renn, 2018).

Unfortunately, researchers found that while smoking may be initiated to cope with stress, it has not been found to reduce the stress among LGBT youth (Rosario, Schrimshaw, & Hunter, 2010).

Seeking Community

Another commonly cited theory about high smoking rates among LGBT youth is the impact of seeking out the community. Unlike youth from other stigmatized populations, LGBT youth rarely have a family member who can help them find other community members. In some high schools, gay-straight alliances (GSAs) serve a key role in introducing LGBT youth to others. For many youth, they seek LGBT community through bars and other high-smoking social venues. Smoking is an easy social lubricant; asking for a light can be a nonthreatening way to begin a conversation. Even with the proliferation of indoor smoking bans, bars can be a place where LGBT youth learn to smoke as LGBT people congregate outside to do so. In Remafedi's study, the most oft-cited reasons encouraging smoking past stress all related to the desire to seek and fit in with the larger community (Remafedi, 2007). When researchers interviewed LGBT leaders about why people smoke, one of their top three reasons was because it is a socialization aid (Jannat-Khah, Dill, Reynolds, & Joseph, 2018).

LGBT youth do not need to be exposed to a traditional smoking environment like a bar to feel the peer pressure to smoke. In a series of LGBT community meetings convened by researchers to talk about smoking, several youth participants emphasized that they had learned to smoke from LGBT youth groups convened at nonprofits: "Everyone would go outside to smoke, even the counselor, so eventually, I followed." In a later community meeting in Arizona, one young adult described another interesting phenomenon: he had stopped buying cigarettes two years prior, but this had had no effect on his smoking. Adult LGBT smokers were eager to give him cigarettes, so his decision to stop buying them did not substantively limit his access. In a large-scale study of young MSM, the odds of being a current smoker were particularly high among young men reporting greater levels of gay community affinity (D'Avanzo et al., 2016).

Smoking is a socially transmitted disease. With the increased prevalence of LGBT adult smoking, it is inevitable that more LGBT youth will also adopt the practice.

Social Environment

There has been increasing evidence that the social or political environmental factors can have a direct correlation on LGBT population health and youth suicide risk. For example, LGB respondents in states without protective policies were almost five times more likely than those in other states to have two or more mental disorders. When states passed constitutional bans on same-sex marriage, mood disorders increased by one-third among their LGB population (only). These factors are very likely to affect smoking rates similarly. Preliminary evidence supports this theory: when researchers stratified Oregon counties by levels of acceptance of LGBT people, they found a positive correlation between this acceptance and lower smoking rates (Hatzenbuehler, Wieringa, & Keyes, 2011). Religious climate has also been directly linked to health behaviors. The same researchers found that youth living in a religious climate supportive of homosexuality had pronouncedly lower odds of alcohol abuse and fewer sexual partners (Hatzenbuehler, Pachankis, & Wolff, 2012).

The conflux of different stressors and stigma leave LGBT youth particularly at risk for smoking. How much of this is attributable to the relatively unwelcoming social environment for LGBT youth in the United States? Insight can be drawn from a study in the Netherlands, where researchers sought to find out how sexual minority youth were faring after 20 years of inclusive policies. They found that social opprobrium is a difficult factor to root out: sexual minority youth were still 2.37 times as likely to smoke as others and to report lower life satisfaction and higher psychosomatic complaints (Kuyper, de Roos, Iedema, & Stevens, 2016).

TOBACCO INDUSTRY TARGETING

An early study by Smith et al. demonstrates that tobacco targeting for LGBT people yields an unexpected response (Smith, Thomson, Offen, & Malone, 2008). While targeting usually generates a community response that varies with the perceived community benefits, in a series of LGBT focus groups, participants judged tobacco targeting by an unusually narrow metric. Aware that LGBT media had often been overlooked by standard advertisers and that Phillip Morris was one of the early advertisers in gay media, the participants generally viewed the targeting positively, taking it as a measure of community viability and legitimacy. The deleterious impact of additional smoking did not measurably concern respondents. No doubt related to this, the participants also did not perceive smoking to be an LGBT health issue. In the words of one participant, when the tobacco industry "specifically address[es] us in our publications [it] makes us very happy. . . . We're not used to that. So we're very vulnerable" (Smith et al., 2008).

In contrast, in similar focus groups conducted with African Americans (no report of their sexual orientation or gender identity), respondents shown evidence of tobacco industry targeting African Americans were primarily upset (Yerger, Daniel, & Malone, 2005). The attitude of gratitude and of relative lack of knowledge of any tobacco disparity is one of the primary challenges in combating tobacco's influence in the LGBT communities.

Smith et al. conducted two additional early studies to further estimate the influence of tobacco ads in LGBT communities. In one, the researchers conducted a content analysis of 20 LGBT community periodicals (Smith, Offen, & Malone, 2005). Slightly over half of all ads found with tobacco content were pro-tobacco or neutral, but these ads took up almost three-quarters of the total ad space, whereas ads negative toward tobacco (mainly ads for cessation programs) took up slightly over one-quarter of the total space. Ads for tobacco products were also much more likely to use imagery, making them more compelling. Interestingly, a significant proportion of the ads using tobacco imagery were not purchased by the tobacco industry—they were from other industries, such as entertainment. The same research team conducted another study analyzing the noncommercial tobacco representations in the same media (Smith, Offen, & Malone, 2006). The authors found that noncommercial reference to or images related to tobacco were predominantly pro-tobacco or neutral. Associating tobacco with celebrities was common, further bolstering the sense that tobacco use was not a health issue.

As noted, the tobacco industry has a long history of seizing the opportunity to advertise in the LGBT press. An early Phillip Morris foray into gay media in 1993 sparked unexpected publicity as news coverage from the *New York Times* to Fox News promoted the move and debated its merits. The *New York Post* headline read, "New cigs aimed at gay smokers" (Smith & Malone, 2003). Phillip Morris quickly backed away from the issue, emphasizing that it did not target gay people.

Project SCUM

Years later, tobacco industry lawsuits would yield more information on its targeting of LGBT people during this era. While the tobacco industry took pains to present itself as a friend to the LGBT communities, one media campaign title belied this attitude. Project Sub Culture Urban Marketing aimed at marketing cigarettes to gay men and homeless people in the Tenderloin region of San Francisco. While the marketers eventually changed their project title, the industry documents have preserved the original title: Project SCUM (R. J. Reynolds, 1995).

Tobacco industry documents yield other insights into the tobacco industry tactics. Typically, it would hire an LGBT community marketing firm to gain access to venues and advise on tactics. Event sponsorship was heavily used at one point as a way to promote specific brands. An excerpt of one internal memo gives an example:

PHILIP MORRIS U.S.A OVERVIEW In 1997, Community Event Marketing commenced its marketing efforts towards Gay and Lesbian adult smokers. Ten events were identified by Spare Parts, Inc. which succeeded in exposing the Benson & Hedges brand to over 300,000 Gay and Lesbian adult smokers and secured 7665 names for the database. (Phillip Morris USA, 1997)

Tobacco industry documents are not available for recent years, so it is difficult to understand how this marketing has changed in the recent decade. But one example from the late 1990s shows particularly clearly how the industry can buy and manipulate LGBT people toward its goals.

Case Study in Targeting

In California in 2016, a looming proposition to raise tobacco taxes was coming up for a population-wide vote. A coalition of tobacco industry representatives banded together to coordinate grassroots opposition. As one step, they hired a person described as "the premier, most credible gay activist in California" who boasted that he had a mailing list of "400,000 to 500,000 registered voters." The activist asserted that while LGBT community members would normally support the tax hike, he could neutralize them into a "no-position" stance. Interestingly, the coalition also decided that "consultants from minority communities will not be retained until later, if at all, to eliminate the notion that the Industry is targeting these groups." The activist then advised them on several very specific strategies, including multiple mailings to the statewide LGBT civil rights list and a "narrow-cast campaign" in the dozens of LGBT papers identified. The activist continued to work with the tobacco industry execs on issue development, urging themes that resonated with the ongoing LGBT civil rights movement: "life-style regulation, government intrusion into personal lives, and removing choice as an option for one's life decisions" (Mixner, 1998).

The evidence showing industry targeting is far from complete. More often, it is only the actions that are seen; rarely do we see a case example this complete of how industry agents directly manipulated LGBT people to further their own ends.

Tailored Advertising

The Web site Trinkets & Trash documents artifacts from the tobacco industry, including ads that have been used to target LGBT communities. While some of the ads run in LGBT publications are generic, there are interesting examples of how little modification is needed to tailor a mainstream ad to appeal to a primarily LGBT audience. The site has an example of a set of Parliament Light ads, one showing a man looking vaguely into a pool where a woman is swimming in the distance. In the LGBT media version of this ad, the designers simply added another man sitting in the sight line of the first and looking back at him. With that small edit, an innocuous mainstream ad now had an overt gay subtext. We see this again in a Newport ad run in 2016: four people are in the ad—a woman in front, a man in back, then another woman, with a man farther back and to her side (Newport Cigarettes, 2016). If this ad were run in a mainstream magazine, it would probably be read as two heterosexual couples. But it ran in a special "black pride" issue of an LGBT community newspaper, where the fact that one of the men was looking intently at the other no doubt contributed to the impression that it was one gay male couple and one lesbian couple.

Civil Rights and Companies That Care

The theme of utilizing LGBT civil rights messages to appeal to the population has surfaced in later tobacco industry ads. Likewise, frequent sponsorship of LGBT and related HIV community events, including high-profile advertising about that sponsorship and supportive hiring practices, continued to cement the image of tobacco companies as allies to the LGBT communities. In 2002, Phillip Morris was selected as one of *Out* magazine's "Companies Who Care."

Examples of ads that use the LGBT civil rights themes include one from Lucky Strike that has one all-caps line on a black background (Lucky Strike, 2001):

WHENEVER SOMEONE YELLS, "DUDE, THAT'S SO GAY," WE'LL BE THERE.

In a similar vein, a later American Spirit ad uses all lowercase letters on a black background to slide tobacco in among all the most salient issues for the LGBT communities (American Spirit, 2005):

freedom. to
speak. to choose. to
marry. to be. to
disagree. to inhale. to
believe. to love. to live.
it's all good.

"How They Get Us to Screw Ourselves"

Also, in 2002, Coalition of Lavender-Americans on Smoking and Health (CLASH) members started an innovative campaign to bring light to the tobacco industry's targeting of LGBT community members. It started by filming a video short entitled "How They Get Us to Screw Ourselves" at the San Francisco Gay and Lesbian Alliance Against Defamation gala. Lucky Strike sponsored the GLAAD awards, including hosting a smoking lounge with spandex-clad models. CLASH members document the response when it points out that indoor smoking is currently illegal in California and asks the industry representatives why they are targeting LGBT people. The film, along with palm cards showing how money for cigarettes is given to tobacco companies, who then spent large amounts supporting antigay legislators, was widely circulated at gay film festivals.

Recent Targeting

Evidence of recent targeting is decidedly scant. There have been multiple reports at community meetings that tobacco company representatives are common fixtures in LGBT bars, often offering some trinket in exchange for allowing them to capture one's home address and contact information. But it is decidedly less common to see open tobacco industry sponsorship of community events as had been common previously. There is also no current access to tobacco industry documents, so researchers cannot document tobacco industry internal targeting efforts.

In 2010, tobacco control advocates reported a surge of ads for RJ Reynolds Snus, a cigarette alternative, in LGBT media across the nation ("Re: [LGBT Tobacco Discussion] Discussion Digest, Vol 51, Issue 13," 2011). Reports of widespread Snus ads persist into 2011. After the Master Settlement Agreement, tobacco advertising fundamentally shifted. Most of it is now focused on point of sale and on capturing individual contact information and then doing direct marketing, which is particularly difficult to track. Trinkets & Trash continues to monitor sporadic advertising in the LGBT publications to this day.

Countermarketing

LGBT tobacco control advocates have become more active in speaking out when there is an uptick in local tobacco advertising or glamorization of tobacco in the LGBT media. As noted, the How They Get Us to Screw Ourselves campaign gained widespread exposure, including coverage in *The Advocate.* In 2007, when *The Advocate* ran a cover glamorizing smoking with a current popular celebrity, the Gay and Lesbian Medical Association countered with a letter denouncing the association, which *The Advocate* later ran. In late 2010 and 2011, the increase in Snus ads met with a similar response: advocates from across the country coordinated a response and sent letters back to editors exposing the link between tobacco ads and our smoking disparity. Unfortunately, community media outlets are often very dependent on advertising, often to the detriment of their commitment to community health. The response to an advocate's complaint about the new tobacco ads in Minneapolis's *Lavender* magazine in Spring 2011 eerily echoes the early tobacco industry messages. The editor is nonplussed by the health risk for LGBT and instead defends his right to take tobacco ads thusly: "Editor's Note: *Lavender* believes in democracy, the essence of which is 'freedom and choice'" (Worthington, 2011).

In recent years, there has been a definite uptick in countermarketing ads in LGBT publications, including notably two overtly LGBT-themed ads from the historic national Centers for Disease Control run Tips from Former Smokers campaign (https://www.cdc.gov/tobacco/campaign/tips/groups/lgbt.html).

COMMUNITY RESPONSE

Lack of Awareness Hinders Response

Considering that every smoker is staged to lose 10 years of life to the disease and at least one in five of every LGBT people smoke, tobacco is overwhelmingly the largest health risk to the LGBT communities. Yet it is much easier to find a project about suicide, HIV, or mental health in many cities than it is to find an LGBT tobacco control project.

One barrier to activating a community response is the relatively low awareness of the LGBT smoking disparity. In a series of needs assessments in Arkansas, Michigan, and Pennsylvania, LGBT people routinely ranked tobacco as one of the lowest health priorities for their communities. This builds on a long history. In 2005, the University of California, San Francisco researchers found that most of the national LGBT leaders surveyed believed that tobacco control was extraneous to their missions and a matter of individual choice that should be respected. In fact, only 24 percent of LGBT considered it one of their top three health issues (Offen, Smith, & Malone, 2008).

Targeting and the high smoking rate likely both play a role in this relative lack of awareness of the toll of tobacco. Another factor is that LGBT people have not routinely been included in mainstream state-level tobacco control campaigns. While Phillip Morris was touting its broad support of community-based LGBT events and organizations, LGBT-targeted tobacco control campaigns were a rare phenomenon in the national tobacco control infrastructure.

Community members have a blind spot when it comes to understanding how tobacco affects the health of LGBT populations. In a recent study in Hawaii, respondents tended to rate their health as "very good" or "excellent" despite higher-than-average smoking rates (Stotzer, Ka'opua, & Diaz, 2014). This is compounded by relative acceptance of tobacco in our media. When researchers asked if community members were familiar with anti-tobacco messages in LGBT media, awareness was quite low (Matthews et al., 2014): a study of media coverage of the tobacco epidemic concluded that it was concentrated in four LGBT blogs and a substantial minority of coverage echoed the conservative argument that smoking was a lifestyle choice (Lee, 2014). Yet, viewers of LGBT movies are bombarded by smoking imagery. One analysis showed that viewers are exposed to depictions of tobacco use once every 15 minutes in LGBT movies (Lee, Agnew-Brune, Clapp, & Blosnich, 2014).

Grassroots Advocates Lead Community Response

Despite the factors that hinder broad community response to tobacco as a health issue, there has been a strong and innovative grassroots-led response. This effort has developed a cadre of networked advocates across the country and has yielded valuable lessons in working in alliance with non-LGBT racial/ethnic leaders as well as advocating for health policy change.

In 2002, one of the CLASH advocates, Bob Gordon, called for the LGBT people attending that year's National Conference on Tobacco or Health to meet in his room. The crowd quickly outgrew his hotel room and moved to a conference room to plan a joint strategy. Attendees identified several priorities: creating a national LGBT action plan, having an LGBT-specific tobacco summit, and conducting joint actions to advance LGBT tobacco control.

The first joint action was implemented at the conference. Approximately 70 participants signed a letter to the head of the second-largest health foundation in the world—Robert Wood Johnson Foundation (RWJ)—urging it to include LGBT groups in its funding. Within a month, the president of RWJ replied, affirming that it would include LGBT grantees in some of its funding streams.

While Gordon's group disbanded, he and other San Francisco–based CLASH members continued the work on another goal, convening a one-day summit about LGBT tobacco to precede the next annual conference on tobacco. In 2003, community members from across the country, with no funding or official structure, created that first daylong LGBT tobacco summit, inviting representatives from several mainstream tobacco control organizations to learn more about this particular disparity. These summits would become a tradition. In 2012, the seventh such summit again preceded the National Conference on Tobacco or Health.

At that summit, another high priority project for the activists was put in motion. Funders were recruited to convene people to create a national LGBT tobacco action plan. By the end of 2003, a diverse group of national leaders had convened to this end, and in 2004, the first *LGBT Communities Tobacco Action Plan* was published (*The National LGBT Communities Tobacco Action Plan: Research, Prevention, and Cessation*, 2004). Volunteer advocates also created and maintained a community-based listserv to share information on LGBT tobacco control issues nationwide.

A few years earlier, LGBT health researchers and policy advocates working in Washington, DC, would start a chain of actions that would ultimately help stabilize and grow the burgeoning volunteer tobacco advocate network into a stable, funded project. As advocates pushed for new LGBT health projects across the range of Department of Health and Human Services agencies, CDC officials used the early reports of LGBT tobacco disparities to respond by funding an LGBT tobacco network among their portfolio of tobacco disparity networks. The first network award was used for a project focused on LGBT community centers, but by 2006, the monies were switched to directly support the community-driven national LGBT Tobacco Action Plan, and the volunteers coalesced into the National LGBT Tobacco Control Network.

By 2011, the National Tobacco Control Network, renamed the Network for LGBT Health Equity, had made substantial inroads in raising awareness of the LGBT tobacco disparity among national leadership while also racking up substantial policy changes at the local and national level. Federal officials have praised the Network specifically for its long-term roles in the following policy advancements: initiating federal LGBT data collection on the National Health Interview Survey; spotlighting LGBT health in Healthy People 2010; and ensuring LGBT inclusion in the cross-HHS tobacco action plan. In 2013, the mission expanded to include cancer and was rebranded as LGBT HealthLink. It continues to be a resource for states and LGBT community centers looking to expand their LGBT engagement today.

Tobacco Opens Closed Doors

The combination of evidence of a dramatic smoking disparity, coupled with the fact that tobacco use is not an illicit or stigmatized activity, results in interesting opportunities. In 2008, the Network reported that 90 percent of state departments of health were interested in expanding LGBT inclusion in their tobacco control work. For some, this would be their first foray into LGBT community engagement on any issue. To put this broad acceptance into political context, this was the same year that California, Florida, and Arizona were newly joining many other states in enacting legislation specifically discriminating against LGBT people, including bans on same-sex marriage.

TREATMENT

As adeptly pointed out by Fagan et al., the total burden of tobacco impact on a population is not measured by smoking rates alone. Ease of access to treatment options affects both ability to quit and the arc of later tobacco-related health problems (Fagan et al., 2007).

Unfortunately, the resistance to including LGBT measures on large health outcome monitoring systems results in a paucity of evidence of the differential impact of tobacco-related health outcomes, such as cancers or cardiopulmonary disease, on this population.

The LGBT communities have a profound access-to-health-care barrier, which no doubt negatively affects both individual access to tobacco treatment as well as the impact of later tobacco-related illnesses.

LGBT-Tailored Tobacco Cessation Groups

A series of community-based LGBT agencies have offered LGBT-tailored tobacco cessation groups. Local cessation programs have often yielded lessons brought to the larger national arena. Bitch to Quit in Chicago pioneered using provocative messaging and imagery to engage clients. The cessation programs run by the New York LGBT Center pioneered cessation for HIV-positive LGBT people. The Last Drag, run by CLASH in San Francisco, provides a model for long-term sustainability. The lessons from a series of national LGBT cessation groups run by Fenway Health (with local partners) in 2004 through 2006 were distilled into a book: *How to Run a Culturally Competent LGBT Smoking Treatment Group* (Scout, Miele, Bradford, & Perry, 2006).

Most LGBT cessation groups use curricula that are slight modifications of mainstream cessation group curricula, such as those offered by American Lung Association or American Cancer Society. There is not enough research on what level of tailoring is needed in order to optimize a cessation group for LGBT participants. Researchers have noted the need for additional research on what factors create a successful LGBT cessation intervention (Baskerville et al., 2017). What evidence there is shows success with LGBT-tailored cessation groups. A review of the longest-standing group in the United States, The Last Drag, found that nearly 60 percent of participants were smoke free at group end, and 36 percent remained smoke free six months after the intervention (Eliason, Dibble, Gordon, & Soliz, 2012). This is remarkably similar to findings from a review of all Australian LGBT smoking cessation groups, where 61 percent of participants were smoke free at group end, and 38.6 percent stayed smoke free at the three-to-six-month mark. In another study on LGBT cessation groups in Chicago, 32.3 percent of attendees reported being smoke free after treatment (Matthews, Li, Kuhns, Tasker, & Cesario, 2013).

When LGBT young adults were asked what would make a compelling cessation intervention, they identified the following desired components:
It should

1.   be LGBTQ+ specific;

2.   be accessible in terms of location, time, availability, and cost;

3.   be inclusive, relatable, and highlight diversity;

4.   incorporate LGBTQ+ peer support and counseling services;

5.   integrate other activities beyond smoking;

6.   be positive, motivational, uplifting, and empowering;

7.   provide concrete coping mechanisms; and

8.   integrate rewards and incentives (Bruce Baskerville et al., 2018)

In a review of all available literature on LGBT cessation interventions, Lee et al. found that community groups showed promise, but no rigorous evaluation of efficacy existed, clinical interventions showed no difference for LGBT and non-LGBT populations, and focus groups suggest that "care is needed in selecting the messaging used in media campaigns" (Lee, Matthews, McCullen, & Melvin, 2014).

Despite the lessons learned in how to conduct an LGBT cessation group, cessation groups are infrequently funded in recent years; state tobacco control programs are more likely to rely on the quitlines as their primary, if not sole, tobacco treatment option.

Quitlines

Every state is funded by the CDC to conduct certain minimal tobacco control activities. One of the basic activities is to operate a tobacco control quitline. These are hotlines where the general public can call and then be linked with a counselor who can walk them through the implementing the best evidence-based strategies for succeeding at quitting smoking. The use of these evidence-based strategies is important, because smokers on average attempt to quit seven times before succeeding. Using the best strategies reduces the number of quit attempts needed.

In 2005, Blue Cross Blue Shield of Minnesota initiated a program to make its quitlines accessible to LGBT people. This multiyear project yielded valuable tools, including tested LGBT measures for surveys, an LGBT cessation booklet for quitline providers to use, and a curriculum for training quitline staff in LGBT cultural competency. Many states use the same providers for their quitlines, so fewer trainings are needed to provide cultural competence for all quitline staff. The report from the Minnesota project yielded the following basic steps to ensure that a quitline was culturally competent:

- Tailor advertising to the LGBT population

- Ask if respondents are LGBT at intake; use tested measure(s). The project included cognitive testing and recommendation of a measure to use for intake.

- Train all quitlines' counseling staff in LGBT cultural competence. Do not presume that LGBT people feel welcome; the history of health care discrimination precludes this. Focus on building counselor skills in demonstrating this welcome and basic strategies for working with LGBT individuals.

- Offer supplemental materials to LGBT quitline callers. The Network for LGBT Health Equity has a generic version of the brochure created for Minnesota that any quitline can use. These materials should focus on building trust in the quitline and raising awareness about LGBT tobacco disparity, not necessarily advising on specific cessation options (Senseman, Havlicek, Cash, & Scout, 2007).

Data from research in Colorado demonstrates the potential gap in quitline efficacy for LGBT people: LGB smokers who intended to quit were 5.2 times more likely than their heterosexual counterparts to "never intend" to call the state quitline (Burns, Deaton, & Levinson, 2011). This is likely due to provider avoidance as a result of adverse experiences, but it could also be related to awareness; one study found fewer gay, bisexual, and transgender men were aware of the quitline than other men (Fallin, Lee, Bennett, & Goodin, 2016).

In 2014, one of the leading quitlines, the National Jewish QuitLine, conducted its second full staff training on LGBT cultural competency. Over the course of those trainings, information about fielding challenges with the current LGBT measures arose. National Jewish QuitLine partnered with Dr. Scout and the National LGBT Tobacco Control Network to develop and field-test an enhanced LGBT measure. Input from the Quit-Line staff was used to identify rough spots in the current measure; a new measure was developed and then field-tested with over 30,000 people. Further modifications were made as a result of field testing; then, the new measure was presented to the North American Quitline Consortium (NAQC). In 2016, the North American Quitline Consortium introduced this new measure to be part of its recommended data set, asking states to comply by mid-2017. As of early 2017, 39 state quitlines measured some form of LGBT status on intake. It is anticipated that this number will rise with the adoption of the new measure.

Quitline intake is essentially an extremely space-constrained survey. Thus, development of an LGBT measure took a different strategy than for some larger and longer surveillance instruments. When space is extremely constrained, the question the researchers faced was: is there any way to create a single measure that accurately captures both the related dimensions of sexual orientation and gender identity? To address this, a combined, check-all measure was tested. Multiple response questions are basically a series of individual true-false questions stacked together under one heading, so this construct lent itself well to the challenges in capturing two intertwined yet distinct social constructs. The original cognitive testing of the multiple response measure in 2005 was successful. The addition of the extensive field testing makes the enhanced measure one of the most thoroughly tested LGBT surveillance measures currently in use. The measure as used by NAQC is presented here:

"Do you consider yourself to be gay, lesbian, bisexual, and/or transgender?"

- ☐ *Yes [continue to prompt below]*
- ☐ *No [skip to next question]*
- ☐ *Refuse [skip to next question]*

[NOTE to Quitline Counselors: If callers show concern about this question, feel free to add the following sentence: "We ask this to determine whether the quitline is serving this population of tobacco users."]

Prompt: "Thank you, please indicate all of the following which apply to you: a) Bisexual, b) Gay or [for a woman] Lesbian, c) Queer, d) Transgender or gender variant."

[NOTE to Quitline Counselor: Please read all response options].

- ☐ *Bisexual*
- ☐ *Gay or [for a woman] lesbian*
- ☐ *Queer*
- ☐ *Transgender or gender variant*

The example of relative widespread adoption of LGBT data collection by quitlines is one of the pronounced successes in LGBT tobacco control. Still, continued attention needs to be paid to LGBT community members' usage of quitlines, especially considering the increased investment in this strategy to the detriment of community-based cessation groups.

Provider Intervention

A main tenet of effective tobacco cessation is having smoking behavior taken as a vital sign at every medical visit and then routine provider encouragement to quit. LGBT community members who have a choice of medical providers are more likely to seek those who are demonstrably welcoming. This means that LGBT health care professionals may have significant numbers of LGBT community members in their patient base. The Gay and Lesbian Medical Association (GLMA), the national convening body of these providers, has long taken leadership on highlighting the role of tobacco disparities and providing resources for their providers to offer the routine interventions that are so important to overall cessation. In 2009, GLMA offered one of the few online LGBT cultural competency programs certified for continuing education credit, an online training about the impact of and best interventions to reduce LGBT smoking (Scout, 2008).

Evidence of efficacy of LGBT clinical interventions is scarce. Avoidance of care is the first barrier. Evidence shows that LGBT patients have good reason to be concerned about provider bias. In a study of first-year medical students, 81 percent exhibited at least some implicit bias against gay and lesbian individuals (Burke et al., 2015). Beyond avoidance, LGBT people experience additional barriers. Researchers found that one-quarter of their LGBT study participants were uncomfortable talking to their doctors about quitting smoking (Levinson, Hood, Mahajan, & Russ, 2012). Life events such as surgery, smoking-related health problems, or transition can often be used to motivate smokers. A study at Boston Medical Center showed the power of an assertive provider counseling strategy combined with hormone initiation for trans people. Its chart reviews showed that 25 percent of the trans male smokers became smoke free since initiating therapy, and fully 64 percent of the trans women became smoke free. The variance is likely due to the increase in thromboembolic events with estrogen therapy (Myers & Safer, 2017).

Educational Campaigns

In 2015, the FDA funded the largest ever LGBT-focused federal initiative—a multiyear tobacco control educational campaign aimed at young adults. The resultant project is entitled This Free Life. It is aimed at reducing tobacco use among LGBT young adults ages 18 to 24 who are on the continuum between occasional and habituated smokers (www .thisfreelife.betobaccofree.hhs.gov). The campaign relies heavily on presenting "authentic and credible messages" from community members encouraging their peers to live tobacco free. To reach the target population, messages are presented through paid and free advertising in a variety of social media channels: YouTube, Instagram, and Facebook, among others. Twelve markets have been identified as intervention sites, and media purchases focus on those sites. Twelve control sites have been matched to the interventions to facilitate evaluation.

The existence of this historic educational campaign has produced resources unlike any other in the history of LGBT tobacco control. High-quality-production videos, shareables, and print ads are being rolled out on a regular basis. For the first time, there is a drumbeat of LGBT tobacco control messaging aimed squarely at a particularly vulnerable section of the LGBT communities. The messaging is edgy and compelling, using themes about blocking what is toxic, staying free of negativity, and living the best life possible to counter the lure of big tobacco. The breadth of the campaign also allows niche marketing the likes of which is relatively unheard of in LGBT health promotion. This Free Life has ads squarely aimed at the bisexual communities, at genderqueers, at LGBT of color, at recently transitioned trans youth, and more.

This Free Life uses social media and popular culture influencers to help make its messages compelling. YouTube influencers are engaged to make videos for the project, and popular drag queens from the *RuPaul's Drag Race* TV show are staples of the ads. One of the leading videos, "Be Known For Your Flawless," has nearly 800,000 views on YouTube (https://www .youtube.com/watch?v=j8GwWzZChno). Anecdotal evidence shows that the influence of these ads goes well beyond the target population base of young adults.

SMOKEFREE AIR

Advocacy efforts to pass policies ensuring "smokefree air" (SA) have long been a component of a broad tobacco control strategy. Their influence in overall health and cessation has grown over recent years. The 2010 Institute of Medicine report demonstrating the enormous link between smoke-free air policies and reduced heart attacks (average reduction of 17 percent) was unusual for public health (Institute of Medicine, 2010). Probably no other single event has demonstrated such a strong link to reducing a dangerous health outcome and the associated health care costs. The surgeon general's report on how tobacco caused disease later that year continued to raise the influence of this single act when at the launch event the surgeon general concluded: "If you walk by a smoker once, I cannot promise you it will not cause cancer, it's that toxic" (Surgeon General, 2010).

Unfortunately, LGBT community members have not always been included in broad strategic partnerships to pass local smokefree ordinances. As community activists were engaged, alliances would sometimes include strongly antigay groups, making it harder to also include LGBT organizations. Through the civil rights efforts in many states, LGBT community organizations and members have built strong skills in policy change, including relationships that could be invaluable to SA ordinance efforts. Unfortunately, this relative disengagement not only limited the addition of these resources to the overall efforts but also sometimes led to basic cultural competency gaffes—like when a major tobacco control group launched an ad using negative images of transgender people to convey a clean-air message.

A few projects have demonstrated the value of engaging LGBT people in clean-air coalitions. In California, an LGBT project to obtain promises from LGBT-friendly legislators not to accept tobacco funding has obtained over 35 commitments from state legislators ("Elected Officials Taking a Stand Against the Tobacco Industry," 2009). In a very specific SA project in Washington, DC, smokefree advocates used the following strategies to activate the LGBT communities around smokefree air and were praised as being key in the ultimate passage of the local legislation (Hitchcock, 2005):

- Obtain LGBT organization endorsement of smokefree air policies;
- Identify LGBT-friendly legislators, educate them directly about the benefits of smokefree air to LGBT communities; and
- Directly counter pro-tobacco messaging in LGBT media and expose if it was funded by the tobacco industry.

Two studies show that LGBT smokers may be particularly impacted by secondhand smoke. In one study, different minority populations were found to be exposed to higher levels of secondhand smoke in their houses than nonminorities (Max, Stark, Sung, & Offen, 2016). In a Missouri study, researchers found a stronger correlation between former LGBT smokers and smokefree-air policies, leading them to conclude that "the SGM [sexual and gender minority] community may collectively accrue greater public health benefits from the adoption of smoke-free policies than the non-SGM community." (Wintemberg, McElroy, Ge, & Everett, 2017)

TRENDS IN MAINSTREAM TOBACCO CONTROL

Mainstream tobacco control programs have undergone a tremendous shift in focus over the last few years. Analysis of evidence has demonstrated irrevocably that individual interventions, such as cessation, are not the most cost-effective path to reducing the smoking rates. The most cost-effective strategies are environmental policy changes. The highest-impact examples of these are smokefree air laws, discussed previously, and increases in tobacco excise taxes. Data show that every 10 percent increase in cigarette prices results in a 4 percent drop in consumption (U.S. Department of Health and Human Services, 2012). Longer-term comprehensive policy initiatives have been shown to be highly cost-effective, returning up to four dollars in savings for every single dollar invested.

Thus, the arena is newly shifting to prioritize broad environmental policy changes over individual interventions such as cessation.

Again, the LGBT communities have a strong base of policy change skills, largely from civil rights battles. Retooling these to advance health is very possible. Several local LGBT tobacco control programs have been building strategies to engage community advocates in the new policy environmental tobacco arena. A project run by The Health Initiative in Atlanta, Georgia (http://thehealthinitiative.org/) is one example of a 12-month project that staged LGBT leaders to engage in tobacco policy. Basic steps used in this project were as follows:

- Fund a community-based organization;
- Assess community tobacco impact through survey;
- Use focus groups to understand facilitators and barriers to policy engagement;
- Use community leaders to engage additional leaders;
- Use community-based priority-setting events to educate and engage leadership, then cull its top priorities for next steps of policy engagement; and
- Distill all evidence into an action plan for tobacco policy engagement.

BEST PRACTICES

Best practices have been collected from LGBT tobacco control work at many levels. At the national level, there are lessons gleaned on the importance and best methods for including LGBT people in data collection. There are also best practices developed for inclusion of LGBT people in funding announcements and strong statements about the importance of such work.

Starting in 2007, the different iterations of the national LGBT tobacco control network have been promulgating best practices for state tobacco control programs. A summary of their current best practices is presented here:

1. Promote LGBT professional safety and leadership in public health;
2. Include LGBT community members in policy-planning steps;

3. Monitor impact of tobacco on LGBT populations;

4. Establish cultural competency standards for statewide programs;

5. Fund community-based programs to help reduce LGBT tobacco disparities;

6. Routinely integrate LGBT tailored efforts into larger wellness/tobacco campaigns; and

7. Disseminate findings and lessons learned.

Over 2011 and 2012, the national LGBT tobacco control network convened a body of experts to solicit evidence to create a national best practices guide for the arena. Many community-based programs lacked rigorous evaluation, which hampered their promulgation across the field. Using a model from the Substance Abuse Mental Health Services Administration, the network used a twin test of theoretical basis and expert review to determine a wide range of promising practices for the field. The final document was based upon the World Health Organization's framework of tobacco control—MPOWER (monitor, prevent, offer cessation, warn, enforce, raise taxes). *MPOWERED: Best and Promising Practices for Tobacco Control and Prevention* can be accessed online at http://www .lgbthealthlink.org/Assets/U/documents/mpowered.pdf.

There have been several robust examples of states using these best practices to move into greater level of LGBT engagement. Due to the relative challenge in identifying accurate state-level data, doing a community-based needs assessment is often one of the first steps to determine local strategy. Missouri, Arkansas, Michigan, and Pennsylvania are all examples of states that have launched community-based, tobacco-focused needs assessments.

Michigan worked with the National LGBT Tobacco and Control Network and the local community-based LGBT centers to adopt a standardized needs assessment instrument and collect data statewide. This approach allows for information to be collected on factors that would not be included in surveillance instruments, such as how often people avoid providers due to fears about lack of acceptance. They used the data collected from this series of surveys to establish the need for and to fund community centers to do educational work in the LGBT population. Idaho leveraged the best practices into a series of LGBT engagement strategies over several years, including ads, blogs, and tailor-made videos highlighting LGBT people who had successfully stopped smoking. The most recent state to enthusiastically pursue LGBT best practices has been Pennsylvania. After launching two regional needs assessments spearheaded by Bradbury-Sullivan LGBT Community Center, they were able to expand the data collection to cover most of the state. Resultant data were persuasive; funders were able to use this basis to launch a statewide educational norming campaign for LGBT tobacco control. The linked community centers across the state work in conjunction with each other to change the social acceptance of smoking in the LGBT communities and build community faith in the state quitline.

CONCLUSION

The LGBT communities experience a profound tobacco disparity. Too many lives are being lost to tobacco use. Too few LGBT community members realize that this disparity exists. Too few funders routinely include LGBT communities in their broad tobacco control plans. Too few measures of LGBT status are added to health-monitoring surveys. Nonetheless, the organization and wherewithal of the community response to this disparity has yielded notable lessons in LGBT health. Community leaders and allies have used ingenuity to address a variety of challenges. Just as HIV programs yielded valuable lessons about health, tobacco control programs are also yielding valuable public health insights—insights that will likely help move other health issues forward over time.

REFERENCES

Agaku, I. T., King, B. A., Husten, C. G., Bunnell, R., Ambrose, B. K., Hu, S. S., . . . Prevention. (2014). Tobacco product use among adults—United States, 2012–2013. *Morbidity and Mortality Weekly Report, 63*(25), 542–547.

Akhtar-Khaleel, W. Z., Cook, R. L., Shoptaw, S., Surkan, P., Stall, R., Beyth, R. J., . . . Plankey, M. (2016). Trends and predictors of cigarette smoking among HIV seropositive and seronegative men: The Multicenter Aids Cohort Study. *AIDS and Behavior, 20*(3), 622–632. doi:10.1007/s10461-015-1099-6

Akhtar-Khaleel, W. Z., Cook, R. L., Shoptaw, S., Surkan, P. J., Teplin, L. A., Stall, R., . . . Plankey, M. (2016). Long-term cigarette smoking trajectories among HIV-seropositive and seronegative MSM in the Multicenter AIDS Cohort Study. *AIDS and Behavior, 20*(8), 1713–1721. doi:10.1007/s10461-016-1343-8

American Spirit. (2005). Freedom to inhale. It's all good. Retrieved from https://trinketsandtrash.org/detail.php?artifactid=4610&page=1

Austin, A., Herrick, H., & Proescholdbell, S. (2016). Adverse childhood experiences related to poor adult health among lesbian, gay, and bisexual individuals. *American Journal of Public Health, 106*(2), 314–320. doi:10.2105/AJPH.2015.302904

Austin, S. B., Ziyadeh, N., Fisher, L. B., Kahn, J. A., Colditz, G. A., & Frazier, A. L. (2004). Sexual orientation and tobacco use in a cohort study of US adolescent girls and boys. *Archives of Pediatrics and Adolescent Medicine, 158*(4), 317–322.

Baskerville, N. B., Dash, D., Shuh, A., Wong, K., Abramowicz, A., Yessis, J., & Kennedy, R. D. (2017). Tobacco use cessation interventions for lesbian, gay, bisexual, transgender and queer youth and young adults: A scoping review. *Preventive Medicine Reports, 6,* 53–62. doi:10.1016/j.pmedr.2017.02.004

Blosnich, J., Lee, J. G., & Horn, K. (2013). A systematic review of the aetiology of tobacco disparities for sexual minorities. *Tobacco Control, 22*(2), 66–73. doi:10.1136/tobaccocontrol-2011-050181

Blosnich, J. R., Gordon, A. J., & Fine, M. J. (2015). Associations of sexual and gender minority status with health indicators, health risk factors, and social stressors in a national sample of young adults with military experience. *Annals of Epidemiology, 25*(9), 661–667. doi:10.1016/j.annepidem.2015.06.001

Blosnich, J. R., & Horn, K. (2011). Associations of discrimination and violence with smoking among emerging adults: Differences by gender and sexual orientation. *Nicotine & Tobacco Research, 13*(12), 1284–1295. doi:10.1093/ntr/ntr183

Blosnich, J. R., Jarrett, T., & Horn, K. (2011). Racial and ethnic differences in current use of cigarettes, cigars, and hookahs among lesbian, gay, and bisexual young adults. *Nicotine & Tobacco Research, 13*(6), 487–491. doi:10.1093/ntr/ntq261

Bruce Baskerville, N., Wong, K., Shuh, A., Abramowicz, A., Dash, D., Esmail, A., & Kennedy, R. (2018). A qualitative study of tobacco interventions for LGBTQ+ youth and young adults: Overarching themes and key learnings. *BMC Public Health, 18*(1), 155. doi:10.1186/s12889-018-5050-4

Buchting, F. O., Emory, K. T., Scout, K. Y., Fagan, P., Vera, L. E., & Emery, S. (2017). Transgender use of cigarettes, cigars, and e-cigarettes in a national study. *American Journal of Preventive Medicine, 53*(1), e1–e7. doi:10.1016/j.amepre.2016.11.022

Buchting, F. S., & Fagan, P. (2008). LGBT of color sampling methodology: Strategies for collecting data in small, hidden, or hard-to-reach groups to reduce tobacco-related health disparities. Retrieved from https://williamsinstitute.law.ucla.edu/wp-content/uploads/LGBTReport-Dec-2008.pdf

Burke, S. E., Dovidio, J. F., Przedworski, J. M., Hardeman, R. R., Perry, S. P., Phelan, S. M., . . . van Ryn, M. (2015). Do contact and empathy mitigate bias against gay and lesbian people among heterosexual first-year medical students? A report from the medical student CHANGE Study. *Academic Medicine, 90*(5), 645–651. doi:10.1097/acm.0000000000000661

Burns, E. K., Deaton, E. A., & Levinson, A. H. (2011). Rates and reasons: Disparities in low intentions to use a state smoking cessation quitline. *American Journal of Health Promotion, 25*(5 Suppl), S59–S65. doi:10.4278/ajhp.100611-QUAN-183

Bye, L., Gruskin, E., Greenwood, G., Albright, V., & Krotski, K. (2004). California lesbians, gays, bisexuals, transgenders tobacco use survey 2004. Retrieved from http://www.dhs.ca.gov/ps/cdic/tcs/documents/eval/LGBTTobacco Study.pdf

Cabrera-Nguyen, E. P., Cavazos-Rehg, P., Krauss, M., Kim, Y., & Emery, S. (2016). Awareness and use of dissolvable tobacco products in the United States. *Nicotine & Tobacco Research, 18*(5), 857–863. doi:10.1093/ntr/ntv212

CDC Winnable Battles. (2011). Retrieved from http://www.cdc.gov/winnable battles/

Coulter, R. W. S., Bersamin, M., Russell, S. T., & Mair, C. (2017). The effects of gender- and sexuality-based harassment on lesbian, gay, bisexual, and transgender substance use disparities. *Journal of Adolescent Health, 62*(6), 688–700. doi:10.1016/j.jadohealth.2017.10.004

Dai, H. (2017). Tobacco product use among lesbian, gay, and bisexual adolescents. *Pediatrics, 139*(4). doi:10.1542/peds.2016-3276

D'Avanzo, P. A., Halkitis, P. N., Yu, K., & Kapadia, F. (2016). Demographic, mental health, behavioral, and psychosocial factors associated with cigarette smoking status among young men who have sex with men: The P18 Cohort Study. *LGBT Health, 3*(5), 379–386. doi:10.1089/lgbt.2015.0128

Dermody, S. S., Marshal, M. P., Cheong, J., Chung, T., Stepp, S., & Hipwell, A. (2016). Adolescent sexual minority girls are at elevated risk for use of multiple substances. *Substance Use & Misuse, 51*(5), 574–585. doi:10.3109/108 26084.2015.1126743

Drope, J., Liber, A. C., Cahn, Z., Stoklosa, M., Kennedy, R., Douglas, C. E., . . . Drope, J. (2018). Who's still smoking? Disparities in adult cigarette smoking prevalence in the United States. *CA: A Cancer Journal for Clinicians, 68*, 106–115. doi:10.3322/caac.21444

Easton, A., & Sell, R. (2004). *Analysis of national longitudinal study of adolescent health*. Palm Springs, CA: Gay and Lesbian Medical Association.

Elected Officials Taking a Stand Against the Tobacco Industry. (2009). Retrieved from http://www.lgbtpartnership.org/officials.html

Eliason, M. J., Dibble, S. L., Gordon, R., & Soliz, G. B. (2012). The last drag: An evaluation of an LGBT-specific smoking intervention. *Journal of Homosexuality, 59*(6), 864–878. doi:10.1080/00918369.2012.694770

Emory, K., Kim, Y., Buchting, F., Vera, L., Huang, J., & Emery, S. L. (2016). Intragroup variance in lesbian, gay, and bisexual tobacco use behaviors: Evidence that subgroups matter, notably bisexual women. *Nicotine & Tobacco Research, 18*(6), 1494–1501. doi:10.1093/ntr/ntv208

Fagan, P., Moolchan, E. T., Lawrence, D., Fernander, A., & Ponder, P. K. (2007). Identifying health disparities across the tobacco continuum. *Addiction, 102* (Suppl 2), 5–29.

Fallin, A., Goodin, A., Lee, Y. O., & Bennett, K. (2015). Smoking characteristics among lesbian, gay, and bisexual adults. *Preventive Medicine, 74*, 123–130. doi:10.1016/j.ypmed.2014.11.026

Fallin, A., Goodin, A. J., & King, B. A. (2015). Menthol cigarette smoking among lesbian, gay, bisexual, and transgender adults. *American Journal of Preventive Medicine, 48*(1), 93–97. doi:10.1016/j.amepre.2014.07.044

Fallin, A., Lee, Y. O., Bennett, K., & Goodin, A. (2016). Smoking cessation awareness and utilization among lesbian, gay, bisexual, and transgender adults: An analysis of the 2009–2010 National Adult Tobacco Survey. *Nicotine & Tobacco Research, 18*(4), 496–500. doi:10.1093/ntr/ntv103

FDA (Producer). (2016, February 27, 2018). FDA takes action against four tobacco manufacturers for illegal sales of flavored cigarettes labeled as little cigars or cigars. [News release] Retrieved from https://www.fda.gov/NewsEvents /Newsroom/PressAnnouncements/ucm532563.htm

Gamarel, K. E., Brown, L., Kahler, C. W., Fernandez, M. I., Bruce, D., Nichols, S., & Adolescent Medicine Trials Network for, H. I. V. A. I. (2016). Prevalence and correlates of substance use among youth living with HIV in clinical settings. *Drug and Alcohol Dependence, 169*, 11–18. doi:10.1016/j.drug alcdep.2016.10.002

Gamarel, K. E., Mereish, E. H., Manning, D., Iwamoto, M., Operario, D., & Nemoto, T. (2016). Minority stress, smoking patterns, and cessation attempts: Findings from a community sample of transgender women in the San Francisco Bay Area. *Nicotine & Tobacco Research, 18*(3), 306–313. doi:10.1093/ntr/ntv066

Gonzales, G., Przedworski, J., & Henning-Smith, C. (2016). Comparison of health and health risk factors between lesbian, gay, and bisexual adults and heterosexual adults in the United States: Results from the National Health Interview Survey. *JAMA Internal Medicine, 176*(9), 1344–1351. doi:10.1001/jamainternmed.2016.3432

Grant, J., Mottet, L., & Tanis, J. (2010). National Transgender Discrimination Survey Report on health and health care. Retrieved from http://transequality.org/PDFs/NTDSReportonHealth_final.pdf

Greenwood, G. L., & Gruskin, E. P. (2007). LGBT tobacco and alcohol disparities. In I. H. Meyer & M. E. Northridge (Eds.), *The health of sexual minorities: Public health perspectives on lesbian, gay, bisexual and transgender populations* (pp. 566–583). New York: Springer.

Gruskin, E. P., Greenwood, G. L., Matevia, M., Pollack, L. M., & Bye, L. L. (2007). Disparities in smoking between the lesbian, gay, and bisexual population and the general population in California. *American Journal of Public Health, 97*(8), 1496–1502.

Hatzenbuehler, M. L., Pachankis, J. E., & Wolff, J. (2012). Religious climate and health risk behaviors in sexual minority youths: A population-based study. *American Journal of Public Health, 102*(4), 657–663. doi:10.2105/AJPH.2011.300517

Hatzenbuehler, M. L., Wieringa, N. F., & Keyes, K. M. (2011). Community-level determinants of tobacco use disparities in lesbian, gay, and bisexual youth: results from a population-based study. *Archives of Pediatrics & Adolescent Medicine, 165*(6), 527–532. doi:10.1001/archpediatrics.2011.64

Hitchcock, D. (2005). *LGBT clean air project.* Paper presented at the National Conference on Tobacco or Health, Chicago.

Huang, J., Kim, Y., Vera, L., & Emery, S. L. (2016). Electronic cigarettes among priority populations: Role of smoking cessation and tobacco control policies. *American Journal of Preventive Medicine, 50*(2), 199–209. doi:10.1016/j.amepre.2015.06.032

Institute of Medicine. (2010). *Secondhand smoke exposure and cardiovascular effects: Making sense of the evidence.* Washington, DC: National Academies Press.

Jamal, A., King, B. A., Neff, L. J., Whitmill, J., Babb, S. D., & Graffunder, C. M. (2016). Current cigarette smoking among adults—United States, 2005–2015. *Morbidity and Mortality Weekly Report, 65*(44), 1205–1211. doi:10.15585/mmwr.mm6544a2

Jamal, A., Phillips, E., Gentzke, A. S., Homa, D. M., Babb, S. D., King, B. A., & Neff, L. J. (2018). Current cigarette smoking among adults—United States, 2016. *Morbidity and Mortality Weekly Report, 67*(2), 53–59. doi:10.15585/mmwr.mm6702a1

James, S. E., Herman, J. L., Rankin, S., Keisling, M., Mottet, L., & Anafi, M. (2016). *A Report of the 2015 U.S. Transgender Survey.* Washington, DC: National Center for Transgender Equality.

Jannat-Khah, D. P., Dill, L. J., Reynolds, S. A., & Joseph, M. A. (2018). Stress, socializing, and other motivations for smoking among the lesbian, gay, bisexual, transgender, and queer community in New York City. *American Journal of Health Promotion, 32*(5), 1178–1186. doi:10.1177/0890117117694449

Jha, P., Ramasundarahettige, C., Landsman, V., Rostron, B., Thun, M., Anderson, R. N., . . . Peto, R. (2013). 21st-century hazards of smoking and benefits of cessation in the United States. *New England Journal of Medicine, 368*(4), 341–350. doi:10.1056/NEJMsa1211128

Johnson, S. E., Holder-Hayes, E., Tessman, G. K., King, B. A., Alexander, T., & Zhao, X. (2016). Tobacco product use among sexual minority adults: Findings from the 2012–2013 National Adult Tobacco Survey. *American Journal of Preventive Medicine, 50*(4), e91–e100. doi:10.1016/j.amepre.2015.07.041

Johnson-Jennings, M. D., Belcourt, A., Town, M., Walls, M. L., & Walters, K. L. (2014). Racial discrimination's influence on smoking rates among American Indian Alaska Native two-spirit individuals: Does pain play a role? *Journal of Health Care for the Poor and Underserved, 25*(4), 1667–1678. doi:10.1353/hpu.2014.0193

Jones, W. J., & Silvestri, G. A. (2010). The Master Settlement Agreement and its impact on tobacco use 10 years later: Lessons for physicians about health policy making. *Chest, 137*(3), 692–700. doi:10.1378/chest.09-0982

King, B. A., Dube, S. R., & Tynan, M. A. (2012). Current tobacco use among adults in the United States: Findings from the National Adult Tobacco Survey. *American Journal of Public Health, 102*(11), e93–e100. doi:10.2105/AJPH.2012.301002

King, B. A., Dube, S. R., & Tynan, M. A. (2013). Flavored cigar smoking among U.S. adults: Findings from the 2009–2010 National Adult Tobacco Survey. *Nicotine & Tobacco Research, 15*(2), 608–614. doi:10.1093/ntr/nts178

Kuyper, L., de Roos, S., Iedema, J., & Stevens, G. (2016). Growing up with the right to marry: Sexual attraction, substance use, and well-being of Dutch adolescents. *Journal of Adolescesnt Health, 59*(3), 276–282. doi:10.1016/j.jadohealth.2016.05.010

Lee, J. G. (2014). Keeping the community posted: Lesbian, gay, bisexual, and transgender blogs and the tobacco epidemic. *LGBT Health, 1*(2), 113–121. doi:10.1089/lgbt.2013.0012

Lee, J. G., Agnew-Brune, C. B., Clapp, J. A., & Blosnich, J. R. (2014). Out smoking on the big screen: Tobacco use in LGBT movies, 2000–2011. *Tobacco Control, 23*(e2), e156–e158. doi:10.1136/tobaccocontrol-2013-051288

Lee, J. G., Griffin, G. K., & Melvin, C. L. (2009). Tobacco use among sexual minorities in the USA, 1987 to May 2007: A systematic review. *Tobacco Control, 18*(4), 275–282.

Lee, J. G., Matthews, A. K., McCullen, C. A., & Melvin, C. L. (2014). Promotion of tobacco use cessation for lesbian, gay, bisexual, and transgender people: A systematic review. *American Journal of Preventive Medicine, 47*(6), 823–831. doi:10.1016/j.amepre.2014.07.051

Levinson, A. H., Hood, N., Mahajan, R., & Russ, R. (2012). Smoking cessation treatment preferences, intentions, and behaviors among a large sample of colorado gay, lesbian, bisexual, and transgendered smokers. *Nicotine & Tobacco Research, 14*(8), 910–918. doi:10.1093/ntr/ntr303

LGBT Tobacco Discussion. *Discussion Digest, 51*(13) (2011, January 5).

Lucky Strike. (2001). Whenever someone yells, "Dude, that's so gay," we'll be there. Retrieved from https://trinketsandtrash.org/detail.php?artifactid=4900&page=4

Martinez, O., Lee, J. H., Bandiera, F., Santamaria, E. K., Levine, E. C., & Operario, D. (2017). Sexual and behavioral health disparities among sexual minority Hispanics/Latinos: Findings from the National Health and Nutrition Examination Survey, 2001–2014. *American Journal of Preventive Medicine, 53*(2), 225–231. doi:10.1016/j.amepre.2017.01.037

Matthews, A. K., Balsam, K., Hotton, A., Kuhns, L., Li, C. C., & Bowen, D. J. (2014). Awareness of media-based antitobacco messages among a community sample of LGBT individuals. *Health Promotion Practice, 15*(6), 857–866. doi:10.1177/1524839914533343

Matthews, A. K., Li, C. C., Kuhns, L. M., Tasker, T. B., & Cesario, J. A. (2013). Results from a community-based smoking cessation treatment program for LGBT smokers. *Journal of Environmental and Public Health, 2013*, 984508. doi:10.1155/2013/984508

Max, W. B., Stark, B., Sung, H. Y., & Offen, N. (2016). Sexual identity disparities in smoking and secondhand smoke exposure in California: 2003–2013. *American Journal of Public Health, 106*(6), 1136–1142. doi:10.2105/AJPH.2016.303071

McCabe, S. E., Hughes, T. L., Matthews, A. K., Lee, J. G. L., West, B. T., Boyd, C. J., & Arslanian-Engoren, C. (2017). Sexual orientation discrimination and tobacco use disparities in the United States. *Nicotine & Tobacco Research*. doi:10.1093/ntr/ntx283

Mixner, D. (1998). Report—Update of progress. Bates No. 2065450170. Retrieved from http://legacy.library.ucsf.edu/tid/vuf73c00

Myers, S. C., & Safer, J. D. (2017). Increased rates of smoking cessation observed among transgender women receiving hormone treatment. *Endocrine Practice, 23*(1), 32–36. doi:10.4158/EP161438.OR

The National LGBT Communities Tobacco Action Plan: Research, prevention, and cessation. (2004). Retrieved from https://www.lgbttobacco.org/files/2004%20LGBT-TobaccoActionPlan.pdf

Newport Cigarettes. (2016). Newport pleasure! Retrieved from https://trinketsandtrash.org/detail.php?artifactid=11175&page=9

Offen, N., Smith, E. A., & Malone, R. E. (2008). Is tobacco a gay issue? Interviews with leaders of the lesbian, gay, bisexual and transgender community. *Culture, Health, & Sexuality, 10*(2), 143–157.

Ortiz, K., Mamkherzi, J., Salloum, R., Matthews, A. K., & Maziak, W. (2017). Waterpipe tobacco smoking among sexual minorities in the United States: Evidence from the National Adult Tobacco Survey (2012–2014). *Addictive Behaviors, 74*, 98–105. doi:10.1016/j.addbeh.2017.06.001

Phillip Morris USA. (1997). CEM's gay and lesbian marketing efforts. Bates No. 2071145104. Retrieved from http://legacy.library.ucsf.edu/tid/dup28d00

Reisner, S. L., Gamarel, K. E., Dunham, E., Hopwood, R., & Hwahng, S. (2013). Female-to-male transmasculine adult health: A mixed-methods community -based needs assessment. *Journal of the American Psychiatric Nurses Association, 19*(5), 293–303. doi:10.1177/1078390313500693

Remafedi, G. (2007). Lesbian, gay, bisexual, and transgender youths: Who smokes, and why? *Nicotine & Tobacco Research, 9*(Suppl 1), S65–S71.

RJ Reynolds. (1995). Project SCUM. Retrieved from http://legacy.library.ucsf.edu/tid/mum76d00

Rosario, M., Schrimshaw, E. W., & Hunter, J. (2009). Disclosure of sexual orientation and subsequent substance use and abuse among lesbian, gay, and bisexual youths: Critical role of disclosure reactions. *Psychology of Addictive Behaviors, 23*(1), 175–184.

Rosario, M., Schrimshaw, E. W., & Hunter, J. (2010). Cigarette smoking as a coping strategy: Negative implications for subsequent psychological distress among lesbian, gay, and bisexual youths. *Journal of Pediatric Psychology, 36*(7), 731–742.doi:10.1093/jpepsy/jsp141 [doi]

Schauer, G. L., Berg, C. J., & Bryant, L. O. (2013). Sex differences in psychosocial correlates of concurrent substance use among heterosexual, homosexual and bisexual college students. *The American Journal of Drug and Alcohol Abuse, 39*(4), 252–258. doi:10.3109/00952990.2013.796962

Scout, M. A. (2008). GLMA plenary Powerpoint presentation. Retrieved from https://www.lgbttobacco.org/files/2008%2010%2024%20-%20GLMA%20 Plenary%2002.ppt

Scout, M. A., Bradford, J., & Perry, D. (2006). Running an LGBT smoking treatment group. Retrieved from http://www.lgbttobacco.org/files/Bible.pdf

Senseman, S., Havlicek, D., Cash, J., & Scout. (2007). *Identifying, reaching and delivering culturally-appropriate telephonic cessation to the GLBT community.* Paper presented at the National Conference on Tobacco or Health, Kansas City, MO. Retrieved from https://www.lgbttobacco.org/files/How%20to%20 reach%20the%20LGBT%20community%20through%20Quitlines.pdf

Shires, D. A., & Jaffee, K. D. (2016). Structural discrimination is associated with smoking status among a national sample of transgender individuals. *Nicotine & Tobacco Research, 18*(6), 1502–1508. doi:10.1093/ntr/ntv221

Smith, E. A., & Malone, R. E. (2003). The outing of Philip Morris: Advertising tobacco to gay men. *American Journal of Public Health, 93*(6), 988–993.

Smith, E. A., Offen, N., & Malone, R. E. (2005). What makes an ad a cigarette ad? Commercial tobacco imagery in the lesbian, gay, and bisexual press. *Journal of Epidemiology and Community Health, 59*(12), 1086–1091.

Smith, E. A., Offen, N., & Malone, R. E. (2006). Pictures worth a thousand words: Noncommercial tobacco content in the lesbian, gay, and bisexual press. *Journal of Health Communication, 11*(7), 635–649.

Smith, E. A., Thomson, K., Offen, N., & Malone, R. E. (2008). "If you know you exist, it's just marketing poison": Meanings of tobacco industry targeting in the lesbian, gay, bisexual, and transgender community. *American Journal of Public Health, 98*(6), 996–1003.

Stall, R. D., Greenwood, G. L., Acree, M., Paul, J., & Coates, T. J. (1999). Cigarette smoking among gay and bisexual men. *American Journal of Public Health, 89*(12), 1875–1878.

Stotzer, R. L., Ka'opua, L. S., & Diaz, T. P. (2014). Is healthcare caring in Hawai'i? Preliminary results from a health assessment of lesbian, gay, bisexual, transgender, questioning, and intersex people in four counties. *Hawaii Journal of Medicine & Public Health, 73*(6), 175–180.

Surgeon General. (2010). *How tobacco smoke causes disease: The biology and behavioral basis for smoking-attributable disease.* Atlanta, GA: Centers for Disease Control and Prevention.

U.S. Department of Health and Human Services. (2012). *Preventing tobacco use among youth and young adults: A report of the surgeon general.* Retrieved from   https://www.surgeongeneral.gov/library/reports/preventing-youth -tobacco-use/index.html

Warren, G. W., Alberg, A. J., Kraft, A. S., & Cummings, K. M. (2014). The 2014 surgeon general's report: "The health consequences of smoking—50 years of progress": A paradigm shift in cancer care. *Cancer, 120*(13), 1914–1916. doi:10.1002/cncr.28695

Watson, R. J., Lewis, N. M., Fish, J. N., & Goodenow, C. (2018). Sexual minority youth continue to smoke cigarettes earlier and more often than heterosexuals: Findings from population-based data. *Drug and Alcohol Dependence, 184,* 64–70. doi:10.1016/j.drugalcdep.2017.11.025

Wintemberg, J., McElroy, J. A., Ge, B., & Everett, K. D. (2017). Can smoke-free policies reduce tobacco use disparities of sexual and gender minorities in Missouri? *Nicotine & Tobacco Research, 19*(11), 1308–1314. doi:10.1093/ntr/ntx078

World Health Organization. (2011). *Research for international tobacco control. WHO report on the global tobacco epidemic.* Geneva, Switzerland: World Health Organization.

Worthington, L. (2011). Letters to the editor. *Lavender Magazine*(April 7–20), 10–11.

Xu, X., Bishop, E. E., Kennedy, S. M., Simpson, S. A., & Pechacek, T. F. (2015). Annual healthcare spending attributable to cigarette smoking: An update. *American Journal of Preventive Medicine, 48*(3), 326–333. doi:10.1016/j .amepre.2014.10.012

Yerger, V. B., Daniel, M. R., & Malone, R. E. (2005). Taking it to the streets: Responses of African American young adults to internal tobacco industry documents. *Nicotine & Tobacco Research, 7*(1), 163–172.

Ylioja, T., Cochran, G., Woodford, M. R., & Renn, K. A. (2018). Frequent experience of LGBQ microaggression on campus associated with smoking among sexual minority college students. *Nicotine & Tobacco Research, 20*(3), 340–346. doi:10.1093/ntr/ntw305

Youatt, E. J., Johns, M. M., Pingel, E. S., Soler, J. H., & Bauermeister, J. A. (2015). Exploring young adult sexual minority women's perspectives on LGBTQ smoking. *Journal of LGBT Youth, 12*(3), 323–342. doi:10.1080/19361653.2015.1022242

8

Intimate Partner Violence in LGBTQ Relationships

Cathy E. Welch

> We all need to keep imagining new community, legal, and social service responses so that we can continue to work toward stopping all forms of violence and abuse, in part by learning how not to force diversely situated people into limited forms of heterosexist gender and sexual identities. (Ristock, 2002)

Most lesbian, gay, bisexual, transgender, and queer (LGBTQ) relationships are nonviolent, respectful, and loving; however, intimate partner violence is part of the fabric of some LGBTQ relationships and is considered an important health issue. Addressing the violence in same-gender relationships has not been easy, and resistance to recognizing relationship violence in LGBTQ communities continues to thrive. This reluctance is perhaps a powerful statement of the extent that homophobia/heterosexism and transphobia continue to operate in our society and the fear of backlash and stigma that persists in our communities.

Violence in relationships is a social phenomenon that is played out in the dynamics between individuals. We cannot talk about violence in LGBTQ relationships without first examining the social forces that contribute to and support relationship violence. LGBTQ intimate partner violence cannot be viewed as distinct from other oppressions, including but not limited to racism, classism, ableism (discrimination based on physical ability), sexism, homophobia/heterosexism, biphobia, and transphobia. A full understanding of intimate partner violence in the lives of LGBTQ people requires that we adopt a view of violence in same-sex/gender relationships as unique, with its own contexts and dynamics distinct and separate from violence in heterosexual relationships (Ristock, 2005). That is, to understand intimate partner violence in the lives of LGBTQ people, we need to move beyond the constrictions of a heteronormative view of violence in relationships that operates within a static model of power and control and a victim/perpetrator paradigm, and allow the complexities of LGBTQ experiences to be heard. As well, it is important to work within a framework of intersectionality (Crenshaw, 1994) where multiple systems of oppression intersect to give meaning to and create vulnerabilities to violence (Hiebert-Murphy et. al., 2011).

Violence in relationships is complex. Attempts to find one model to account for the wide range of experiences and to develop a broader understanding of violence can run the risk of simplifying and homogenizing individual experiences. There are many inherent problems in assuming that violence in relationships is the same for all LGBTQ people. As well, considering all violence to be the same in its context, intent, and impact is fraught with multiple problems. There is no one LGBTQ community; rather, lesbians, gays, bisexuals, trans, and queer communities are diverse yet share a common identity based on our shared experiences of being marginalized based on our gender and sexuality. This makes it difficult to develop a common understanding of intimate partner violence in the lives of LGBTQ, because the experiences of lesbians are different from those of gay men or bisexuals, and trans folks do not often identify as being lesbian or gay and thus do not necessarily consider themselves as being in same-sex relationships (Durish, 2007). The majority of the studies of violence in same-sex/gender relationships have looked at the experiences of women in lesbian relationships. To a lesser extent, the experiences of gay men have been explored. Very few studies have considered bisexual men and women and trans men and women in same-sex or opposite-sex partnerships. In this chapter, I attempt to discuss the commonalities of our experience and to go beyond that to highlight and speak to the diversity and complexities of intimate partner violence in the lives of LGBTQ people.

TROUBLING LANGUAGE

Understanding and acknowledging violence in queer relationships is hampered by language and the perception that many of the terms that are used to refer to violence in intimate relationships do not reflect the experiences of LGBTQ people. A variety of diverse and varied language has been used to refer to violence in LGBTQ relationships, with no one consistent language that fully reflects the experience of LGBTQ people. Many terms that are used to describe relationship violence are seen by many LGBTQ people to be more representative of a heterosexual experience of violence. For instance, the term "domestic violence" is commonly used and, while this is done in an attempt to be more inclusive and less specific to heterosexual women's experience of violence, it is interpreted by some LGBTQ groups to refer to the gender-based power imbalance found in predominately relationships between white heterosexuals (Chung & Lee, 1999) and to situate the violence in the private sphere of the "home" (Holmes, 2009). Even the more recently used term "intimate partner violence" (IPV), which also attempts to be gender neutral and more inclusive of LGBTQ experiences of violence, for some, it continues to reflect and embody a heterosexual perspective of violence in relationships. Janice Ristock (2011, pp. 4–5) aptly articulates this dilemma in the following statement: "Considering how best to frame and conceptualize intimate partner violence then requires us to think critically about the assumptions embedded in our language and requires us to be more aware of the limitations of what we are able to see and know as a result of our framings."

As well lumping lesbians, gay men, bisexuals, trans, and queer-identified people in to one category, "LGBTQ" also has its dangers in that it can lull us into thinking that violence in all gender-variant and sexual minority lives is the same and misleads us into believing that one response and one service model fits all.

In this chapter, I use the language of intimate partner violence and violence in same-sex/gender relationships but remain fully cognizant of the troubling nature of the terms and the ways that language can minimize, discount, and even obliterate individual experiences (or even the experiences of whole segments of the population).

PREVALENCE AND SILENCE

The prevalence of violence in same-gender relationships has been difficult to determine because of the inability to collect information from a purely random sample, as well as difficulties in determining if the violence reported was solely in the context of LGBTQ relationships (Davis & Glass, 2011). Conducting a truly independent study to determine the overall incidence of violence in LGBTQ relationships is fraught with many obstacles. Often, research has relied on self-disclosure of participants, and many studies have targeted participants in counseling or support services, where the incidence of experiences of violence in relationships might be expected to be higher than that in the general population. Studies often vary in size and scope and in their definition of what constitutes relationship violence, and they often ask questions about violence in relationships generally, not specific to LGBTQ relationships. As well, the vast majority of studies have focused on white, middle-class, urban, able-bodied participants. While some researchers have attempted to address the experiences of people of color, immigrants, and Aboriginal people, most have not.

However, survey results have ranged from between 11 and 52 percent of respondents indicating that they have experienced violence in an intimate same-gender relationship. Greenwood et al. (2002) found that one in five gay men in their study were battered by an intimate partner and that the rates were higher for HIV-positive men. Rohrbaugh (2006), reviewing prevalence rates, speaks of the difficulty in obtaining accurate data on the prevalence of violence in same-gender relationships. In her review, she focuses on several larger health studies that ask a variety of questions about general health and in which violence in relationships is one aspect of the studies, not the sole focus. In these studies, the incidence of lesbian intimate partner violence is relatively lower (11 to 12 percent) than in many of the studies whose focus is solely on violence in relationships (Rohrbaugh, 2006). Few large-scale studies have explored the incidence of violence in gay male relationships. However, Bryant and Demian's 1994 study of 506 gay male couples reported that 11 percent of men reported violence in their relationships. Results of the National Violence Against Women Survey in the United States (Tjaden & Thoennes, 2000) where 8,000 women and 8,000 men were surveyed as to their experiences of violence in hetero-sexual and same-sex relationships, indicated that 11 percent of women reported being raped, physically assaulted, or stalked by a female partner compared to nearly 25 percent of heterosexual women who reported being raped and/or physically assaulted by a male partner. About 15 percent of men living with a male partner reported being raped, physically assaulted, and/or stalked by a male intimate partner.

The Survivor Project (Courvant & Cook-Daniels, 1998) showed that 50 percent of trans and intersex people report being assaulted or raped by a romantic partner. These statistics do not, however, specify if these rates relate to violence in same-gender relationships where one or both of the partners is trans or in opposite- gender relationships. Relatively few stud-ies have looked at violence in the relationships of transgender people (see Brown, 2011; Courvant & Cook-Daniels, 1998; and FORGE, 2005). The kinds of violence and the dynamics of violence in relationships where one or both of the partners is trans contain elements that are unique to the experience of being trans in a transphobic society. While there are simi-larities with violence in same-sex/gender relationships and heterosexual relationships, the distinct aspects of being trans require that we consider the context of the lives of transgender people when developing and providing service to trans survivors of violence in relationships (Goldberg & White, 2011).

Few studies have considered the prevalence of violence in the lives of LGBTQ youth or young adults, although some of the highest incidences of relationship violence occur in dating relationships and for youth and young adults (regardless of sexual orientation) between the ages of 16 and 34 (see "Family Violence in Canada: A Statistical Profile," 2010 and Mahony, 2008). Freedner and colleagues (2002) reported on a study of 632 adolescents between the ages of 13 and 22. While this study had many of the same difficulties that plague other prevalence studies, there are some interesting results that require further consideration. This study found that of the 101 males who identified as gay, 44 (43.6 percent) reported some form of violence by a male partner; 39.8 percent of females experienced abuse by a female partner; and for bisexual youth, the rates of violence were higher than for either gay or lesbian youth (57.1 percent as opposed to 41.5 percent for gay/lesbian youth) and that the violence was equally perpetrated by same- and opposite-gender partners.

There are many factors that contribute to the continued silence surrounding violence in LGBTQ relationships. Ongoing societal oppression of LGBTQ people and the resulting myths about who we are and what our relationships are like have resulted in a climate where it is difficult to talk about the realities and complexities of our lives and especially to admit to issues of violence in relationships for fear of fueling these harmful stereotypes and prejudices. As well, gender stereotypes of women being caring, gentle, and nonviolent and that men cannot be victimized discount the fact that some women are violent and that gay men can be victims.

As a result, it is difficult for individuals and communities to identify and respond to violence in intimate relationships, and this can manifest in the following ways:

- Relationship violence and sexual assault are thought of as male violence against women
- Social preconceptions that undermine the seriousness of same-sex/gender relationship violence
- Fear of being "outed"
- Fear of losing LGBTQ friends and/or community
- Fear of calling the police given historical homophobia, heterosexism, transphobia, and racism within the criminal justice system
- People in small communities being reluctant to come forward for fear of being ostracized, or of outing themselves and their partners

- Normalization of abusive behavior by the perpetrator
- Fears that exposing such violence will fuel LGBTQ phobia
- The attitude that it's "just fighting," that "it's mutual," and that if it happens, it's rare
- Fear of disturbing the notion of "lesbian utopia"
- Limited resources for help for the victim and perpetrator because of homophobia and transphobia and lack of culturally appropriate resources in anti-violence services
- Isolation in homo/bi/transphobic society
- Shame and self-blame

FORMS OF VIOLENCE

Conflict is a normal part of all relationships. It can be expressed in healthy, unhealthy, or abusive ways. Healthy conflict involves working through disagreements using negotiation and mutually beneficial compromise. Unhealthy conflict arises when there is a difficulty in discussing or reaching a mutually beneficial outcome. In abusive conflict, there is no mutually beneficial discussion or resolution of disagreements. It is not always easy to tell the difference between unhealthy conflict and abusive behavior. Unhealthy conflicts are sometimes misconstrued as abuse, although it is more common for abusive behavior to be minimized, viewed as normal, or excused.

What Is Abuse?

Violence in LGBTQ relationships entails the conscious effort to control another person through the use of "threats, humiliation, coercion, and/or force" (Ristock, 2005). The intent is to undermine, hurt, humiliate, manipulate, punish, coerce, or degrade another person. Abusive behaviors can include subtle or covert harm as well as life-threatening acts of violence, creating a situation where one person attempts to isolate, dominate, and intimidate their partner. Abuse may take many forms in LGBTQ relationships and includes emotional, financial, verbal, physical, and sexual violence (Ristock, 2002; Toppings, 2004).

Below is a table that depicts some of the tactics that an abusive person may use toward their intimate LGBTQ partner. Many of these tactics are similar to the kinds of violence that is found in abusive heterosexual relationships (e.g., general verbal abuse, pushing, shoving, etc.), and others are unique to same-sex/gender relationships by virtue of the broader context of homophobia, heterosexism, transphobia, and biphobia surrounding

LGBTQ relationships. Sexual assault in intimate relationships often goes unrecognized, and many LGBTQ people may not acknowledge that what they are experiencing is sexual violence. The language of rape or sexual assault may not fit or accurately describe what gay men, lesbians, bisexuals, or trans people experience (Ristock, 2002).

Intimate partner violence can result in significant impacts on the health and well-being of survivors, including physical injuries and emotional impacts (Table 8.1; Ristock, 2002). Physical injuries can include

Table 8.1   Examples of the Different Forms of Intimate Partner Violence and Some of the Tactics Used in Abusive LGBTQ Relationships

Emotional Abuse	Financial Abuse	Physical Violence	Sexual Violence
verbal abuse (yelling, name-calling, verbal insults, humiliation)	creating debt	pushing	forced nonconsensual sex, rape
threats, including homophobic or transphobic threats: –threatening to disclose your sexual or gender identity to family, friends, work, immigration, child welfare; –threatening to infect you with HIV; –threatening to disclose HIV status; –threatening to harm or deny you access to children and/or pets; –threats to immigration status; –threats of suicide; –threats to kill	restricting access to funds needed for hormones, sexual reassignment surgery, and medications	shoving	intentional use of certain sexual acts that deny/assault one's trans/intersex identities
using the social marginalization and invisibility of LGBTQ people to increase isolation	controlling finances	restraining	making demeaning sexual comments

(continued)

Table 8.1   (Continued)

Emotional Abuse	Financial Abuse	Physical Violence	Sexual Violence
encouraging shame and self-hatred about being LGBTQ, including deliberate attempts to undermine a person's identity	denying contributions or rights to family assets	hitting, biting	verbal and/or psychological attacks on who you are as a sexual being
controlling clothing; controlling access to surgery, hormones, electrolysis, etc.	running up credit cards	hitting/ punching walls	raping someone with an object or weapon
denying parental rights as a co-parent	stealing money	throwing things	coercive unprotected sex
denying the existence of the relationship to you or the community		physically harming pets	mutilation of body parts
stalking, harassing		destroying property	insulting of body parts
controlling or limiting a partner's behavior or actions, including who their friends are and what activities and community events they can attend		touching body parts in ways or in places that have been set off-limits	
constantly interrupting someone's sleep		choking, strangling	
jealousy, manipulation, and other treatment intended to inflict pain		attacking specific body parts	
terrorizing		use of weapons	
racist attacks		lethal use of force	

bruises, cuts, broken bones, burns, and the health-related effects of physical violence, including chronic pain and chronic injuries. The emotional responses to experiences of violence are individual and can include depression, anxiety, anger, fear, shame, suicidal ideation, post-traumatic stress, and a variety of stress-related syndromes. Freedner et al. (2002), in their study of lesbian, bisexual, and gay adolescents, found that those reporting experiences of dating violence were more likely to show higher rates of substance use, forced sexual contact, sexually risky behaviors, teen pregnancy, eating disorders, and higher rates of suicidality than their peers.

RELATIONSHIP DYNAMICS

The dominant understanding of violence in relationships has focused on a gender-based power-and-control model of abuse in heterosexual relationships that assumes that there is one perpetrator (male) and one victim (female) and that the violence occurs in a cyclical fashion that increases in frequency and intensity over time. While this model accounts for the violence in many heterosexual relationships, it does not fit all (Pense & Dasgupta, 2006) and cannot account for the differing contexts and dynamics in same-sex/gender relationships (Ristock, 2005; Durish, 2007; Poon, 2011; Brown, 2007). As a construct, the power-and-control model of violence in relationships has conceptualized the perpetrator as holding all the power and victims as powerless, passive, and with little agency.

The impact of this conceptualization has been particularly troublesome for gay men, as the "social construction of masculinity depicts men as being independent, self-reliant and emotionally in control" and thus can make it difficult for them to identify themselves as being abused (Poon, 2011). Similarly, this model doesn't account for fighting back, acting in self-defense, or retaliating and has led to the belief that violence in same-sex/gender relationships is "mutual" or "just fighting," which assumes "equal power, motivation and intention to harm" (Ristock, 2002). As well, the "rigid victim-perpetrator dichotomy . . . helps maintain systems of oppression by ignoring the violence experienced by large groups of people on a daily basis" (Ristock, 2002). Power and the abuse of power is a part of intimate partner violence, but that power is not static or fixed; nor does it lie solely with the perpetrator. Our understanding of power and control in intimate partner violence needs to encompass the reality that someone can be both a victim and a perpetrator of violence.

Various authors have identified a range of dynamics in abusive same-sex/gender relationships. These include:

• Power-and-control dynamics where there is one perpetrator and one victim and where the violence resembles a cyclical or spiral pattern that intensifies over time (Island & Letellier, 1991; Renzetti, 1992; Ristock, 2002);

• Situations where the violence is less frequent or sporadic and does not seem to follow a pattern (Ristock, 2002);

- Fighting back or self-defense and retaliation; some researchers have reported that there is a higher tendency for lesbians or gay men to fight back in self-defense or even to retaliate for violence they experience from their partner. (Ristock, 2002; Ristock, 2005; Durish, 2007; Marrujo & Kreger, 1996; Poon, 2011). In Ristock's study (2002), 37 percent of the lesbians spoke of fighting back as a way of coping with the violence, as a way of resisting, and as a way of intentionally causing harm and/or as a self-defense reaction; and

- Shifting power—where the power shifts back and forth between the partners over time or moves back and forth depending on the situation, and uniquely to that relationship (Ristock, 2002). One of the women in Ristock's study (2002) talked about getting tired of being controlled by her partner and fighting back and then moving into the role of abusing her partner.

Clearly, relationship dynamics are complex, generally are not static, and can shift or change throughout the course of a relationship. Relationship dynamics can be influenced by a wide variety of social and individual factors, such as the level and comfort with one's sexuality and being "out"; internalized homophobia and heterosexism; racism, sexism, transphobia, etc. They can also be influenced by personal experiences of violence and trauma—for example, childhood experiences of abuse/violence, witnessing or exposure to relationship violence, past experiences of homophobic/hate violence, and violence in previous relationships.

SOCIAL CONTEXT OF RELATIONSHIP VIOLENCE

The varying contexts that surround LGBTQ lives expose how violence is sanctioned by social structures that create isolation and enable inequality and vulnerability, which may contribute to the risk of experiencing or perpetrating violence. Research has highlighted the impact of such contexts to include homophobia/heterosexism/transphobia; the experience of first relationships; experiences of being bisexual; experiences of social isolation; experiences of immigration; racism and other -isms; the normalization of a lifetime of violence; dealing with of HIV/AIDS; experiences of transitioning; alcohol and drug use; and the combined effects of multiple oppressions. This is not a definitive list, and these contexts may overlap with one another, but it is presented to enhance our understanding of the complexities at play in the lives of LGBTQ people. It is important to recognize that while these contexts may enhance the probability that violence may occur, it does not mean that they cause violence.

Context of Homophobia/Heterosexism/Transphobia

We live in a society where difference is often met with suspicion, discrimination, prejudice, and societally condoned violence. As LGBTQ people, we are inundated with messages that imply, explicitly or implicitly, that we are abnormal, sick, and deviant. The everyday threat of homophobia, biphobia, transphobia, and heterosexism has fostered a climate where, as a queer community and therefore as individuals, we often feel the need to portray our relationships as strong, healthy, happy, and nonviolent. This has made it difficult for the community to effectively respond to both the person who experiences violence and the person who uses violence and has resulted in increased isolation, fear of speaking up, and barriers to accessing service. This increased isolation, vulnerability to being outed, and the lack of services can be exploited by an abusive partner.

Talking about the abuse, especially to mainstream services, police, and social workers means "coming out" and also outing one's partner, which for some people is unthinkable, thus further increasing isolation. Loyalty and not wanting to be subjected (or to subject another) to homophobic/transphobic discrimination is often given as a reason for not seeking help (Ristock, 2002).

Even though there has been an increase in acceptance and visibility of LGBTQ, some people remain closeted and continue to hide their sexuality and gender identity, in at least certain aspects of their lives. As well, those living in rural and remote communities may be especially vulnerable to threats of being outed by an abusive partner.

It is only recently, and in major urban cities, that programs for people who use violence in intimate LGBTQ relationships have been developed. Fears of being ostracized by the community have created barriers to coming forward about one's use of violence and seeking help. Research into the motivating factors for violence in same-sex relationships has indicated that the impact of the stress of homophobia, heterosexism, and the internalization of homophobia (minority stress) has accounted for the use of physical violence in intimate gay male relationships (Mendoza, 2011).

Context of First Relationships

In her research, Janice Ristock (2002) identified that nearly 60 percent of the lesbians she interviewed talked about the abuse occurring in their first lesbian relationship. This speaks to the vulnerability of coming out, not being out, and the isolation of not being connected to many other gay/lesbian/queer people or communities—which may increase the risk of violence. The violence may be normalized as a part of being in a same-sex/

gender relationship and may play on the abused person's fears of losing a relationship that confirms one's newfound identity.

Context of Bisexuality

Bisexuals often face discrimination and marginalization from both the heterosexual and lesbian/gay communities—vulnerabilities that can be exploited by an abusive partner. According to Freedner et al. (2002), bisexual adolescents are less accepted by both lesbian/gay and heterosexual peers, making them more vulnerable to threats of outing. In their study, adolescent bisexual males and bisexual females were far more likely to report being threatened with outing by a partner than were either lesbians or gay male adolescents. Bisexual females were twice as likely as heterosexual females to report sexual abuse (Freedner et al., 2002). Few studies specifically examine the experiences of violence in relationships for bisexual men and women. Often, their experiences are included with those of lesbians or gay men or heterosexuals (depending on whether the abuse occurred in a same-gender or opposite-gender relationship) or are discounted altogether.

Context of Social Isolation/Immigration

Rural Communities

Studies suggest that LGBTQ people living in small, rural communities may be particularly vulnerable to violence because of fears of experiencing discrimination when revealing one's sexual and/or gender identity, increased isolation, lack of services, and an increased prevalence of firearms (Ristock, 2005).

Social Isolation of Dislocation

Moving to a New Community: Moving to a new community to find community or to escape homophobic environments creates a vulnerability due to the isolation of not knowing anyone or having any contacts in the new community. Similar to the experiences of first relationships and of the isolation of homophobia and being in the closet, such a vulnerability that can be exploited by an abusive partner.

Recent Immigration

Cultural and language barriers combined with anti-immigrant sentiments create social isolation and can make it difficult to leave abusive LGBTQ relationships. New immigrants may have few supports other than an intimate partner and may be dependent on the partner for information and/or financial support. Abusive people can use their partner's immigration status, language barriers, and lack of knowledge about the legal system against them and threaten to expose them as being in a same-sex relationship. As well, an abusive person can use their partner's racial or cultural background against them to make them feel inferior (Ristock, 2005).

Context of HIV/AIDS

HIV/AIDS still carries with it much social stigma and can be a factor in any relationship, but it is of particular concern to bisexual and gay men given its high incidence (65 percent of those infected with HIV are gay or bisexual men [Pantalone, Lehavot, Simoni, & Walters, 2011]). Some of the ways in which HIV status has been found to be a part of the violence in gay and bisexual men's lives include:

* The withholding of medication or threat of doing so (Letellier, 1996);

* Threatening to reveal HIV status;

* Reluctance of those who are positive to leave the relationship, especially if they have limited supports other than the abusive partner;

* Fears of becoming sick or dying as a major factor in remaining in a relationship with an abusive person (Merrill & Wolfe, 2000);

* In cases where both partners are positive, they may depend on each other financially, and to leave the relationship would mean putting themselves and their partner at significant risk; and

* When the abusive partner is positive, the victim may feel guilty about reporting or leaving, or they may feel that they are abandoning their partner (Cruz, 2003).

Context of Transitioning/Transphobia

Trans People as Victims

Specific Vulnerabilities:

* Transphobia sets the stage where trans people are vulnerable to abuse in both individual and institutional ways.

* Beliefs that few men are interested in trans women as partners can lead to engaging in high-risk sexual activities within intimate partnerships.

* Barriers to accessing services for trans people and sometimes gaining entry to services means "passing" as the gender for which the service is intended. Trans people living in poverty or on low income may be

particularly discriminated against in this manner because they do not have the financial means to afford surgeries, electrolysis, makeup, etc. that would facilitate passing (Namaste, 2000).

- Trans men in need of safe housing may face the stigmatizing experience of passing as female to access women's shelters or risk potential violence in the men's shelter system.

- For many trans people, involving the police is simply not an option due to the historical difficulties with being victimized by police when seeking help, concerns of not being taken seriously, and a lack of respect from the justice system. As well, the use of birth names in legal proceedings can create barriers to seeking help.

- Seeking medical attention following an assault is fraught with fear of exposure and can be retraumatizing and make it harder for trans people to seek treatment (Goldberg, 2003).

Examples of Abusive Tactics for Exploiting and Undermining Trans Identity:

- Deliberately using wrong pronouns;

- Ridiculing body parts or touching them in ways or places that are off-limits;

- Destroying means by which trans people communicate gender (i.e., clothing, makeup, hormones, wigs, etc.);

- Demeaning partners by implying that they are not "real" men/women; manipulating behavior by suggesting that "this is what 'real' men/ women do";

- Threatening to out partners to friends, family, employers, landlords;

- Exploiting isolation and lack of resources;

- Facilitating or encouraging drug or alcohol use;

- Incorporating the lack of safety in trans people's lives into the abuse tactics—reinforcing that shelters are transphobic, that police won't believe them, etc.;

- Rationalizing control over partner as being caring and protective;

Trans People as Perpetrators of Violence

Little is known about trans people as perpetrators of violence. Brown (2011) reports on her earlier research of cis women in relationship with trans men. In this research, 5 of the 20 women she interviewed identified experiencing abuse in their relationships with trans men. Several of these women stated that they did not identify what they were experiencing as violence until after they left the relationship. While this is a very small sample, it does shed some light on the kinds of vulnerabilities and abuse tactics that were at play in these relationships.

Specific Vulnerabilities:

- Nontrans partner's guilt around transphobia and privilege of being cisgender was exploited by the abusive trans partner;
- Dependence on partner for information about trans identity, community, and what is "normal" in relationships with trans men coming from the abusive partner who normalized and dismissed violence (this is similar to the context of first relationships discussed above);
- Isolation due to transphobia and fears of fueling transphobia if exposing the abuse; and
- Perceived low likelihood of the nontrans partner to be the victim of abuse (e.g., one woman thought that her partner was "so powerless in a societal sense that there was no way that he could have enough power to be abusive" [Brown, 2011]).

Examples of Abuse Tactics:

- Hormones blamed as reason for abusive behaviors;
- Questions about transition expenses or timing met with accusations of nonsupport;
- Abusive behaviors framed as a function of transitioning or transphobia;
- Using traditional gender role conceptualization to account for abusive behavior; and
- Stress of being an oppressed person (minority stress) used as an explanation for behavior.

Context of Alcohol and Drug Use

The use of substances can create a climate where violence is normalized or is triggered in relationships. Alcohol or drug use is a common element in the escalation of violence. In some cases, women reported being violent only when using alcohol or drugs (Smith, 2011). This is not to say that substance use was the causal factor for the violence, but it definitely was part of the context of the violence in these situations, and some abusive women blamed their abusive behavior on the use of drugs and alcohol (Ristock, 2002). As well, women who experienced violence reported using alcohol to numb themselves and to cope with their experiences. Pantone et al. (2011)

reported that the men in their study shared similar experiences and that alcohol and drug use was intertwined with violence in their relationships.

Context of Normalization of Violence

Historical experiences of violence are not uncommon in the lives of LGBTQ people. For example, Ristock (2002) reported that 48 percent of the women she interviewed had previous experiences of violence, including childhood abuse, sexual assaults, and violence in previous heterosexual and/or same-sex relationships. In her study, women also spoke of experiences of racist violence and the impact of colonization. Rothman et al. (2011), in their review of 75 different studies that looked at the prevalence of sexual assault in the lives of lesbians, gays, and bisexuals, found that the lifetime sexual assault for lesbians and bisexual women ranged from 15.6 to 85.0 percent and 11.8 to 54.0 percent for gay and bisexual men. Fifty-nine percent of the gay and bisexual men reported experiencing childhood sexual assault. They also found that lesbian and bisexual women were more likely to report childhood sexual assault, adult sexual assault, lifetime sexual assault, and sexual assault in intimate relationships than were gay or bisexual men. Gay and bisexual men were more apt to report hate crimes.

As well, experiences of violence based on sexual orientation or gender identity are prevalent in our lives. Herek and colleagues (1997) showed that 20 percent of women and 25 percent of men experienced some form of violence based on their sexual orientation. Moran and Sharpe (2004) found that 60 percent of trans people had experienced some form of hate-motivated violence. Lombardi and colleagues (2001) found that over 50 percent of the transgender people in their study reported experiencing some form of violence and discrimination throughout their lives.

Clearly, experiences of violence can be a factor in of the lives of LGBTQ people and can set the backdrop for violence in intimate relationships. These experiences play out in the dynamics of a relationship in numerous ways for both those who use violence and those who experience violence in intimate partnerships. For instance, abusive dynamics in adult relationships can mirror or replicate the dynamics and experiences of childhood, creating a situation where the abuse feels familiar and perhaps inevitable in relationships (Ristock, 2002). Feelings of anger and engaging in controlling behaviors are normal responses to being violated (Welch, 2007) and can be triggered in intimate LGBTQ relationships where one or both of the partners are survivors of childhood abuse.

Several authors have talked about a person being abused in one intimate relationship and then being abusive in another relationship (Renzetti, 1992; Ristock, 2002; Hamlett, 1998) in a sort of self-protection to ensure that they don't repeat the experiencing of violence from the past. The use of violence is thus seen as a strategy for keeping oneself safe from further victimization. I do not mention this to excuse abusive behavior but rather to bring forward the complexities and varying contexts operating in people's lives and relationships.

Context of Multiple Oppressions (Racism, Classism, and Violence)

As discussed above, intimate partner violence is just one of numerous forms of violence that may be present in the lives of some LGBTQ people. In addition to multiple experiences of violence, we need to consider how racism, including the colonization of indigenous peoples, and colonialism, classism, sexism, and homophobia shape people's lives and their relationships in different ways. Connecting our analysis of violence in intimate LGBTQ relationships to all systems of oppression allows us to take a both/and approach and, for instance, to hold people who use violence accountable for their actions and to see the ways that the needs of those who use violence are intertwined with the needs of those who experience violence, especially in small, diverse communities (Ristock, 2005; Kanuha, 1990). When we consider the context of multiple oppressions in the lives of LGBTQ people, the neat categories of victim and perpetrator become blurred. As well, we become aware that we miss much of the complexities of people's lives when we narrowly define intimate partner violence (Taylor & Ristock, 2011).

By examining the contexts within which violence exists in people's lives, we can begin to recognize the diversity of ways that violence occurs and how intimate partner violence is linked to larger systems of oppression.

RESPONDING TO INTIMATE PARTNER VIOLENCE IN THE LIVES OF LGBTQ PEOPLE

For an LGBTQ person experiencing abuse or violence in a same-sex/gender relationship, reaching out for help can be difficult and fraught with numerous barriers and obstacles. One of the impacts of the context of homophobia, biphobia, and transphobia and heterosexism is the multiple barriers that arise when accessing support. As discussed earlier (see section on Troubling Language), identifying one's experiences as being abusive can be difficult because of the silence and misconceptions about violence in same-sex/gender relationships. Fears of confirming the negative stereotypes of LGBTQ identity as being unhealthy can create barriers to identifying violence in relationships and seeking help and in receiving appropriate interventions. Talking about the abuse means coming out and also outing one's partner, which is unthinkable for some people, especially in approaching mainstream services, police, social workers, and medical professionals; this may increase a person's vulnerability and isolation. As responders, we cannot underestimate the power that loyalty and not wanting to be subjected to (or to subject another person to) homophobic/transphobic discrimination can have on one's decisions to reach out for help.

Complex power dynamics and a tendency for higher rates of fighting back or retaliating for past violence in some same-sex/gender relationships can make it difficult to talk about the violence one has experienced, especially if that person has also used violence. It can be hard to sort out what is happening in the relationship and to know where to turn for help. As well, for service providers, it can be confusing and problematic to provide the appropriate interventions without an analysis and understanding of complex ways that power operates in relationships.

Any service or service provider who works with LGBTQ people who have experienced violence in relationships needs to have at least a basic understanding of the impacts of homophobia, biphobia, transphobia, and heterosexism in the lives of LGBTQ. It is important for service providers to engage in ongoing anti-oppression training that addresses sexual and gender diversity. As well, agencies need to have clear policies that address issues of discrimination and harassment based on sexual orientation and gender diversity for clients, staff, and volunteers. It is essential that agencies work to create services that are open and welcoming of LGBTQ people and that this is communicated in all correspondence and advertising through the use of nonheterosexist, LGBTQ-inclusive language. This may require a critical examination of policies and practices for ways they inadvertently (or not) create barriers and gaps to providing service to LGBTQ people. For example, services that define violence in relationships as gendered violence (i.e., male violence against women) exclude the violence that LGBTQ people in same-sex relationships experience and the experiences of trans men in heterosexual relationships.

Effective responses to violence in same-sex/gender relationships need to incorporate a range of community responses; programs and services should be flexible, address a wide range of related issues, and meet the needs of diverse communities. There need to be services that can provide support and information that includes information on legal options and assistance with the justice system, counseling services for those who experience violence and for those who use violence; information on housing; medical concerns; and issues of child welfare, as well as programs that address prevention and community development. Workshops and programs that focus on building healthy relationships and healthy communication skills are also important.

It is not always realistic to expect that every service can address all of these needs, but it is important for there to be some sort of a coordinated community response that, as a minimum, establishes a network of services and coordinates referrals across agencies.

Janice Ristock (2002) suggests that exploring the following questions can help make us more accountable and may help to illuminate what we may not fully understand:

- Who benefits from the way we currently talk about relationship violence, and what difference does that make?

- Whose voices are heard and not heard when we use the categories heterosexual domestic violence, family violence, violence against women, LGBTQ relationship violence, etc.? And what difference does that make?

- Who is telling me their story, from what social location, and in what social context?

- How can we think outside the gender binary system?

- What does a framework of intersectionality bring to my work?

Examples of Innovative Approaches

A wide variety of programs, services, and community development initiatives have created innovative projects and programs that work to overcome the barriers and gaps in services that continue to create challenges in addressing intimate partner violence in LGBTQ lives. I have highlighted a few examples below.

Since identifying and acknowledging violence in same-sex/gender relationships is met with a multitude of challenges, many communities have developed programs that, while ultimately working with issues of violence in relationships, provide supports, education, and advocacy in ways that do not necessarily directly address the issues of violence in relationships. For example, in responding to limited participation in support groups designed specifically for lesbians who experienced violence in their relationships, the Safe Choices Support and Education Program (www.endingviolence. org) developed a series of healthy queer relationship workshops "intended to provide queer women with opportunities for connection, dialogue, exchange of information and resources, and skill building about healthy relationships." As well, the Queer Asian Women's Shelter in San Francisco has hosted potluck dinners designed to strengthen friendship networks and community ties through discussions about relationships in an informal and nonthreatening atmosphere.

There are other programs, such as the Northwest Network for Bi, Trans, Lesbian, and Gay Survivors of Abuse (www.nwnetwork.org), that have developed an innovative initiative, and the Pink Martini Project provides posters, matchbooks, and resource cards with information about LGBTQ relationship violence to queer bars in Seattle. The initiative, while bringing awareness of violence in queer relationships, also engages queer bars in taking a stance against violence in LGBTQ communities.

Web-based information and webinars have been used to increase awareness of LGBTQ intimate partner violence. Another program, located in a small community serving a predominantly rurally based population, developed a series of webinars to provide education and information about healthy queer relationships as well as general information about violence in queer relationships.

Group programs for survivors of violence and those that address the use of violence are an important aspect of the continuum of services that are need to address LGBTQ intimate partner violence. Many programs have focused on supports for survivors of violence, while others have recognized the need to address services for both survivors and for those who use violence. For example, the LA Gay and Lesbian Center offers services to court-mandated perpetrators of violence while maintaining an emphasis on the safety of survivors. The Northwest Network advocates for services that provide self-determination and safety for survivors and that focus on accountability for those using abusive behavior.

Mendoza and Dolan-Soto (2011) reviewed group programs in New York (New York City Gay and Lesbian Anti-Violence Project) and Toronto (Toronto David Kelley Services' Partner Assault Program) and have made several recommendations for group programs for perpetrators of violence in LGBTQ relationships, including the need for staff training and the need for separate groups for men and women; programs should see violence in same-sex relationships as both a health issue and a criminal justice issue; and the goals of groups need to focus on the "promotion of behaviour change towards healthy conflict and that the responsibility for violence lies with the perpetrator."

The majority of the programs that I have discussed above are programs designed and delivered by LGBTQ services within the communities they serve. While it is important for LGBTQ communities to create opportunities for LGBTQ people to access services in their own communities, it is equally important for mainstream agencies and services to be able to address issues of LGBTQ intimate partner violence with similar levels of support as they provide for dominant heterosexual culture. This is particularly true in small rural areas where social services are limited to begin with, let alone offering specialized services to LGBTQ individuals.

CONCLUSION

There remains much that we do not know about intimate partner violence in the lives of LGBTQ. Violence in LGBTQ relationships has to be viewed through the context of multiple oppressions and different experiences that define the lives of LGBTQ people. It is essential that we remain cognizant of the political nature of violence in LGBTQ relationships and to understand how it can be used against LGBTQ people. Our analyses and responses need to take into consideration people's differing experiences and contexts of relationship violence within a broader framework of intersectionality, where the nature of identity and systems of power and privilege are part of the context of intimate partner violence in queer lives.

REFERENCES

Brown, N. (2007). Stories from outside the frame: Intimate partner abuse in sexual-minority women's relationships with transsexual men. *Feminism & Psychology, 17*(3), 373–393.

Brown, N. (2011). Holding tensions of victimization and perpetration: Partner abuse in trans communities. In J. Ristock (Ed.), *Intimate partner violence in LGBTQ lives* (pp. 153–168). New York: Routledge.

Bryant, A. S., & Demian. (1994). Relationship characteristics of gay and lesbian couples: Findings from a national survey. *Journal of Gay and Lesbian Social Services, 1*, 101–117.

Chung, C., & Lee, S. (1999). *Raising our voices: Queer Asian women's response to relationship violence.* San Francisco: Family Violence Prevention Fund.

Courvant, D., & Cook-Daniels, L. (1998). Trans and intersex survivors of domestic violence: Defining terms, barriers, and responsibilities. Survivor Project. Retrieved from http://www.survivorproject.org/defbarrresp.html

Crenshaw, K. W. (1994). Mapping the margins: Intersectionality, identity politics, and violence against women of color. In M. A. Fineman & R. Mykitiuk (Eds.), *The public nature of private violence* (pp. 93–118). New York: Routledge.

Cruz, J. M. (2003). "Why doesn't he just leave?" Gay male domestic violence and the reasons victims stay. *Journal of Men's Studies, 11*(3), 309–324.

Davis, K., & Glass, N. (2011). Reframing the heteronormative constructions of lesbian partner violence. In J. Ristock (Ed.), *Intimate partner violence in LGBTQ lives* (pp. 13–36). New York: Routledge.

Durish, P. (2007). Honouring complexity: Gender, culture and violence in the lives of lesbian, gay, bisexual, transgender, queer individuals. In A. Yuen & C. White (Eds.), *Conversations about gender, culture, violence and narrative practice* (pp. 125–134). Richmond, Australia: Dulwich Centre.

Family violence in Canada: A statistical profile. (2010). Statistics Canada. Retrieved from www.statcan.gc.ca/pub/85-224-x/85-224-x2010000-eng.htm

FORGE. (2005). Transgender Sexual Violence Project. FORGE. Retrieved from http://www.forge-forward.org/transviolence/docs/FINAL_Graphs.pdf

Freedner, N., Freed, L. H., Yang, Y. W., & Austin, S. B. (2002). Dating violence among gay lesbian and bisexual adolescents: Results from a community survey. *Journal of Adolescent Health, 31*, 469–474.

Goldberg, J. M. (2003). *Trans people in the criminal justice system: A guide for criminal justice personnel.* Vancouver, BC: Justice Institute of BC and the Trans Alliance Society.

Goldberg, J. M., & White, C. (2011). Reflections on approaches to trans anti-violence education. In J. Ristock (Ed.), *Intimate partner violence in LGBTQ lives* (pp. 56–80). New York: Routledge.

Greenwood, G. L., Relf, M. V., Hung, B., Pollack, L. M., Canchola, A., & Catania, A. (2002). Battering victimization among probability-based sample of men who have sex with men. *American Journal of Public Health, 92*, 1964–1969.

Hamlett, N. (1998). *Women who abuse in intimate relationships.* Minneapolis, MN: Domestic Abuse Project.

Herek, G., Gillis, R., Cogan, J. C., & Glunt, E. K. (1997). Hate crime victimization among lesbians, gay and bisexual adults: Prevalence, psychological correlates, and methodological issues. *Journal of Interpersonal Violence, 1*(12), 195–215.

Hiebert-Murphy, D., Ristock, J. L., & Brownridge, D. A. (2011). The meaning of "risk" for intimate partner violence among women in same-sex relationships. In J. L. Ristock (Ed.), *Intimate partner violence in LGBTQ lives* (pp. 37–55). New York: Routledge.

Holmes, C. (2009). Destabilizing homonormativity and the public/private dichotomy in North American lesbian domestic violence discourses. *Gender, Place & Culture, 16*(1), 77–95.

Island, D., & Letellier, P. (1991). *Men who beat the men who love them: Battered gay men and domestic violence.* Haworth gay & lesbian studies. New York: Haworth.

Kanuha, V. K. (1990). Compounding the triple jeopardy. In L. S. Brown & M. P. P. Roots (Eds.), *Diversity and complexity in feminist therapy.* New York: Haworth.

Letellier, P. (1996). Twin epidemics: Domestic violence and HIV infection among gay and bisexual men. In C. Renzetti & C. Miley (Eds.), *Violence in lesbian and gay domestic partnerships* (pp. 69–82). New York: Haworth.

Lombardi, E., Emilia, L., Wilchins, R. A., Priesing, D., & Malouf, D. (2001). Gender violence: Transgender experiences with violence and discrimination. *Journal of Homosexuality, 42*, 89–101.

Mahony, T. H. (2008). Police-reported dating violence in Canada, 2008. Retrieved from www.statcan.gc.ca/pub/85-002-x/2010002/article/11242-eng.htm

Marrujo, B., & Kreger, M. (1996). Definition of roles in abusive lesbian relationships. In C. Renzetti & C. N. Miley (Eds.), *Violence in gay and lesbian domestic partnerships* (pp. 23–34). New York: Harrington Park.

Mendoza, J. (2011). The impact of minority stress on gay male partner abuse. In J. L. Ristock (Ed.), *Intimate partner violence in LGBTQ lives* (pp. 169–181). New York: Routledge.

Mendoza, J., & Dolan-Soto, D. R. (2011). Running same-sex batterer groups: Critical reflections on the New York City Gay and Lesbian Anti-Violence

Project and the Toronto David Kelley Services' Partner Assault Response Program. In J. L. Ristock (Ed.), *Intimate partner violence in LGBTQ lives* (pp. 274–300). New York: Routledge.

Merrill, G. S., & Wolfe, V. A. (2000). Battered gay men: An exploration of abuse, help-seeking and why they stay. *Journal of Homosexuality, 39*(2), 1–30.

Moran, L. J., & Sharpe, A. N. (2004). Violence, identity and policing: The case of violence against transgender people. *Criminal Justice, 4*(4), 395–417.

Namaste, V. K. (2000). *Invisible lives: The erasure of transsexual and transgendered people.* Chicago: The University of Chicago Press.

Pantalone, D. W., Lehavot, K., Simoni, J. M., & Walters, K. L. (2011). I ain't never been a kid: Early violence exposure and other pathways to partner violence for sexual minority men with HIV. In J. L. Ristock (Ed.), *Intimate partner violence in LGBTQ lives* (pp. 182–208). New York: Routledge.

Pense, E., & Dasgupta, S. D. (2006). *Re-examining "battering": Are all acts of violence against intimate partners the same?* Duluth, MN: Praxis International.

Poon, M. K. L. (2011). Beyond good and evil: The social construction of violence in intimate gay relationships. In J. L. Ristock (Ed.), *Intimate partner violence in LGBTQ lives.* (pp. 102–130). New York: Routledge.

Renzetti, C. M. (1992). *Violent betrayal: Partner abuse in lesbian relationships.* Newbury Park, CA: Sage Publications.

Ristock, J. (2005). Relationship violence in lesbian/gay/bisexual/transgender/queer (LGBTQ) communities: Moving beyond a gender-based framework. *Violence Against Women Online Resources.* Retrieved from http://www.mincava.umn.edu/documents/

Ristock, J. L. (2002). *No more secrets: Violence in lesbian relationships.* New York: Routledge.

Ristock, J. L. (Ed.). (2011). *Intimate partner violence in LGBTQ lives.* New York: Routledge.

Rohrbaugh, J. B. (2006). Domestic violence in same-gender relationships. *Family Court Review, 44*(2), 287–299.

Rothman, E. F., Exner, D., & Baughman, A. L. (2011). The prevalence of sexual assault against people who identify as gay, lesbian or bisexual in the United States: A systemic review. *Trauma, Violence & Abuse, 12*(2), 55–66.

Smith, C. (2011). Women who abuse their female intimate partner. In J. L. Ristock (Ed.), *Intimate partner violence in LGBTQ lives* (pp. 131–152). New York: Routledge.

Taylor, C. G., & Ristock, J. L. (2011). "We are all treaty people": An anti-oppressive research ethics of solidarity with Indigenous LGBTQ people living with partner violence. In J. L. Ristock (Ed.), *Intimate partner violence in LGBTQ lives* (pp. 301–320). New York: Routledge.

Tjaden, P., & Thoennes, N. (2000). *Full report of the prevalence, incidence, and consequences of violence against women: Findings from the National Violence Against Women Survey.* Washington, DC: Department of Justice.

Toppings, P. (2004). *Removing barriers + building access: A resource manual on providing culturally relevant services to lesbian, gay, transgender and bisexual victims of violence.* Vancouver, BC: The Centre.

Welch, C. (2007). Challenging our assumptions: Working with women's anger and use of violence. In *Freedom from violence: Tools for working with trauma, mental health and substance use*. British Columbia Association of Specialized Victim Assistance and Counselling Programs (currently known as the Ending Violence Association of British Columbia). Retrieved from www .endingviolence.org/publications

9

Cardiovascular Health and the LGBT Community

Rebecca Allison

Cardiovascular disease, which includes heart disease and stroke, is the leading cause of death both worldwide and in the United States. For the year 2004, the World Health Organization reported 7.2 million deaths worldwide from coronary heart disease, representing 12.2 percent of all deaths reported; and 5.71 million deaths from stroke and other cerebrovascular disease, representing 9.7 percent of all deaths reported (World Health Organization, 2008). In the United States, statistics for the year 2007 reported heart disease as the leading cause of death, with 616,067 deaths, representing 25.4 percent of all deaths reported. Cerebrovascular disease accounted for 135,952 deaths, or 5.6 percent of all deaths reported, ranking third behind heart disease and cancer (all forms) (Xu, Kochanek, Murphy, & Tejada-Vera, 2010, p. 5). Overall mortality from heart disease and stroke has been declining over the past 50 years (Xu et al., 2010, p. 9), suggesting that there have been improvements in both prevention and treatment of cardiovascular disease.

RISK FACTORS FOR CARDIOVASCULAR DISEASE

Since 1948, the landmark Framingham Heart Study has tracked the cardiovascular health of thousands of residents of Framingham,

Massachusetts, over multiple generations. The study has generated hundreds of research publications and has provided information on the causes of heart disease and stroke, which has defined the modern practice of cardiology (Levy, 2005).

While there are genetic factors that predispose persons to develop cardiovascular disease, there are other factors that can be treated or prevented, greatly reducing a person's cardiovascular risk. These treatable factors include cigarette smoking, hypertension, diabetes mellitus, and hyperlipidemia (abnormal blood cholesterol) (McGill, 2005).

Tobacco Use

The American Lung Association's publication *Smoking Out a Deadly Threat: Tobacco Use in the LGBT Community* identifies higher rates of cigarette smoking for gay men, who were up to 2.4 times as likely to be smokers as heterosexual men (Blatt, 2010). For lesbians, the incidence of smoking is also up to 2.0 times as likely as for heterosexual women. A further analysis suggested that smoking rates are significantly higher in younger lesbians, particularly those who self-identify as "butch," or a woman with a masculine gender expression (Lee, Griffin, & Melvin, 2009). Bisexual men and women have very high rates of smoking—as high as 39 percent in some studies (Blatt, 2010). In a recently released report from the National Center for Transgender Equality, 33 percent of transgender men and 29 percent of transgender women reported current tobacco use, compared with 23 percent of men and 18 percent of women in the general population (Grant, 2010).

The tobacco industry has for many years advertised in publications for the LGBT community, with ad content specifically targeting gay and lesbian populations.

Smoking increases blood pressure, reduces levels of HDL (good) cholesterol, and reduces a person's capacity for physical exercise. Nicotine constricts blood vessels and may produce spasm of the coronary arteries. Smoking greatly increases a person's risk for peripheral arterial disease (PAD), a major cause of disability. Furthermore, passive inhalation of cigarette smoke has a cumulative effect similar to that of active smoking (Tonkin, Beauchamp, & Stevenson, 2009).

After smoking cessation, the risk of coronary heart disease is reduced to that of a nonsmoker within about five years. Surveys repeatedly show that many smokers would like to quit smoking but have been unable to do so on their own. In every state, there are public health resources available to help smokers quit. A comprehensive list of national and local resources is available at the National LGBT Tobacco Control Network (http://lgbttobacco.org).

Medications to help with smoking cessation may be useful for some persons. Each of these medications has its own potential side effects and should be used for short-term treatment only.

Nicotine replacement is available without prescription as skin patches, gum, or lozenges; or as prescription nasal spray or oral inhaler. Combinations, such as patch and inhaler, have reported success rates of near 20 percent after one year. Persons using nicotine replacement must be prepared to completely stop smoking because of the significant increase in heart attack risk if they smoke and use nicotine replacement.

Bupropion is an antidepressant unrelated to the major categories of tricyclics and selective serotonin reuptake inhibitors. Bupropion has been found to aid in smoking cessation and is marketed as Zyban for this purpose. Initial success rates of as high as 50 percent are encouraging, but the long-term success rates are about 20 percent. Bupropion may be given long term, unlike nicotine replacement, but it is contraindicated in persons with a history of seizures, bulimia, or anorexia nervosa. Some reports of depression and suicidal thoughts occurring in persons taking bupropion have prompted the Food and Drug Administration to issue a "black box" warning about these dangers.

Varenicline (Chantix) is a "nicotine receptor partial agonist" that appears to have a success rate similar to bupropion (23 percent at one year) (Jorenby et al., 2006). Common side effects include nausea, headache, and insomnia; concerns have been reported about depression and suicidal thoughts occurring in persons taking varenicline. Previously, a "black box" warning was ordered by the Food and Drug Administration for this drug. More recently, based on newer studies, this warning was removed.

Obesity

A survey of over 5,500 U.S. adults, conducted by the Centers for Disease Control and Prevention, revealed that in 2007 to 2008, 32.2 percent of men and 35.5 percent of women were obese, with a body mass index (BMI) greater than 30 (Ogden, 2006). Obesity is associated with increased incidence of diabetes mellitus, hypertension, and hyperlipidemia, as well as with reduced levels of physical activity. Obesity is therefore a condition that increases the risk of coronary heart disease and cerebrovascular disease.

Increased prevalence of obesity in lesbian and bisexual women has been well documented (Yancey, Cochran, Corliss, & Mays, 2003). Lesbian women of color appear to have an especially high likelihood of obesity (Cochran et al., 2001). A prospective evaluation from the Pittsburgh Men's Study from 1999 to 2006 found rates of overweight (BMI 25.0 to 29.5) to be 33.8 percent and obesity (BMI over 30) to be 22.4 percent in men who have sex with men (Guadamuz, Lim, Marshall, Friedman, & Silvestre, 2008).

As in the general population, weight loss through dietary measures is challenging and requires long-term commitment. The results seen with the various forms of bariatric surgery can be impressive and can provide the patient with motivation to maintain calorie restriction. Bariatric surgery is generally performed on patients who are morbidly obese (100 or more pounds over ideal body weight, or body mass index [BMI] greater than 40). Laparoscopic forms of surgery, including the adjustable gastric band and sleeve gastrectomy, have a very low rate of complications; even the gastric bypass procedure has a mortality rate of 0.5 percent. Postoperatively, the study found improvement or complete resolution of diabetes, hypertension, hyperlipidemia, and obstructive sleep apnea in over 70 percent of patients (Buchwald et al., 2004).

Hypertension

As noted in the 2017 Guidelines from the American College of Cardiology and the American Heart Association, blood pressure elevations of greater than 130 systolic and 80 diastolic have been associated with increased risk of cardiovascular disease, including congestive heart failure, myocardial infarction (heart attack), stroke, aneurysm of the aorta, and cardiac arrhythmias (especially atrial fibrillation).

The National High Blood Pressure Education Program (Chobanian, 2003) discusses in detail the indications for treatment of hypertension and the various classes of antihypertensive drugs. However, it is common to observe failure of these prescribed medications to control hypertension, even at maximum doses. A likely explanation for this failure is nonadherence with the medication. Since hypertension is an asymptomatic condition until its late stages, it is difficult to persuade a patient to take a medication that will produce unpleasant symptoms. In particular, gay men are unlikely to comply with a medication that may produce erectile dysfunction, as many antihypertensive medications do. The process of finding the right medication combination requires patience and knowledge of the potential risks of each drug.

As mentioned in the discussion of obesity, blood pressure lowering may be improved by significant weight loss. Also effective as dietary measures are sodium restriction, which involves not just table salt but seasonings such as monosodium glutamate (MSG); and the Dietary Approaches to Stop Hypertension (DASH) eating plan, especially when combined with regular exercise (Blumenthal et al., 2010).

Diabetes Mellitus and Lipid Disorders

Adult-onset (type 2) diabetes mellitus is estimated to occur in 2.6 percent of adults in the United States ages 20 to 39. For ages 40 to 59, the prevalence is 10.8 percent, and for persons age 60 and over, 23.1 percent (Kenny, Aubert, & Geiss, 1995). Adults with a BMI greater than 40 have a risk of diabetes that is seven times greater than those who are not obese (Mokdad et al., 2003). Similarly, elevations of LDL cholesterol and triglycerides occur with increased frequency in obese children and adults. The risk of coronary heart disease is especially increased in the so-called "metabolic syndrome" consisting of abdominal obesity, hypertension, diabetes, and lipid abnormalities, including elevated triglycerides and low levels of HDL cholesterol (Grundy, 2005). The metabolic syndrome is not uncommon in gay, lesbian, bisexual, and transgender persons. Management of this syndrome requires individual management of each abnormality.

In 2014, the American College of Cardiology and the American Heart Association published a Guideline on the Treatment of Blood Cholesterol to Reduce Atherosclerotic Cardiovascular Risk in Adults (Stone, 2013). These guidelines, based on randomized, controlled trials of cholesterol-lowering drugs, provide indications for primary prevention of atherosclerotic cardiovascular disease in various categories of risk as well as secondary prevention of adverse cardiovascular events in persons with a history of atherosclerosis.

Sexually Transmitted Infections and the Cardiovascular System

Dilated cardiomyopathy (enlargement and weakness of the heart) has been reported in persons infected with the human immunodeficiency virus (HIV). The prevalence is approximately 8 percent of patients and is more common in persons with a CD4 count of less than 400 cells per cubic millimeter (Barbaro, DiLorenzo, Grisorio, & Barbarini, 1998). It is uncertain whether the dilated, weakened heart muscle is due to direct viral infection or to immunologic causes. Most patients are asymptomatic, but rare cases of severe acute heart failure have been reported (Fingerhood, 2001). Management of HIV cardiomyopathy includes standard treatment of congestive heart failure, with beta blockers, angiotensin-converting enzyme inhibitors, and diuretics as the possible choices for initial therapy.

Highly active antiretroviral therapy (HAART) has been successful in suppressing viral load and maintaining a stable clinical condition for many years. With increased longevity for patients with HIV infection, the likelihood of cardiovascular disease related to standard risk factors is increased. Furthermore, there are unique effects of some antiretroviral drugs that may impact the cardiovascular system.

The combination of metabolic and structural body changes called "HIV lipodystrophy" is seen with antiretroviral treatment, including protease inhibitors (PI), nucleoside reverse-transcriptase inhibitors (NRTI), and non-nucleoside reverse-transcriptase inhibitors (NNRTI) (Kotler, 2009).

In interpreting the metabolic effects of HAART, it is important to realize that total cholesterol and LDL cholesterol levels may be very low prior to the initiation of HAART. The rise in levels that occurs may only bring the levels back into the normal range. Still, there are reported cases of significant elevation of LDL cholesterol and, especially, triglyceride levels. When these levels are high enough to merit drug treatment, caution must be exercised in the choice of lipid-lowering drugs. In general, fibrates (gemfibrozil, fenofibrate) are considered safer than the statin drugs, but if a statin is necessary, simvastatin and lovastatin should be avoided because their effects and toxicities are greatly enhanced by the use of HAART. Other statins, such as atorvastatin and rosuvastatin, appear safer (Gometz, 2006).

Of note, when studies have been adjusted to allow for other risk factors (primarily cigarette smoking), there has been no evidence for an increased incidence of coronary artery disease in persons with HIV, regardless of what therapy they are receiving.

Gonorrhea is a common sexually transmitted infection which produces infection usually localized to the genital area. If untreated, approximately 1 to 2 percent of patients will develop disseminated gonococcal infection (DGI), which may manifest as dermatitis, septic arthritis, meningitis, or endocarditis. Gonococcal endocarditis more often affects the aortic valve than the mitral valve and is more common in men. It produces typical symptoms of fever, chills, sweats, and malaise. The presence of a heart murmur helps make the diagnosis, which can be confirmed by echocardiography and blood cultures. If untreated, gonococcal endocarditis can be fatal.

Syphilis, if untreated over many years, may produce very late ("tertiary") complications, including an inflammation of the aorta in the chest, called aortitis. Syphilitic aortitis is associated with chronic scarring of the outer layers of the aorta, gradually producing a thickening and a narrowing of the lumen, or inside area of the aorta. Syphilitic aortitis typically does not produce symptoms and is diagnosed when a chest x-ray made for an unrelated reason demonstrates an enlarged aorta. There is no specific treatment other than treating the actual infection, but after so many years, the structural changes in the aorta will not return to normal.

DRUG EFFECTS ON THE CARDIOVASCULAR SYSTEM

Since 1998, several related drugs have been found to improve symptoms of erectile dysfunction in many persons. These drugs include sildenafil (Viagra, Revatio), tadalafil (Cialis), and vardenafil (Levitra). Sildenafil was initially studied in England as a drug to treat high blood pressure, but when its effects on penile erection became known, it was marketed for that indication. These drugs are now some of the most prescribed medications in the United States.

In rare instances, these drugs can cause a severe drop in blood pressure that may cause fainting. In persons with preexisting heart disease, heart attacks have been reported. These cases have usually occurred when persons were taking some form of nitroglycerin (pills or patches) or using other forms of nitrites such as amyl nitrite ("poppers") (Romanelli & Smith, 2004). Patients are routinely advised not to use any nitrite-containing drugs when taking sildenafil, tadalafil, or vardenafil. These medications are contraindicated in persons with symptomatic coronary artery disease.

Cocaine

Cocaine use in the LGBT community, especially among gay and bisexual men, remains common. Cocaine use can be considered in two major forms: nasal inhalation ("snorting") of powdered cocaine, and "crack" cocaine, a solid form that is heated and smoked. Compared to powdered cocaine, crack has a faster onset of action and longer duration of action. Its effects include euphoria, a heightened sense of self-esteem, increased short-term strength and endurance, and enhanced sexual performance. Cocaine has a short duration of action (about an hour when snorted, 15 minutes or less when smoked).

Cocaine produces a rapid release of dopamine into the circulation, resulting in elevations of heart rate and blood pressure that are sometimes dramatic. Cardiac arrhythmias may be life-threatening. Deaths from cardiac arrest, presumably due to ventricular fibrillation, have been reported. Extreme elevation of blood pressure may result in a stroke.

Acute cardiac complications are managed as any other cardiovascular emergency. Community education about the dangers of cocaine use is essential to eliminate continuing risk of toxicity.

Methamphetamine

For many years, methamphetamine has been a drug of choice for gay and bisexual men. It produces stimulant effects similar to cocaine; users report more sustained enhancement of libido and sexual performance. Unlike the short duration of action of cocaine, the effects of methamphetamine may persist for 12 to 24 hours. A significant danger of these effects is that the meth user experiences such euphoria that he may disregard safe-sex practices and may be more likely to acquire any sexually transmitted disease, including HIV.

The cardiovascular effects of methamphetamine are similar to those of cocaine: elevated blood pressure, elevated pulse rate, cardiac arrhythmias, and increased risk of heart attack or stroke with short-term use; and enlargement, inflammation, and scarring of the heart muscle with chronic use (Robinson, 2005). At times, the chronic effects may be irreversible and produce a chronic cardiomyopathy, with weakness of the heart muscle and congestive heart failure. The cardiomyopathy increases the risk of arrhythmias, which can be life-threatening.

Management of heart damage from cocaine or from methamphetamine is dependent on stopping the use of the drug. In the past decade, community education has been effective in reducing the prevalence of stimulant use in the gay community, but the need for continuing education and prevention will always remain important as young people enter the community and are exposed to the opportunities for drug use.

CARDIOVASCULAR HEALTH AND TRANSGENDER PATIENTS

As a group, transgender persons are more likely to postpone seeking medical care, whether primary care for disease prevention or urgent care for acute symptoms. There are multiple reasons for this failure to access the health care system, including fear of discrimination, refusal of care by health care providers, and lack of ability to afford health care (Grant, 2010). The result is that risk factors for cardiovascular disease may go unrecognized and untreated until an acute cardiac or cerebrovascular event occurs.

The effects of hormone therapy on cardiovascular risk have been evaluated in large studies of nontransgender patients. The Women's Health Initiative (WHI) Study included a clinical trial that evaluated postmenopausal hormone therapy. Over 27,000 women participated in this study and were randomly assigned to three groups: estrogen (as conjugated estrogens) alone, estrogen plus progestin, or placebo. The study was stopped before its scheduled date of completion due to findings of increased risks in women taking estrogen, with or without progestin. It was found that women taking the combination had a 24 percent overall increased risk of developing coronary artery disease and a 31 percent increased risk of embolic stroke compared to women taking no hormone replacement. Women taking estrogen alone also had a higher risk of stroke, but their risk of coronary artery disease was not significantly increased, and in women younger than age 60, the risk of coronary disease was slightly reduced (Rossouw et al., 2002). In the WHI and several other studies, the cardiovascular risk was greatest in the first year after starting hormone therapy. Numerous studies have indicated that estrogen increases the risk of thromboembolic disease or clotting problems, including deep vein thrombosis and pulmonary embolism (Hulley & Grady, 2004). The cardiovascular risks of estrogen therapy are increased significantly in persons who smoke cigarettes (Wilson, Garrison, & Castelli, 1985).

The effects of testosterone on the cardiovascular system are less well studied. Testosterone is known to increase the blood level of LDL cholesterol. Polycystic ovary syndrome (PCOS) is common in female-to-male transgender patients (Baba et al., 2007) and is associated with insulin-resistant diabetes, obesity, and elevated testosterone levels.

It has been suggested that transdermal hormone therapy may be less likely than oral therapy to increase cardiovascular risk (Scarabin et al., 1997). Other routes of administration that have been used include intramuscular injection and sublingual absorption (for nonenteric-coated tablets).

Recommendations for Cardiovascular Evaluation of Transgender Patients

Prior to beginning hormone treatment, patients should be aware of the potential risks of hormone therapy. Smokers should be strongly urged to stop smoking. Persons with additional cardiac risk factors (hypertension, hyperlipidemia, diabetes) and/or are over 45 years old should be considered for cardiac stress testing for further risk assessment.

Persons with cardiac risk factors should consider taking aspirin, 81 milligrams daily, to reduce the risk of heart attack and stroke. There is no data to support anticoagulation with warfarin in persons without a history of thromboembolic disease or other specific indications for anticoagulation.

Consider transdermal hormone therapy for both female-to-male and male-to-female transgender persons who have additional cardiovascular risk factors. Other options include intramuscular injection of long-acting estrogen or testosterone. Estradiol can be taken sublingually, and so it may be preferable to conjugated estrogens. The use of progesterone may carry increased cardiovascular risk. If an androgen antagonist is used for a male-to-female patient, spironolactone may be valuable for its diuretic and antihypertensive properties.

Other cardiovascular risk factors are managed as they are in the general population. Persons being treated with spironolactone, who need additional antihypertensive treatment, should be monitored closely for potassium and sodium levels, especially if they are taking angiotensin converting enzyme (ACE) inhibitors or angiotensin receptor blockers (ARB).

Monitoring of liver function tests, as well as a lipid profile, should be done once a year in patients on transgender hormone therapy. A complete blood count should be performed in persons taking testosterone.

Finally, a regular exercise program can be very helpful for transgender (and lesbian, gay, and bisexual) patients. Inactivity can increase the risk of obesity, diabetes, and thromboembolic events. Exercise is especially important for persons preparing for major elective surgery. The positive psychological benefits of exercise can be significant in a population at increased risk for depression. Once an appropriate risk assessment has been completed and the patient is not at significantly increased cardiovascular risk, both aerobic exercise and weight training may be initiated safely.

SUMMARY

Cardiovascular disease (heart disease and stroke) is a major cause of illness and death among lesbian, gay, bisexual, and transgender persons. Young LGBT persons who practice healthy habits (maintain ideal body weight; exercise regularly; avoid tobacco, cocaine, and methamphetamine; and practice safe sex) are more likely to escape the health problems of cardiovascular disease later in life. All LGBT persons should make the effort to find a health care provider who is supportive of their unique health issues and skilled in their management. A strong relationship with a health care provider will improve adherence to such healthy habits.

REFERENCES

ACC/AHA/AAPA/ABC/ACPM/AGS/APhA/ASH/ASPC/NMA/PCNA guideline for the prevention, detection, evaluation, and management of high blood pressure in adults: A report of the American College of Cardiology/American Heart Association Task Force on Clinical Practice Guidelines. (2018). *Journal of the American College of Cardiology, 71*(19), e127–e248.

Baba, T., Endo, T., Honnma, H., Kitajima, Y., Hayashi, T., Ikeda, H. ... Saito, T. (2007). Association between polycystic ovary syndrome and female-to -male transsexuality. *Human Reproduction, 22*(4), 1011–1016.

Barbaro, G., DiLorenzo, G., Grisorio, B., & Barbarini, G. (1998). Incidence of dilated cardiomyopathy and detection of HIV in myocardial cells of HIV -positive patients. *New England Journal of Medicine, 339*(16), 1093–1099.

Blatt, B., et al. (2010). *Smoking out a deadly threat: Tobacco use in the LGBT community.* Washington, DC: American Lung Association.

Blumenthal, J. A., Babyak, M. A., Hinderliter, A., Watkins, L. L., Craighead, L., Lin, P. H., . . . Sherwood, A. (2010). Effects of the DASH diet alone and in combination with exercise and weight loss on blood pressure and cardiovascular biomarkers in men and women with high blood pressure: The ENCORE study. *Archives of Internal Medicine, 170*(2), 128–136.

Buchwald, H., Avidor, Y., Braunwald, E., Jensen, M. D., Pories, W., Fahrbach, K., & Schoelles, K. (2004). Bariatric surgery: A systematic review and meta -analysis. *JAMA, 292*(14), 1724–1737.

Chobanian, A. V., Bakris, G. L., Black, H. R., Cushman, W. C., Green, L.A., Izzo, J. L., Jr., . . . National High Blood Pressure Education Program Coordinating Committee. (2003). The seventh report of the joint national committee on prevention, detection, evaluation, and treatment of high blood pressure:

The JNC 7 report. *Journal of the American Medical Association, 289*(19), 2560–2572.

Cochran, S. D., Mays, V. M., Bowen, D., Gage, S., Bybee, D., Roberts, S. J., et al. (2001). Cancer-related risk indicators and preventive screening behaviors among lesbian and bisexual women. *American Journal of Public Health, 91*, 591–597.

Fingerhood, M. (2001). Full recovery from severe dilated cardiomyopathy in an HIV-infected patient. *The AIDS Reader, 11*(6), 333–335.

Gometz, E. D., Grimm, D., King, M., et al. (2006). *Association of lipid changes in HAART-treated individuals with apolipoprotein genotypes.* Presented at the 13th Conference on Retroviruses and Opportunistic Infections; February 5–8, 2006; Denver, CO, Abstract 768.

Grant, J., et al. (2010). *National transgender discrimination survey report on health and health care.* National Gay and Lesbian Task Force and National Center for Transgender Equality.

Grundy, S. M., Cleeman, J. I., Daniels, S. R., Donato, K. A., Eckel, R. H., Franklin, B. A., . . . Costa, F. (2005) Diagnosis and management of the metabolic syndrome: An American Heart Association/National Heart, Lung, and Blood Institute scientific statement. *Circulation, 112*(17), 2735–2752.

Guadamuz, T. E., Lim, S. H., Marshall, M. P., Friedman, M. S., & Silvestre, A. (2008). *Are gay men getting fatter? Prevalences and trends of overweight and obesity among a cohort of men in Pittsburgh.* Presented at the American Public Health Association Annual Meeting, 2008.

Hulley, S. B., & Grady, D. (2004). The WHI estrogen-alone trial—Do things look any better? *JAMA, 291*(14), 1769–1771.

Jorenby, D. E., Hays, J. T., Rigotti, N. A., Azoulay, S., Watsky, J., Williams, K. E., . . . Reeves, K. R. (2006). Efficacy of varenicline, an alpha4beta2 nicotinic acetylcholine receptor partial agonist, versus placebo or sustained-release bupropion for smoking cessation: A randomized controlled trial. *JAMA, 296*(1), 56–63.

Kenny, S. J., Aubert, R. E., & Geiss, L. S. (1995). Prevalence and incidence of non-insulin-dependent diabetes. In M. I. Harris, C. C. Cowie, M. P. Stern, E. J. Boyko, G. E. Reiber, & P. H. Bennett (Eds.), *Diabetes in America* (2nd ed., pp. 47–68). Bethesda, MD: National Institutes of Health

Kotler, D. P. (2009). HIV and antiretroviral therapy: Lipid abnormalities and associated cardiovascular risk in HIV-infected patients. *Journal of Acquired Immune Deficiency Syndromes, 49*(2), S279–S285.

Lee, G. L., Griffin, G. K., & Melvin, C. L. (2009). Tobacco use among sexual minorities in the USA: 1987 to May 2007: A systematic review. *Tobacco Control, 18*(4), 275–282.

Levy, D., & Brink, S. (2005). *A change of heart: How the people of Framingham, Massachusetts, helped unravel the mysteries of cardiovascular disease.* New York: Knopf.

McGill, H. C., & McMahan, C. A. (2005). Risk factors: Established, emerging, and controversial. In V. Fuster E. J. Topol, & E. G. Nabel (Eds.), *Atherothrombosis and coronary artery disease* (p. 24). Philadelphia, PA: Lippincott Williams & Wilkins.

Mokdad, A. H., Ford, E. S., Bowman, B. A., Dietz, W. H., Vinicor. F., Bales, V. S., & Marks, J. S. (2003). Prevalence of obesity, diabetes, and obesity-related health risk factors, 2001. *JAMA, 289*(1), 76–79.

Ogden, C. L., Carroll, M. D., Curtin, L. R., McDowell, M. A., Tabak, C. J., & Flegal, K. M. (2006). Prevalence of overweight and obesity in the United States, 1999–2004. *JAMA, 295*(13), 1549–1555.

Robinson, M. R. (2005). Chronic methamphetamine use linked to cardiomyopathy. *Poster presentation at 2005 Scientific Session of the American Heart Association.*

Romanelli, F., & Smith, K. M. (2004). Recreational use of sildenafil by HIV-positive and -negative homosexual/bisexual males. *Annals of Pharmacotherapy, 38*(6), 1024–1030.

Rossouw, J. E., Anderson, G. L., Prentice, R. L., LaCroix, A. Z., Kooperberg, C., Stefanick, M. L., . . . Writing Group for the Women's Health Initiative Investigators. (2002). Risks and benefits of estrogen plus progestin in healthy postmenopausal women: Principal results from the Women's Health Initiative randomized controlled trial. *JAMA, 288*(3), 321–333.

Scarabin, P. Y., Alhenc-Gelas, M., Plu-Bureau, G., Taisne, P., Agher, R., & Aiach, M. (1997). Effects of oral and transdermal estrogen/progesterone regimens on blood coagulation and fibrinolysis in postmenopausal women. *Arteriosclerosis, Thrombosis, and Vascular Biology, 17*(11), 371–378.

Stone, N. J., et al. (2014). 2013 ACC/AHA guideline on the treatment of blood cholesterol to reduce atherosclerotic cardiovascular risk in adults. *Circulation, 129*(Suppl 2), S1–S45.

Tonkin, A. M., Beauchamp, A., & Stevenson, C. (2009). The importance of extinguishing secondhand smoke. *Circulation, 120*(14), 1339–1341.

Wilson, P. W. F., Garrison, R. J., & Castelli, W. P. (1985). Postmenopausal estrogen use, cigarette smoking, and cardiovascular morbidity in women over 50—The Framingham Study. *New England Journal of Medicine, 313*(17), 1038–1043.

World Health Organization. (2008). *Fact Sheet 310.* Geneva, Switzerland: World Health Organization.

Xu, J. Q., Kochanek, K. D., Murphy, S. L., & Tejada-Vera, B. (2010). Deaths: Final data for 2007. *National Vital Statistics Reports, 58*(19), 5.

Yancey, A. K., Cochran, S. D., Corliss, H. L., & Mays, V. M. (2003). Correlates of overweight and obesity among lesbian and bisexual women. *Preventive Medicine, 36*(6), 676–683.

10

When a Welcoming Health Care Environment Matters Most

Diane Bruessow, Henry Ng, and Amy Wilson-Stronks

LGBT individuals and families are often faced with a number of challenges when accessing health care. These challenges include navigating assumptions—from what is in the patient registration forms through the clinical interaction, the patient satisfaction questionnaire, and the lack of tracking of our health outcomes—that LGBT individuals are heterosexual and cisgender (Bruessow, 2011).

A welcoming health care environment provides an opportunity for disclosure of information that is important to care, including sexual identity, sexual behavior, sexual attraction, assigned sex at birth, and gender identity. There are four critical opportunities related to the delivery of health care services when disclosure matter most:

- Patient registration and intake should allow LGBT patients to ensure their legal rights in visitation, advance directives, preferred name, and so forth;
- The clinical interaction requires history taking that is patient centered and appropriately incorporates sexual attraction, behaviors, and identity, as well as gender identity–assigned sex at birth;

- Patient satisfaction evaluations should capture the experiences of LGBT patients; and

- Health outcomes of LGBT patients should be tracked and improved. (Bruessow & Poteat, 2018)

MAKING IT SAFE TO DISCLOSE

Although many LGBT-inclusive nondiscrimination policies and practices are now mandated by federal regulation and required for hospital accreditation, fear of discrimination can inhibit LGBT patients from making these important disclosures. It is unethical for a health care provider to refuse to serve or deny care to a patient on the basis of sexual orientation or gender identity.

Section 1557 of the Patient Protection and Affordable Care Act (ACA) prohibits discrimination in health programs and activities on the basis of race, color, national origin, sex, age, or disability. This is the first law to prohibit sex discrimination in the delivery of health care, and it has been interpreted to include discrimination on the basis of sexual orientation and gender identity (Office of Civil Rights, U.S. Department of Health and Human Services, 2016).

It has been applied to health insurance issuers, health care providers (including pharmacies and health clinics), and some group health insurance plans. The law applies even if just one insurance plan or program receives any federal funds from the U.S. Department of Health and Human Services (HHS) (Office of Civil Rights, U.S. Department of Health and Human Services, 2017a).

One illustration of how HHS Centers for Medicare and Medicaid Services (CMS) supports nondiscrimination in health care is by enforcing the rights of patients—including same-sex partners—to designate their person of choice to make medical decisions on their behalf should they become unable to make their own decisions. This role is sometimes referred to in various federal, state, and local jurisdictions as a surrogate medical decision maker, health care proxy, or medical power of attorney.

CMS also has a policy implementing the recommendations of the Memorandum on Hospital Visitation from 2010, which states that hospitals that participate with CMS should allow patients to designate visitors regardless of sexual orientation, gender identity, or any other non-clinical factor (The White House, 2010). As of January 18, 2011, all hospitals that accept payment from Medicare and Medicaid must

> have written policies and procedures regarding the visitation rights of patients, including those setting forth any clinically necessary or reasonable restriction or limitation that the hospital may need to place on such rights and the reasons for the clinical restriction or limitation. A hospital must

meet the following requirements: (1) Inform each patient (or support person, where appropriate) of his or her visitation rights, including any clinical restriction or limitation on such rights, when he or she is informed of his or her other rights under this section. (2) Inform each patient (or support person, where appropriate) of the right, subject to his or her consent, to receive the visitors whom he or she designates, including, but not limited to, a spouse, a domestic partner (including a same-sex domestic partner), another family member, or a friend, and his or her right to withdraw or deny such consent at any time. (3) Not restrict, limit, or otherwise deny visitation privileges on the basis of race, color, national origin, religion, sex, gender identity, sexual orientation, or disability. (4) Ensure that all visitors enjoy full and equal visitation privileges consistent with patient preferences.

Shortly thereafter, the Joint Commission, an independent, nonprofit organization that accredits and certifies health care organizations and facilities in the United States, updated its accreditation standards to also prohibit discrimination in hospital visitation on the basis of sexual orientation and gender identity (The Joint Commission, 2011).

Both CMS and the Joint Commission have patient-friendly Web sites where individuals may file complaints against health care staff and institutions (Office of Civil Rights, U.S. Department of Health and Human Services, 2017b; Joint Commission International, n.d.).

BEFORE ACCESSING HEALTH CARE

The quality of health care for LGBT individuals and families can be enhanced with a few simple strategies and resources. Before individuals and families access health care, it may be helpful to jot down any questions that they may have for their providers. Patient-oriented health resources such as Medlineplus.gov, which is a joint program of the National Library of Medicine and the National Institutes of Health, were created specifically for patients and may help individuals and families to formulate their questions ahead of time. MedlinePlus content is available in multiple languages and at various reading levels.

During the health care encounter, it may be helpful to make notes on the experience—With whom did the patient or family members speak? What tests were done? What treatments were ordered or given? Bringing a trusted friend or family member (referred to as a patient advocate) to health care appointments and any hospital-based encounters can provide another layer of support. Information regarding whom to contact if there are any concerns may be especially useful, such as internal resources (patient advocates, social workers, chaplaincy services, grievance procedures, etc.) or external resources, such as those mentioned throughout this chapter.

Patient advocacy training may be helpful to improve the quality of health care outcomes achieved by LGBT individuals and families. If there are no training opportunities available in your area, the Joint Commission's Speak Up campaign has a series of award-winning animated videos and infographics (The Joint Commission, 2002).

Patient Registration Process

Most people think that the forms they fill out during their first appointment in a new health care setting are only for billing purposes. However, these forms also serve as an opportunity to ensure an individual and family's legal rights.

Intake forms should provide an opportunity to identify a patient's preferred name, gender identity, and sex assigned at birth in addition to other information such as age, racial and ethnic identity, spiritual identity, family composition, and employment. Electronic health records are becoming more LGBT inclusive. Some intake processes have been amended to update options in the parent/guardian section of the registration process to have the ability to add the same relationship multiple times (i.e., two mothers or two fathers); some allow a system flag as a reminder to use a patient's preferred name and pronouns; and some allow for assigned sex at birth as well as gender identity. Presenting this information during the patient registration process should help mitigate assumptions that all patients are heterosexual and cisgender. Questions about sexual attraction, behavior, and identity are not typically part of the registration process and are usually deferred until the clinical encounter.

Advance directives are written statements to ensure the individual's wishes are carried out should the person be unable to communicate them at a later date. These directives provide individuals with a proactive opportunity to communicate their wishes to family, friends, and health care professionals and may help to avoid confusion later on. Without written advance directives, when patients are unable to make their own health care decisions, health care providers will follow their health system's protocol for determining which family member will be asked to make your decisions. While access to marriage has mitigated many of the barriers faced by same-sex couples, many states still have barriers to adoption for same-sex couples that could result in a legally unrecognized parent or guardian being left out of their minor child's care.

There are different types of advance directives. A living will provides instructions concerning medical treatments, while a medical power of attorney or health care proxy allows a trusted person to be designated as a surrogate medical decision maker who is authorized to make medical decisions when someone is unable to make their own decisions.

Advance directives are recognized throughout the United States. The terminology used to describe advance directives varies, as laws defining advanced directives vary from state to state. Depending on what state you are living in, advanced directives may include a living will, medical power of attorney, medical directive, a directive to physicians, declaration regarding health care, designation of health care surrogate, patient advocate designation, or health care proxy. Legal experts recommend that LGBT individuals and families complete advance directives for each state they spend a significant amount of time in. The American Hospital Association provides templates of advanced directives for personal and family use by individuals for every state and the District of Columbia, as well as instructions (American Hospital Association, n.d.).

Visitation directives, as mentioned earlier in this chapter, may not be included in advance directives. Visitation directives allow each individual to define who they want to allow access to visit them while they hospitalized. Visitation directives also provide an opportunity to name individuals who are not allowed to visit. When LGBT individuals and families are estranged from their biological relatives, it can be helpful to signal to hospital staff who matters most. These exclusions can be named individually or by referring to biological relatives in general (Human Rights Campaign, n.d.).

After one has completed all of these advance directives, he, she, or they should distribute copies to loved ones as well as to the primary care provider. There are also companies that provide electronic access service for health care directives. These companies make health care documents instantly available in an emergency through an automated fax or secure Web page.

A welcoming health care environment provides opportunities to ensure that an individual and associated loved ones are recognized and that one's wishes are legally protected in writing.

THE CLINICAL ENCOUNTER

Regardless of the setting—whether an encounter is for an office visit, a visit to the emergency room, or a health care professional is coming to a home, one can expect to be asked a series of questions and experience some level of physical examination. In a welcoming environment, health care providers seek patient input on affirming language to describe their partners, their anatomy, and themselves.

The Health History

Access to a new health care provider is always expected to take longer than after a patient relationship is established. One reason for this is the quantity of historical information that needs to be communicated.

Creating and maintaining a personal health record or patient health record (PHR) can help ensure that nothing of importance is overlooked during transfer of care to a new provider or during emergency care. The information to include within the PHR may include the patient's name, birth date, blood type, emergency contact information, date of last physical exam, dates and results of tests and screenings, all major illnesses and surgeries with dates, all vaccinations with dates; a list of medications and supplements, their dosages, and how long they've been taken; any allergies and the reactions they cause; any chronic diseases; and any history of illnesses in one's biological parents, siblings, and children.

Once the patient's historical health information has been gathered, there are different ways to maintain a PHR: paper files can be placed in a folder, the information can be scanned and saved on a password-protected flash drive, and there are also Web-based applications designed for this purpose (Office of the National Coordinator for Health Information Technology, 2013).

Beyond a patient's historical health information, heath care providers are trained to explore the patient's health complaint and the history of their present illness or injury. Patients will be asked questions about their current state of health and any other symptoms they might have.

Health care providers are also trained to explore the many other factors that can influence health and wellness, specifically the patient's thoughts, behaviors, and environment. This is referred to as the psychosocial history and is where sexual attraction, sexual behavior, sexual identity, and gender identity are most commonly discussed. Other areas of concern can include the environments (e.g., school, work, and home), behaviors (e.g., with regard to seatbelts, bike helmets, or condom use, as well as tobacco or alcohol use), among others. Sometimes a health history will also include questions about the patient's thoughts and feelings. How these questions are asked can be as important as what is being asked.

In a welcoming environment, health care providers are forthcoming about the relevance of their questions and how any sensitive information will be recorded. When this is not the case, it is appropriate to raise these questions to the provider.

There is a health care theory referred to as "cultural humility" that suggests that cultural competence is not something that can be fully achieved. Cultural humility suggests that providers should not make any assumptions about or based on a patient's identities. To illustrate cultural humility: a provider would not assume that a self-identified gay or lesbian patient has had sexual attraction to or sexual behavior with only people of the same gender, or the anatomy or gender of their partners. Nor would a provider assume that a man who has sex with men identifies as gay or bisexual. Given the diversity within LGBT communities, approaching patients with cultural humility allows for a more comprehensive inquiry and meaningful communication between providers and their LGBT patients beyond asking, "Do you have sex with men, women, or both?"

The Physical Examination

With the exception of life-saving treatment being delivered at the scene of an accident, all patients should expect a respectful level of privacy to include draping (covering of parts of the body that are not being examined), limiting the number of people present to essential personnel, and conversations at an appropriate volume to maintain privacy and confidentiality. One exception is a requirement for many health care institutions to have a chaperone in the room during sensitive physical examinations such as breast and genital exams.

Patients are encouraged to ask all personnel involved in their care to identify themselves and their roles. Patients should be given the opportunity to accept or decline engagement by anyone not directly responsible for their care (e.g., students), and patients may request to have a patient advocate of their choosing in the room.

Just as patients have the right to limit those present during their physical exam to the professionals who are responsible for their care, they also might choose to inquire about the relevance of the breadth of the physical exam to the possible diagnoses that are being considered. In a welcoming environment, health care providers are forthcoming about the relevance of sensitive aspects of the physical exam. When this is not the case, a patient may choose to decline to allow the examination until these questions are answered to their satisfaction. The caveat to this recommendation is that some illnesses and injuries require timely identification and treatment.

In a welcoming environment, health care providers are responsive to affirming language to describe each patient and their anatomy. A health care provider in a welcoming environment will appreciate this opportunity to help their patient be at ease. This is especially important for affirming a patient's gender identity (e.g., referring to chest or breasts based on patient preference.)

Screenings and Diagnostic Testing

In a welcoming environment, health care providers answer all questions about the testing being recommended. There are some circumstances where the rules regarding nondiscrimination on the basis of sexual orientation and gender identity may be incongruent with medical necessity if it is for the purpose of "doing no harm" or intended for early detection of cancer or other illness. In other words, testing can sometimes be incongruent with our identities. One such scenario might involve requesting a pregnancy test from a person who was assigned female at birth whose uterus is intact, regardless of their gender identity, as well as someone assigned female at birth who identifies as a lesbian. Another such scenario may include a person who was assigned male at birth who identifies as female may benefit from cancer screenings of the prostate. A person who was assigned female at birth and identifies as male may benefit from cervical cancer screening; however, sending this patient to a gynecologist located within a women's health pavilion would be an incongruent environment to their gender identity. The chapters on cancer discuss this in more detail. Another illustration would be the criteria for fertility treatments that are relevant to heterosexual, cisgender couples may not be relevant to same-gender couples (e.g., 12 months of actively trying to conceive).

Referrals

Some third-party payors (insurance companies) require the identification number of the specialist to be included on the referral at the time the referral is processed. In this situation, a patient may not have an opportunity to research whether that specialist is knowledgeable of LGBT health. Sometimes there is only one specialist within a health insurance plan. It is common to not have anyone within a plan that is experienced in gender-affirming procedures. Each insurer has a written process for filing a grievance or appeal of a coverage decision.

Refer to other sections of this chapter regarding recommendations before you access health care, resources to ensure your rights, where to file complaints involving providers and insurers, and finding a provider who is knowledgeable of LGBT health.

PATIENT SATISFACTION

Patient satisfaction surveys provide an opportunity for patients to have a direct impact on the health systems and health care professionals who provide care. Patients who complete satisfaction surveys help to keep health care professionals and institutions accountable and even have an influence how much a health care provider will be paid for the services they provided.

Patient satisfaction surveys are also sometimes used to define value in health care delivery in the United States. There is increasing utilization of a fee-for-value model of health care delivery, where providers are paid based on patient outcomes. In the value-based model, patient satisfaction is one of the metrics being measured and used to define value. This is a one of the differences from the current fee-for-service model, where providers are paid based on the services a patient receives, regardless of outcomes.

A welcoming health care environment provides an opportunity for patients to identify themselves as LGBT within the satisfaction survey and will respond to trends in patient satisfaction affecting LGBT patients.

HEALTH OUTCOMES

Health outcomes focus on the results of health care activities—specifically, how much better or worse a patient's illness or injury became from the physical, mental, and social perspective. It doesn't focus on the activity per se, but on the results of the activity. Health outcomes can be measured individually or in groups.

HHS has identified objectives within the following topic areas as being of particular importance to health outcomes for LGBT adolescents and adults. These topic areas include binge drinking and alcohol use, breast cancer screening, bullying among adolescents, cervical cancer screening, condom use, educational achievement, health insurance coverage, HIV testing, illicit drug use, mental health and mental illness, nutrition and weight status, tobacco use, and having a usual source of health care (Office of Disease Prevention and Health Promotion, 2018).

Health experts will sometimes say they cannot improve what is not measured. Measurement also allows efforts that improve the health of our communities to be identified so that they may be more widely implemented. Improving health outcomes for LGBT individuals and families means first being able to identify LGBT patients, monitor their health outcomes, and contrast their health outcomes with all other patients. Many health care systems have taken the first step by including sexual identity, assigned sex at birth, and gender identity as part of their intake process (IOM, 2013).

A welcoming health care environment provides an opportunity for patients to identify themselves as LGBT and monitors for trends in health outcomes affecting LGBT patients.

FINDING A PROVIDER

Some LGBT individuals seek care in specialized environments at LGBT community health clinics (Centers for Disease Control and Prevention, 2014). Others turn to resources like the provider directories offered by

GLMA, the World Professional Association for Transgender Health (WPATH), RAD Remedy, My Trans Health, or Out Care Health (GLMA, n.d.; World Professional Association for Transgender Health, n.d.; RAD Remedy, n.d.; My Trans Health, n.d.) However, these options are not accessible everywhere, so LGBT individuals and families need to be prepared to serve as our own advocates.

Becoming aware of institutional policies and practices is another important step. The Human Rights Campaign Foundation in partnership with GLMA launched the Healthcare Equality Index (HEI) in 2007. HEI is a national LGBT benchmarking tool that evaluates health care facilities' policies and practices related to the equity and inclusion of the LGBT patients, visitors, and employees. It is the only tool of its kind in the United States to explore institutional policies on an annual basis and to present findings to the public through a user-friendly Web portal. There are four core criteria, including inclusive and nondiscrimination policies specifically for LGBT patients, families, and employees, as well as training for all staff to ensure policies are implemented into practice (Human Rights Campaign Foundation, n.d.).

CONCLUSION

There has been remarkable progress in the development of legal and regulatory protections for LGBT individuals and families, and thanks to efforts like the HRC Foundation's Healthcare Equality Index and the Joint Commission's accreditation standards, institutional policies and provider competencies are moving forward as well. This chapter has shared best and promising practices regarding welcoming health care environments, including how LGBT individuals and family may prepare before accessing care; finding a provider; where and when disclosure of sexual identity, sexual behavior, sexual attraction, assigned sex at birth, and gender identity matters most; as well as where to submit grievances when health care isn't caring. Health care has been more dynamic in the last 5 years than it has been in the last 50 years, and this chapter's authors anticipate that changes will continue to occur after the publication of this handbook.

REFERENCES

American Hospital Association. (n.d.). Put it in writing. Retrieved February 2018 from https://www.aha.org//2017-12-11-put-it-writing

Bruessow, D. (2011). Keeing up with LGBT health: Why it matters to your patients. *JAAPA, 24*(3), 14.

Bruessow, D., & Poteat, T. (2018). Primary care providers' role in transgender healthcare. *JAAPA, 31*(2), 8–11.

Centers for Disease Control and Prevention. (2014). LGBT health. Retrieved from http://www.cdc.gov/lgbthealth/health-services.htmhttp://bit.ly/fV5e9Z

Gay and Lesbian Medical Association. (n.d.). Find a provider. Retrieved March 2018 from http://bit.ly/SGhd1O

Human Rights Campaign. (n.d.). Protecting your visitation and decision-making rights. Retrieved from https://www.hrc.org/resources/protecting-your -visitation-decision-making-rights

Human Rights Campaign Foundation. (n.d.). Healthcare equality index. Retrieved March 2018 from http://www.hrc.org/hei

Institute of Medicine. (2013). *Collecting sexual orientation and gender identity data in electronic health records: Workshop summary.* Washington, DC: The National Academies Press.

The Joint Commission. (2002). Speak Up initiatives. Retrieved from https://www .jointcommission.org/speakup.aspx

The Joint Commission. (2011a). *Advancing effective communication, cultural competence, and patient- and family-centered care for the lesbian, gay, bisexual, and transgender (LGBT) community: A field guide.* Retrieved from https:// www.jointcommission.org/assets/1/18/LGBTFieldGuide.pdf

The Joint Commission. (2011b). Requirements related to CMS patient visitation rights: Conditions of participation. Retrieved from https://www.jointcom mission.org/assets/1/6/20110701_Visitation_Rights_HAP.pdf

Joint Commission International. (n.d.). Report a quality and safety issue with a JCI-accredited organization. Retrieved from https://www.jointcommission international.org/contact-us/report-a-quality-and-safety-issue/

Office of Civil Rights, U.S. Department of Health and Human Services. (2016). OCR enforcement under Section 1557 of the affordable care act sex discrimination cases. Retrieved from https://www.hhs.gov/civil-rights /for-individuals/section-1557/ocr-enforcement-section-1557-aca-sex -discrimination/index.html

Office of Civil Rights, U.S. Department of Health and Human Services. (2017a). Section 1557 of the patient protection and affordable care act. Retrieved from https://www.hhs.gov/civil-rights/for-individuals/section-1557

Office of Civil Rights, U.S. Department of Health and Human Services. (2017b). How to file a civil rights complaint. Retrieved from https://www.hhs.gov /civil-rights/filing-a-complaint/complaint-process/index.html

Office of Disease Prevention and Health Promotion. (2018). Healthy people 2020. Retrieved from https://www.healthypeople.gov/2020/topics-objectives /topic/lesbian-gay-bisexual-and-transgender-health/objectives

Office of the National Coordinator for Health Information Technology. (2013). What is a personal health record? Retrieved from https://www.healthit .gov/providers-professionals/faqs/what-personal-health-record

RAD Remedy. (n.d.). Find a provider. Retrieved March 2018 from https://rad remedy.org/

The White House. (2010). Presidential memoranda. Retrieved from https://obama whitehouse.archives.gov/the-press-office/presidential-memorandum -hospital-visitation

World Professional Association for Transgender Health. (n.d.). Find a provider. Retrieved March 2018 from http://bit.ly/2HUUutO

11

LGBT Health beyond North America

Megan C. Lytle, Travis P. Sherer, and Vincent M. B. Silenzio

In order to thoughtfully examine the health concerns of lesbian, gay, bisexual, and transgender (LGBT) individuals across the globe, it is essential to consider the roots from which laws and policies related to sexual orientation and gender identity stem. The intersection of religious and cultural traditions has led to the criminalization and practice of pathologizing LGBT individuals for not fitting into societal constraints. As a result, the mental and physical health needs of LGBT individuals have been relatively overlooked, and laws and policies that prevent LGBT individuals from receiving basic rights (e.g., health care) persist. Although the medical and mental health fields in most developed nations have evolved significantly over the past 40 years, barriers to accessing services, concerns about receiving optimal care, and legalized discrimination continue to impact LGBT health in and beyond North America.

Therefore, this chapter will begin with an overview of laws and policies specific to LGBT individuals; we will examine LGBT mental and physical health concerns; and last, we will explore the status of LGBT rights and health concerns across the world. Recommendations and resources are also provided.

LAWS AND POLICIES FROM ANTIQUITY THROUGH PRESENT DAY

The laws and policies regarding LGBT rights have evolved throughout history. In the patriarchy of ancient Greece and Rome, there were no laws regarding same-sex behaviors and relationships among men (Simon & Brooks, 2009); however, there were expectations about social status. Same-sex relationships between men of equal status were not socially acceptable, whereas relationships between men of different social strata, such as relations with male slaves, were tolerated. Until the rise of Christianity, most Roman emperors had male lovers. Indeed, Roman Emperor Nero was reported to have had at least one marriage to another man. According to Stewart (2010), same-sex relationships between women were not uncommon in China during the Ming dynasty. In Japan during the 1800s, hierarchical relationships between boys and men were typical, and during the Middle Ages, same-sex marriages between men were legally recognized in parts of Europe (Stewart, 2010). However, religiously based views of sodomy (regardless of sexual orientation) became prevalent during the Middle Ages and resulted in the criminalization of male homosexuality, which was punishable by death (Benkov, 2000; Simon & Brooks, 2009). In ancient Greece and Rome, same-sex relationships between women were not permitted. Although there are fewer historical accounts of lesbianism during the Middle Ages, same-sex behaviors between women eventually resulted in capital punishment (Greenberg, 1990; Benkov, 2000). However, by the 18th century, some European countries had started to decriminalize homosexuality and/or reduced the punishment (Greenberg, 1990).

Aside from religious and legal sanctions against same-sex relationships, reports of medical remedies for homosexuality were developed as early as medieval times. Practices such as cauterization (i.e., to burn tissue) were used to treat women who had sexual desires for other women (Benkov, 2000). By the late 19th and early 20th centuries, physicians began to consider homosexuality a medical disorder, and some practitioners started advocating against laws that criminalized homosexuality, citing that it was not volitional (Minton, 2002). Even before homosexuality was labeled a mental illness in the first *Diagnostic and Statistical Manual of Mental Disorders* (DSM), physicians were suggesting that same-sex behaviors should be treated with self-acceptance (Minton, 2002). Yet, the medical field varied greatly in how its members viewed homosexuality and whether it could be cured (Minton, 2002).

The term "homosexuality" originated in 1869 (Minton, 2002), and in 1910, sexologists and physicians started to examine the differences between gender identity and sexual orientation. Moreover, self-labels for identifying sexual orientation and gender identity have continuously progressed and vary greatly between cultures. Transgender individuals may identify as female-to-male (i.e., experiencing a gender transition), whereas others identify as male-to-male (i.e., experiencing a consistent gender). Some individuals identify as men who have sex with men (MSM), women who have sex with women (WSW), or queer instead of LGBT; however, the laws and policies that impact LGBT health usually focus on behavior rather than identity and are relevant across cultures. Further, due to the intersection between gender and sexual identities, lawmakers have overlooked the needs of transgender individuals.

In 2007, the *Yogyakarta Principles: Principles on the Application of International Human Rights Law in Relation to Sexual Orientation and Gender Identity* were introduced at the United Nations Human Rights Council. Although the Yogyakarta Principles have influenced the United Nation's (UN's) stance toward LGBT rights, this is not an official UN document; nor is it legally binding (Arus Pelangi, 2009). In 2011, the Office of the High Commissioner for Human Rights (OHCHR) released a report about violence and discrimination against LGBT individuals. In addition to demanding that LGBT individuals are guaranteed basic human rights, these documents suggest that due to laws and policies across the world, the health care needs of LGBT individuals have not been adequately addressed. Specifically, the UN's report mentioned that discrimination against LGBT individuals has resulted in harmful and medically unnecessary treatments such as reparative therapy and sexual reassignment surgery (SRS) for intersex children (OHCHR, 2011). The Yogyakarta Principles (2007) go beyond arguing for optimal mental and physical health care and contend that LGBT individuals must be protected from medical abuse, both mental and physical.

LGBT HEALTH

Mental Health

Over the years, the mental health field has shifted from pathologizing homosexuality toward trying to understand the experiences of LGB persons, and in 2011, the American Psychological Association (APA) updated its guidelines for working with LGB individuals. Although clinicians and scholars still tend to focus on negative experiences such as oppression and stigma, more recently, they have started to examine the strengths and positive attributes of LGB individuals. Conversion therapy used to be a standard of care for treating sexual minorities (Dworkin, 2003; Minton, 2002) until 1973, when homosexuality was removed from the DSM; and in 1992, the World Health Organization (WHO) declassified it as a mental illness (Dworkin, 2003). However, even today, some clinicians still provide this "treatment," although it is viewed as deleterious, and in 1998, the APA posted a position statement citing that reorientation therapy was unethical and harmful. Recently, the American Psychiatric Association (2013) replaced Gender Identity Disorder (GID) with Gender Dysphoria in the DSM-5 as a step toward decreasing stigma without limiting access to care, regardless of transition status. The term "disorder" was replaced because gender nonconformity is not considered a mental illness, but since insurance coverage is contingent on a diagnosis, Gender Dysphoria was included in the manual.

According to Meyer (2003), the discrimination and stigma (i.e., minority stress) that LGBT persons continue to face has resulted in higher incidence of mental health concerns. Below are just some of the mental health concerns that LGBT individuals across the world may experience. Thus, until there are dramatic changes with public policy and societal prejudice, practitioners must acknowledge their own biases, receive cultural competency training, and recognize barriers that prevent LGBT individuals from seeking care.

Anxiety and Depression. Given the levels of discrimination, prejudice, and stigma toward LGBT individuals, it is not surprising that they tend to report higher levels of anxiety and depression. Sandfort and colleagues (2001) reported that gay men have a three-times-greater prevalence of being diagnosed with an anxiety or mood disorder, while lesbians were twice as likely to have a lifetime prevalence for mood disorders. Although LGB individuals tend to have higher rates of mental health disorders, these discrepancies were insignificant after controlling for psychosocial factors (Safren & Heimberg, 1999). For instance, the International Gay and Lesbian Human Rights Commission (IGLHRC, 2003) reported that lesbian women in India who concealed their identities were more isolated and at risk of depression, substance use, and suicide. Similarly, Polders and colleagues (2008) found that lower levels of self-esteem and higher levels of hate speech predicted depression among South African sexual minorities.

Substance Use. Lesbian and bisexual women frequently report higher rates of substance use. Specifically, lesbian and bisexual women have substance use rates that ranged from three to four times greater than heterosexual women, while the odds of gay and bisexual men reporting substance misuse were approximately two times greater than heterosexual men (King et al., 2008). Moreover, Ortiz-Hernández and colleagues (2009) found that Mexican LGB youth (15 to 24 years old) reported greater odds of smoking and drinking alcohol compared to heterosexuals, with lesbian and bisexual women having the highest prevalence of substance use. Further, the current and lifetime use of alcohol and tobacco were mediated by family violence, crimes, and violated rights, suggesting that discrimination and violence against LGBT individuals explains part of these discrepancies (Ortiz-Hernández et al., 2009).

Suicide. In 2008, King and colleagues completed a systematic review of the mental health concerns among LGB individuals and reported that the odds of LGB individuals attempting suicide (i.e., over 12 months) was twice that of heterosexuals, with gay and bisexual men reporting a lifetime prevalence of suicide attempts that was four times greater than that of heterosexuals. Moreover, researchers have started to demonstrate that LGB individuals with multiple minority statuses may report higher rates of suicide attempts. For instance, black, Latino, and older LGB individuals had greater odds of reporting suicide attempts than white and younger LGB people (Meyer, Dietrich, & Schwartz, 2008; O'Donnell, Meyer, & Schwartz, 2011). Clements-Nolle, Marx, and Katz (2006) conducted one of the few studies about suicidal behavior in the transgender population. Almost one-third of their sample had attempted suicide, and approximately half of the respondents under the age of 25 had attempted suicide. From a global perspective, LGBT individuals face additional challenges beyond discrimination and violence that impact suicidal thoughts and behaviors. For example, due to the laws and policies that criminalize homosexuality, some countries have bolstered their asylum policies, and there have been reports of LGBT asylum seekers committing suicide after their applications were denied (Cviklová, 2012).

Physical Health

In conjunction with the mental health approaches that attempt to cure homosexuality and gender nonconformity, the medical model has used a number of methods (e.g., electroshock convulsive therapy, lobotomies, and castration) to treat LGBT individuals (Meem, Gibson, & Alexander, 2010). Early in the 20th century, doctors started to develop gender affirmation surgery (GAS) methods for transgender individuals, and until recently, sex reassignment surgery was used to treat intersex individuals, often without permission (Meem et al., 2010). Over time, the American Medical Association (AMA, 2013) has developed policies for LGBT physicians, students, and patients in order to prevent discrimination and to improve the quality of treatment for LGBT individuals. Aside from mental health and sexually transmitted illnesses such as HIV/AIDS, research and training focusing on the health concerns of LGBT individuals has lagged behind, resulting in inadequate health care.

Cancer. For various reasons, LGBT individuals may have a greater risk for certain types of cancer. Due to stigma from medical providers, lesbians are less likely to seek treatment, thus increasing their odds of having a delayed diagnosis of breast or cervical cancer. Specifically, Ben-Natan and Adir (2009) found that only 22 percent of Israeli lesbians in their sample had ever had a Pap smear. Conversely, providers may not check lesbian patients for cervical cancer, based on the assumption that lesbians do not have sex with men (Katz, 2011). Yet, an international literature review suggested that lesbian women, regardless of their sexual histories, may be at risk of cervical cancer. Additionally, gay men may have higher rates of anal cancer depending on their sexual behaviors, but again, providers assume that all gay men have an equal risk of anal cancer rather than asking about their sexual health for clarification (Katz, 2011). An Australian study found that a low percentage of MSM were aware of their risk for anal cancer and human papillomavirus; therefore, they did not seek preventive treatments (Pitts, Fox, Willis & Anderson, 2007). While bisexual men and women have been understudied, similar risks still apply.

Heart Disease. Elevated substance use, hormone treatments, and minority stress are among the risk factors that may result in hypertension and high blood pressure among LGBT individuals (Boehmer & Bowen, 2007). According to the Committee on Lesbian, Gay, Bisexual, and Transgender Health Issues and partners (2011), few international research studies that have investigated the risk of coronary disease among LGBT individuals, since most researchers focus on people living with HIV/AIDS (PLWHA) or individuals undergoing hormone treatments. Due to contradictory findings, additional research examining the prevalence of heart disease among LGBT individuals in comparison to non-LGBT individuals is needed.

HIV Status and Immigration. In 2010, the U.S. Citizen and Immigration Services overturned their ban that prevented PLWHA from gaining admission to the United States. According to the UNAIDS policy brief (2008), approximately 60 countries have bans that prevent PLWHA from immigrating to their nations, citing health and economic reasons. The medical care, confidentiality, and stigma toward PLWHA vary between countries; thus, being diagnosed with HIV/AIDS during the immigration process may lead to deportation back to a country without adequate treatment (UNAIDS, 2008). While some nations do not protect PLWHA from legalized discrimination, others use HIV to justify laws against homosexuality. Either scenario has the potential to exacerbate stigma and violence toward LGBT individuals and PLWHA.

LGBT HEALTH, LAWS, AND POLICIES ACROSS THE GLOBE

Africa

Cameroon. Homosexuality is against the law in Cameroon, and due to stigma, most lesbian and gay individuals identify as bisexuals (Gueboguo, 2010). International reports describe how LGBT individuals are often denied medical care in prison or forced to have medical anal examination to obtain evidence of sodomy (Alternatives Cameroun, Centre for Human Rights, & IGLHRC, 2010). The prejudice is so rampant that individuals can be arrested based on perceived sexual orientation, and individuals are often detained for extended periods of time. Indeed, the HIV rate in the general population is 5.4 percent, whereas the estimated prevalence in the LGBT community is 18 percent (Gueboguo, 2010), and the government has used HIV rate discrepancies to support the criminalization of LGBT individuals rather than develop HIV prevention for this community (Alternatives Cameroun, et al., 2010). Although legalized and societal discrimination limits the rights of LGBT individuals, there are some organizations, such as Alternatives Cameroun, that provide legal, medical, and financial aid to LGBT individuals (Gueboguo, 2010).

Malawi. Although the recent change in leadership holds promise that the status of LGBT individuals in Malawi will improve, increased homophobia in Africa remains a barrier. In 2009, due to pressure from the United Nations secretary-general, President Mutharika pardoned two men who were arrested for "gross indecency" after their marriage; however, in 2011, the law against consensual same-sex behaviors was expanded to include women (Center of Development of People, Center for Human Rights, & IGLHRC, 2011). Since President Banda took office, she ambivalently discussed overturning the sodomy laws, and in October of 2012 she officially suspended them (Ugwu, 2012).

Another concern is the government's control over HIV/AIDS testing and the lack of confidentiality regarding test results. According to the Center of Development of People (CDP), Center for Human Rights (CHR), and IGLHRC (2011), some groups have been forced to have HIV/AIDS tests, with the results published in the newspaper. Although the barriers to LGBT health in Malawi remain, there has been progress. In December 2011, the Fenway Institute was involved with HIV prevention training programs geared toward MSM (Kapila, 2012). Local health care providers received training about sexually transmitted illnesses and HIV, while peer educators were given psychoeducation about internalized homophobia and safe-sex practices.

South Africa. There are discrepancies between the legal rights of LGBT individuals and deep-rooted social prejudice in South Africa. The 1996 revised constitution protected the rights of LGBT individuals, and by 2003, marriage equality, the right to joint adoptions, and equal opportunity in employment were granted (Butler & Astbury, 2005). Although LGBT individuals enjoy legal freedoms, violence and harassment toward them have increased. Mieses (2009) reported on the occurrence of "corrective rape," in which lesbians are sexually assaulted as a punishment for their sexual orientation or an attempt to change their sexual identity. To make matters worse, few perpetrators have been convicted, none of these offenses were labeled as hate crimes, and, aside from traumatizing women, it puts them at risk for such sexually transmitted illnesses (STIs) (Mieses,

2009). Although corrective rape is associated with South Africa, there have been reports of this crime across the globe, including in Uganda, Jamaica, and the United Sates (Pillay, 2011).

Due to social stigma, LGBT individuals have reported varying levels of satisfaction with their health care providers. White LGBT individuals have reported higher levels of satisfaction with their doctors since they can afford to meet with private physicians, whereas black LGBT individuals tend to consult government providers and are less likely to be satisfied with their health care (Wells, 2006). Regardless of how LGBT individuals view their doctors, Wells (2006) found that almost two-thirds reported being tested for HIV. Compared to most African states, LGBT individuals in South Africa have more rights and better access to health care.

Uganda. In Uganda currently, homosexuality is punishable with life imprisonment, but the government has proposed to increase this sentence to the death penalty (Freedom and Roam Uganda [FARUG] & IGLHRC, 2010) and plans to make the promotion of homosexuality illegal (i.e., funding or sponsoring LGBT organizations, disseminating LGBT materials, or community events supporting LGBT individuals) (Amnesty International, 2012). Aside from legalized discrimination, the media targets LGBT individuals. Newspapers and television networks list the names, photos, addresses, and car descriptions of people who are assumed to be LGBT, and these media outlets have called for Ugandans to attack and/or murder LGBT individuals (FARUG & IGLHRC, 2010). Additionally, the health care system exacerbates the stigma and fear that LGBT individuals live with, since individuals are subjected to unauthorized medical procedures, threatened if they disclose their sexual orientation or gender identity, and cannot always access the care they need (FARUG & IGLHRC, 2010).

Asia

China. In 1997, China decriminalized homosexuality, and by 2001, it was no longer considered a mental disorder; however, LGBT individuals still face discrimination and police harassment (Mountford, 2009). While homosexuality is no longer considered a psychiatric diagnosis, in 2011, the Hong Kong government sponsored a workshop promoting reparative therapy (Cho & Chan, 2011). Stigma against LGBT individuals in China has been exacerbated by the government's censorship of the media, which prohibits LGBT content in television programs, film, print, and Web sites, aside from health-related materials (Mountford, 2009). Specifically, the HIV/AIDS epidemic in China has resulted in government sponsored HIV/AIDS education and prevention programs targeted toward MSM (Chen et al., 2012). In a study comparing MSM who engage in high-risk sexual behaviors to a MSM control group, the high-risk group was more likely to be married, have suicidal ideations, and drink more, suggesting that stigma may have a negative influence on sexual minorities in China.

While transgender individuals have the right to undergo GAS, there are numerous social barriers that prevent people from receiving this medical procedure. For instance, to qualify for GAS, transgender individuals must prove that their family members are aware of the potential surgery, are required to live and work as the other gender, cannot be married, and cannot be under criminal investigation (Mountford, 2009). Unfortunately, this creates a potentially inescapable situation, since transgender individuals often struggle to find work due to prejudice, and if they are prosecuted for sex work they cannot qualify for surgery.

India. As a British colony, India was forced to enact a law making homosexuality illegal (Misra, 2009), which had an additional consequence of prohibiting safe-sex education, since nongovernmental organizations (NGOs), activists, and advocates faced arrest if they distributed condoms and educational brochures. As a result, LGBT persons were less likely to come out. The first attempt to fight Section 377 was in 1994, when a group of physicians tried to distribute condoms to inmates engaging in same-sex behaviors, but they were unsuccessful, since they were perceived as condoning a criminal act (Misra, 2009). Again in 2001, activists tried to fight Section 377 after a group of activists were harassed by police, but the petition was dismissed. In 2009, India decriminalized consensual sex between same-sex individuals (Misra, 2009), but this law was reinstated in 2013 (Wu, 2016). Thus, additional advocacy is needed to legally prevent discrimination and provide LGBT individuals with mental and physical health care.

Indonesia. King Oey (Arus Pelangi, 2009) reported that although there are no laws that criminalize LGBT people based on sexual orientation or gender identity, there are laws that have been used against LGBT individuals. The Indonesian definition of prostitution includes sex acts outside of marriage regardless of whether money was exchanged for them (Arus Pelangi, 2009). Similarly, the definition of pornography goes beyond the general meaning and includes same-sex behaviors, among other nonprocreational forms of intercourse. While legal discrimination against LGBT individuals remains prevalent, by 1983, homosexuality was no longer listed as a psychiatric disorder (Arus Pelangi, 2009). Unfortunately, recent anti-LGBT campaigns have resulted in the only Islamic school for transgender individuals closing down; the psychiatric association has called for LGBT individuals to be cured, and one government official has encouraged Indonesians to kill gay people (BBC, 2016). Thus, Indonesia has lost some of its gains.

Thailand. Although Thailand performs the most GAS in the world (IGL-HRC & Iranian Queer Organization, 2011), LGBT individuals continue to face legal and societal discrimination (Likhitpreechakul, 2009). While the Thai constitution protects LGBT individuals from discrimination, the legal system does not protect them. For instance, when a political group prevented the 2009 Chiang Mai Pride parade, police stood by and refused to intervene (Likhitpreechakul, 2009). Contrary to reports from LGBT Thai activists, Williams (2010) reported that Thailand has a reputation of accepting LGBT individuals. However, Williams acknowledged that the Thai government has a history of prohibiting LGBT individuals from working in certain professions, such as education and military ("It's time," 2010). Though Thailand offers basic services to all, this does not cover advanced care. Therefore, the government developed HIV/AIDS prevention programs and provides free condoms (Williams, 2010).

Australia

Australia. Between 1973 and 1997, all of the Australian territories decriminalized homosexuality (Corleto & Sullivan, 2010), and over time, the government has taken steps to provide LGBT individuals and their families more rights (Gay and Lesbian Rights Lobby, 2009). Along with social change, the Australian government has recognized the need for and promotes equity in LGBT health care (Corleto & Sullivan, 2010).

According to McNair and colleagues (2001), the Ministerial Advisory Committee on Gay and Lesbian Health was developed to learn about LGBT health concerns and barriers to care. Although LGBT individuals have a greater prevalence for some types of cancer, among other mental and physical health concerns, they seek out health services at a lower rate. LGBT individuals also have an increased risk for STIs due to insufficient sex education and myths (e.g., "lesbians are immune to STI"). Therefore, McNair and colleagues suggested that medical professionals, other service providers, and educators should learn about the LGBT community, address the discrimination and stigma toward LGBT individuals, and develop LGBT-specific health promotion programs. Further, the Australian Human Rights Commission (AHRC, 2009) started the sex-and-gender diversity project to examine discrimination against LGBT individuals and then made recommendations to improve the legal process of changing one's sex identity. Among the AHRC's recommendations was to expand the definition of gender affirmation treatment beyond GAS, to include counseling and hormone treatments.

Europe

Bosnia and Herzegovina. In Bosnia and Herzegovina, LGBT individuals are protected from discrimination to varying degrees. The 1995 constitution explicitly protects the rights of most minority groups and indirectly protects those of "other status." The 2003 Gender Equity law protects individuals from discrimination based on their gender and sexual orientation, but none of these laws directly protect gender identity (Global Rights & International Rights Clinic, 2006a). While discrimination based on sexual orientation is against the law, employers have not been charged after firing their employees based on their sexual orientation (Global Rights & International Rights Clinic, 2006). Therefore, it is not surprising that less than 33 percent of LGBT individuals are out to their families, less than 30 percent are out to their doctors, and the majority of LGBT individuals do not believe that their medical providers are aware of LGBT health concerns (Quinn, 2006).

Further, intersex and transgender individuals in Bosnia and Herzegovina do not have access to GAS or hormone treatment, and many medical professionals have limited knowledge of the mental and physical health needs related to gender identity (Quinn, 2006). Though the government does not have standardized procedures for changing the gender on legal documentation, some transgender individuals have been able to change their legal identification (Quinn, 2006). As a candidate for the European Union, Bosnia and Herzegovina needs to develop procedures for transgender individuals to access GAS and medical treatment as well as develop standardized policies for transgender individuals to legally change their identities (Global Rights & International Rights Clinic, 2006).

Italy. Italy provides LGBT individuals freedom from discrimination and refugee status if homosexuality was outlawed in their country of origin, and transgender individuals can receive financial assistance for GAS (Cartabia, 2008). However, until July 2011, transgender individuals who had GAS were sterilized (IGLA-Europe, 2011a). While discrimination is prohibited, the Italian law does not include LGBT individuals as a protected group in their hate crime legislation (Cartabia, 2008).

Romania. According to a 2008 report developed by ACCEPT-Romania, IGLHRC, and European Region of the International Lesbian and Gay Association (ILGA-Europe), Romania provides protection against discrimination based on sexual orientation but not gender identity. Although stigma persists in Romania, there have been some successful fights against discrimination. For instance, ACCEPT successfully helped to repeal a ban against allowing LGBT individuals to teach, and they received government support in fighting for and winning the right to have an LGBT march (ACCEPT, IGLHRC, & IGLA-Europe, 2008).

In terms of health care, Romania provides standardized procedures for HIV/AIDS protection, treatment, and confidentiality, and there is a national strategy to prevent HIV/AIDS that includes provisions for preventing HIV among MSM (Quinn, 2008). Transgender individuals are able to receive medical treatment for their gender identity (i.e., hormone treatment and GAS); however, medical guidelines for GAS have not been developed, and the process for changing one's identity on legal documents has not been streamlined (ACCEPT, IGLHRC, & IGLA-Europe, 2008). While Romania is a member of the WHO, some mental health care providers believe that homosexuality is an illness that can be cured, and the current Mental Health Law includes a statement that gives providers the right to prevent "unnatural sexual behaviour" from spreading (Quinn, 2008). Thus, LGBT Romanians are somewhat protected by the law and have access to basic health care but may not receive appropriate mental health treatment.

Russia. Although homosexuality was decriminalized in 1993, LGBT individuals do not receive equal rights, they are not legally protected from discrimination, and the government uses morality to repress their rights (IGLHRC, 1995). In 2006, some regions began adopting laws banning "homosexual propaganda" to protect the morality of minors; by 2013, there were federal laws that prevented same-sex propaganda, and the 2016 proposed guidelines call for treatment of gender dysphoria and measures to prevent homosexuality (ILGA-Europe, 2012, 2013, 2016). There has since been an increase in hate crimes against LGBT individuals (ILGA-Europe, 2012, 2013). Due to these laws, LGBT organizations are rarely allowed to hold public meetings, there are restrictions on disseminating information, and these policies are used as legal defense for attacking LGBT individuals (ILGA-Europe, 2013). Moreover, Russia has passed a number of regulations (i.e., the federal agent and treason laws) that criminalize human rights advocacy.

Aside from limiting the rights of LGBT individuals, the aforementioned policies have significant implications on health and health care. These laws prohibit psychoeducation on safe sex, reproductive health, and prevention services (ILGA-Europe, 2012). Though the first federal study on HIV among gay men and sex workers in Russia was expected to begin in 2014 ("Government," 2013), it is unclear how information from will be utilized.

United Kingdom. In comparison to some parts of Europe, LGBT individuals in the United Kingdom enjoy freedom and protection from discrimination. According to the IGLA-Europe (2011b), both sexual orientation and gender identity are protected from discrimination, and the court system has a history of supporting LGBT rights. Specifically, a civilian was fined and a politician was suspended for homophobic remarks, and a mental health clinician who used conversion therapy was suspended from practice until she completes additional training (IGLA-Europe, 2011b). Further, the government developed an action plan for transgender equality that focuses on discrimination at work, transgender-specific health care, access to mental health services, and suicide prevention (Home Office, 2011). Thus, it appears the United Kingdom is actively examining issues that impact LGBT individuals, and the government has taken action to improve their quality of life.

Islamic States

Sharia is the moral code developed by the Islamic Ottoman Empire, and it still has influence over the legal systems in Muslim countries (Peters, 2005). Islamic law prevailed from the 16th through the 18th century, and by the 19th century, colonialism and westernization started to impact the penal code. For instance, under sharia law, same-sex intercourse was punishable by death, but in the 1871 revised penal code, the penalty for unlawful sex was flogging (Peters, 2005). After the Ottoman Empire collapsed, some nations returned to Islamic law. Once again, same-sex intercourse became punishable by death, and as of today, the following countries continue to use the death penalty: Iran, Mauritania, northern Nigeria, Saudi Arabia, southern Somalia, Sudan, and Yemen (Itaborahy, 2012).

Iran. In 2011, contributors to the IGLHRC and the Iranian Queer Organization (IRQO) submitted a report to the UN about the human rights violations against LGB individuals. Specifically, same-sex intercourse is punishable by death in Iran regardless of consent, and for women, the issue is compounded by strict patriarchy. LGB individuals are at risk of arbitrary arrests and torture, and they may be forced to have medical anal exams to determine their sexual orientation (IGLHRC & IRQO, 2011). Iran also has stern dress codes that put transgender individuals at risk, despite official sanctions approving of GAS. Moreover, LGB advocates are also at risk of false charges and harassment to prevent them from being agents of change.

Najmabadi (2008) described how the fatwa (i.e., religious ruling) originally intended for intersex individuals also applies to transgender individuals. Even though these surgeries are legally and medically viewed as a cure, they can empower transgender individuals. In addition, for those who are religious, the GAS is viewed as a means to reconcile their sexual orientation and religious beliefs (Najmabadi, 2008).

GAS in Iran is based on heterosexism (i.e., bias that everyone is heterosexual) and cisgenderism (i.e., bias that everyone's gender identity is aligned with their assigned sex) and originated as a way to force intersex individuals into the gender binary (IGLHRC & IRQO, 2011; Najmabadi, 2008). Iranians who pursue GAS must go through months of therapy to confirm that they are not LGB individuals trying to pass as transgender, and afterward, they receive certification and benefits (e.g., health care, housing assistance, and military exemption). GAS has also been used in some courts as a more lenient punishment for homosexuality than the death penalty (Carter, 2011). Needless to say, the health care needs of LGB individuals in Iran are not and cannot be addressed until religious and legal policies change.

Kyrgyzstan. In Kyrgyzstan, LGBT individuals are not legally protected from discrimination, and this is compounded by prejudice in the medical community (Sexual Health and Rights Project, 2007); hence, LGBT individuals do not receive adequate health care. Due to confidentiality concerns, most LGBT individuals prefer private medical professionals to state medical care, but few can afford private physicians (Sexual Health and Rights Project, 2007). Additionally, government IDs are required prior to receiving medical care; thus, transgender individuals are more likely to avoid professional health care.

Turkey. According to SPoD, Kaso GL Association, and IGLHRC (2012), LGBT Iranian refugees who want asylum often move to Turkey but continue to face discrimination and harassment. Moreover, Turkey only permits asylum status to individuals from Europe; thus, LGBT individuals from Africa and Asia need assistance from the UN High Commissioner for Refugees (UNHCR) and have to move to a third country before receiving refugee status (Grungras, Levitan, & Slotek, 2009). While asylum seekers wait months, even years, to become refugees, they do not have equal access to housing, work, or health care, which is often exacerbated by police discrimination (Grungras et al., 2009).

Although same-sex intercourse is legal in Turkey, LGBT individuals are not protected from discrimination or hate crimes. SPoD, Kaso GL Association, and IGLHRC (2012) reported that the legal defense of "family honor" and "unjust provocation" for murdering LGBT individuals often results in reduced prison sentences. Similarly, LGBT asylum seekers usually refuse to go to the authorities for protection against discrimination and violence due to police harassment (Grungras et al., 2009). At best, LGBT individuals are told by the police to express their gender and sexual identity based on social norms or to be more cautious.

North America

Canada. In the 1980s, Canada abolished discrimination based on sexual orientation. By 2005, Canadians obtained marriage equality, and some provinces have started to provide protection based on gender identity (Chamberland et al., 2010; The Court, 2012). However, the Canadian Rainbow Health Coalition (2004) reported that due to homophobia and heterosexism, LGBT individuals face a number of health disparities. The rates of suicide, smoking, depression, unemployment, violence, homeless, and sexually transmitted illness are all higher among LGBT individuals than in the general population.

Mulé and colleagues (2009) reported that mental and physical health concerns experienced by LGBT individuals should be addressed by health promotion policy and suggested that these efforts go beyond focusing on HIV/AIDS prevention. Among the LGBT health concerns that need to be better examined are medical and mental health disparities, barriers to care, and the needs of intersex individuals. Mulé and colleagues (2009) went on to provide guidelines for educational systems, communities, families, health care systems (i.e., mental and physical health), and researchers to develop more inclusive and affirming policies that address the biopsychosocial needs of LGBT individuals.

Mexico. Although Mexico has not explicitly offered protection from discrimination based on sexual orientation or gender identity, there is a general sanction against discrimination, and in 2003, the government provided sexual minorities protection from workplace discrimination (Global Rights, IGLHRC, & International Human Rights Clinic [IHRC], 2010). Regardless of the legal protections, LGBT individuals in Mexico frequently face prejudice, stigma, and violence. According to Global Rights, IGLHRC, & IHRC (2010), more than 75 percent of LGBT individuals have been physically assaulted, 20 percent of these assaults are by the police, and for 80 percent of the LGBT individuals who were murdered, there have been no convictions. Among all of this unrest and violence, Mexico City is one of the few places that provide LGBT individuals any rights. For example, in Mexico City, LGBT individuals were granted marriage equality, and transgender individuals have the right to change their identity on legal documents.

Native Americans. Until colonization, reservations, and Christian missionaries challenged their traditions and values, Native Americans had a history of more accepting attitudes toward sexual orientation and gender identity. For instance, the term "two-spirit" refers to the fluidity of gender and suggests that some individuals have both feminine and masculine spirits (Balsam, Huang, Fieland, Simoni, & Walters, 2004). Two-spirited individuals used to be revered and often played a role in Native American spiritual traditions (Tafoya, 1997). Similarly, the term "berdarche," now considered archaic, incorrectly referred to men who take a passive role during intercourse but actually denotes individuals who live as the other gender (Bronski, 2011). Over time, as Native Americans were forced to assimilate into the developing American culture, many of their affirming traditions have eroded, and many LGBT Native Americans experience internalized homophobia (Balsam et al., 2004).

United States. Unlike international LGBT advocacy that often uses a human rights approach, LGBT advocacy in the United States tends to focus on civil rights (Mertus, 2007). The beginning of the LGBT civil rights movement started with the Human Rights Society in 1924, the

Kinsey reports, the Mattachine Society in 1950, and Evelyn Hooker's revolutionary work about gay men (Marcus, 2002; Wolfe, 2000). Meanwhile, Senator Joseph McCarthy started to blacklist people for homosexuality and communism, and police raids on lesbian and gay bars began to intensify (Marcus, 2002; Wolfe, 2000). By the 1970s, the lesbian and gay civil rights movement became active, and over the next 20 years, gay and lesbian groups organized around the AIDS epidemic. Eventually, these groups expanded to include bisexuals and transgender individuals. In 2003, the Supreme Court ruled sodomy laws unconstitutional (Mertus, 2007), and even today, legalized discrimination against LGBT individuals exists, since the rights of LGBT individuals are not protected at the federal level. The denial of access to rights related to the legal recognition of same-sex relationships ended with the landmark Supreme Court ruling in 2015.

South America

Brazil. Brazil decriminalized homosexuality late in the 20th century (Bottassi & Fernandes, 2000); by 2004, the government launched a national campaign to fight against discrimination and to promote the LGBT community, and another LGBT affirming action plan started in 2009 (Carrara, 2012). Further, the Brazilian government has been proactive in training educators about LGBT individuals and adjusted the guidelines for SRS to make it more accessible (Carrara, 2012). Brazil's involvement in the LGBT movement began with the AIDS epidemic and intensified after the 1993 UN Human Rights Conference highlighted the atrocities that LGBT individuals faced across the globe (Marsiaj, 2011).

Chile. The indigenous people of Chile tend to be more open about sexuality and gender roles than Chilean society. Indeed, women and men in the Mupuche culture were equal, and male spiritual leaders often dressed in feminine clothing—whereas the Inca people revered homosexuality, and sexual minorities were accepted (Galgani, 2010). Not until the 16th century, when the Spanish conquered Chile, was homosexuality outlawed (Galgani, 2010). By 1999, the Chilean government decriminalized homosexuality and has slowly started to address some of the human rights violations made against LGBT individuals (Global Rights & IHRC, 2007). LGBT organizations such as the Movimiento Unificado de Minorías Sexuales and the Movimiento de Integración y Liberación Homosexual have fought for LGBT human rights and have helped to change how the public views LGBT individuals (Galgani, 2010). Although the situation in Chile has improved, human rights violations such as police abuse, expelling students from school based on sexual orientation, the denial of medical treatment, and mandatory medical exams to determine sexual orientation persist (Global Rights & IHRC, 2007).

In terms of health care, all Chileans have universal access to basic medical care, and there are regulations for HIV/AIDS treatment and prevention. Specifically, the government requires confidential and voluntary HIV/AIDS testing and covers the cost of antiretroviral medications (Global Rights & IHRC, 2007). Aside from HIV/AIDS awareness, the mental and physical health care needs of LGBT individuals in Chile are not sufficiently addressed. According to Global Rights and IHRC (2007), unauthorized GAS and unnecessary psychological exams have been performed on intersex children. Thus, additional activism, training, and guidelines are still needed in order to improve the health care for LGBT individuals.

Guatemala. Although Guatemala decriminalized homosexuality, there are no laws that protect sexual orientation or gender identity, and stigma is pervasive. The Organización Trans Reinas de la Noche, Red Latinoámericana y del Caribe de Personas Trans, IGLHRC, Heartland Alliance for Human Needs and Human Rights, and IHRC (2012) found that the prevalence of HIV/AIDS among LGBT individuals increased while the general population's risk decreased, and LGBT individuals have been denied access to health care, forced out of school, and denied employment. Due to patriarchy and prejudice, criminal offenses against LGBT individuals and women are rarely prosecuted, and even fewer cases result in convictions. Guatemalan LGBT individuals are still fighting for their basic rights, let alone adequate health care.

However, LGBT organizations like Organización de Apoyo a Una Sexualidad Integral frente al SIDA (OASIS) offer support to LGBT individuals. OASIS staff provides outreach to homeless LGBT youth and psychoeducation about safe sex, and it promotes employment opportunities (AsylumLaw.Org, 2010). While OASIS is a safe haven for some, racism and cisgenderism within the LGBT community has resulted in a turnover at OASIS. Once OASIS started to reach out to transgender and indigenous individuals, some Latinos walked away. Currently, LGBT organizations are supported by international NGOs and are often required to have police presence for their safety (AsylumLaw.Org, 2010).

Honduras. Though Honduras does not have laws that criminalize homosexuality; there are laws against "morality and decency," which are used to target LGBT individuals (Global Rights & IHRC, 2006b; Wilets, 2010). Similarly, there are no laws that prevent discrimination against LGBT individuals; thus, Hondurans can be fired based on their sexual orientation, gender identity, and/or HIV/AIDS status (Global Rights & IHRC, 2006b). Needless to say, there are no laws to protect the rights of people living with HIV/AIDS, let alone their confidentiality. In addition to legalized discrimination and insufficient health care, LGBT individuals are often targets for violent crimes (Wilets, 2010).

RECOMMENDATIONS

First and foremost, it is essential that governments, LGBT organizations, and NGOs continue working together in the fight for LGBT rights. Although the UN was hesitant to grant LGBT NGOs consultative status in 1991, by 1993, the UNHCR stated that sexual minorities were eligible for refugee status, and more recently, the UN released a report calling for an end to discrimination and violence toward LGBT individuals (OHCHR, 2011). Indeed, OHCHR started the Free & Equal campaign to promote equal rights for LGBT individuals (UN News Center, 2013) and the current UN secretary-general, Ban Ki-moon, has been actively advocating for LGBT individuals (UN Free & Equal, 2013). Now that international support for LGBT rights is more widespread, there is a need for binding international laws that protect LGBT individuals. Currently, there are binding international treaties to protect racial minorities, women, children, and political rights; however, an additional treaty to protect LGBT individuals is needed to deal with human rights violations (OHCHR, 2013).

Based on the UN's Universal Declaration of Human Rights (2013), everyone has the right to receive adequate health care. However, if health providers are not aware of the unique health care needs of LGBT individuals, then these individuals may not receive adequate health care, let alone optimal care. According to Mayer and colleagues (2008), four barriers to care impact the health of LGBT people: unwillingness to disclose sexual orientation and gender identity to providers; few providers have the competency to adequately treat LGBT individuals; insurance policies that limit LGBT health care options; and an insufficient number of culturally focused prevention programs. With advocacy and awareness, these barriers can be addressed. Specifically, if medical and mental health training programs were mandated to include LGBT health within cultural competency programs, there would be more awareness. If providers were more aware, trained to inquire about sexual orientation and gender identity, and offered educational materials for LGBT individuals, the issue of cultural mistrust might slowly decrease. Further, these changes would help LGBT individuals recognize the relationship between their health and their identities, and they could selectively disclose their sexual orientation and gender identity when medically relevant. In addition to improving training programs, additional research is needed to better understand the current health care needs of LGBT individuals and to stay informed as these needs may change over time.

RESOURCES

Amnesty International, LGBT Rights
- http://www.amnestyusa.org/our-work/issues/lgbt-rights

IGLHRC
- http://www.iglhrc.org/cgi-bin/iowa/home/index.html

IGLHRC, Asylum Resources
- https://outrightinternational.org/content/asylum-resources

LGBT Asylum Support Task Force
- http://www.lgbtasylum.org/

Organization for Refugee, Asylum, and Migration
- http://oramrefugee.org/

State-sponsored homophobia: A world survey of laws prohibiting same sex activity between consenting adults
- https://ilga.org/ilga-state-sponsored-homophobia-report-2017

UN Free & Equal
- https://www.unfe.org/#

UN report on discriminatory laws and practices and acts of violence against individuals based on their sexual orientation and gender identity.
- https://www.ohchr.org/documents/issues/discrimination/a.hrc.19.41 _english.pdf

UNHCR
- http://www.unhcr.org/cgi-bin/texis/vtx/home

World Professional Association for Transgender Health
- http://www.wpath.org

Yogyakarta Principles
- http://www.yogyakartaprinciples.org/

CONCLUSIONS

Across the globe, the laws and policies regarding sexual orientation and gender identity impact the health and well-being of LGBT individuals. While some nations have enacted laws to protect the rights of LGBT individuals; there are numerous states that continue to criminalize same-sex behaviors and gender expression that is outside of gender norms. Moreover, some nations still use capital punishment for same-sex behaviors. Therefore, it is the responsibility of developed nations to reexamine their legal systems, ensure that their LGBT citizens are guaranteed basic human rights (e.g., health care), and move toward providing LGBT individuals with equal rights. With the dire needs of LGBT individuals in some African states, more countries need to revise their asylum systems in order to facilitate the needs of LGBT refugees.

In some parts of the world, optimal health care for LGBT individuals is more of an aspiration until their basic human rights violations are addressed, and every nation has some work to do in terms of improving policies, laws, and perceptions of LGBT individuals. A first step toward improving the health care services provided to LGBT individuals is to ensure that medical providers receive training to recognize how their own biases impact treatment, learn about the unique needs for LGBT individuals, and to make sure that educational resources address the needs of LGBT people. In addition, it is essential to understand the barriers that prevent LGBT individuals from seeking care and exploring ways to improve access.

REFERENCES

ACCEPT-Romania, International Gay and Lesbian Human Rights Commission, & European Region of the International Lesbian and Gay Association. (2008). *Romania: Human rights and LGBT people in Romania—Submission to the UN universal periodic review.* Retrieved from http://www.iglhrc.org/cgi-bin/iowa/article/publications/reportsandpublications/176.html

Alternatives Cameroun, Centre for Human Rights, & International Gay and Lesbian Human Rights. (2010). *The status of lesbian, gay, bisexual, and transgender rights in Cameroon: A shadow report.* Retrieved from http://www.iglhrc.org/cgi-bin/iowa/article/publications/reportsandpublications/1488.html

American Medical Association. (2013). AMA policies on GLBT issues. Retrieved from http://www.ama-assn.org/ama/pub/about-ama/our-people/member-groups-sections/glbt-advisory-committee/ama-policy-regarding-sexual-orientation.page

American Psychiatric Association. (2013). Gender Dysphoria. Retrieved from http://www.dsm5.org/Documents/Gender%20Dysphoria%20Fact%20Sheet.pdf

American Psychological Association. (2011). Practice guidelines for LGB clients. Retrieved from http://www.apa.org/pi/lgbt/resources/guidelines.aspx

Amnesty International. (2012). Uganda: Further information: Ugandan anti-homosexuality bill not tabled. Retrieved from http://www.amnesty.org/en/library/info/AFR59/010/2012/en

Arus Pelangi. (2009). What to do with the Yogyakarta Principles. Retrieved from http://www.google.com/url?sa=t&rct=j&q=&esrc=s&source=web&cd=1&ved=0CDIQFjAA&url=http%3A%2F%2Fwww.oocities.org%2Farus_pelangi%2Fstatement%2Fwhat_todo_with_yogyaprinciples.pdf&ei=nsoSUaqTNouO0QGM2YDwBQ&usg=AFQjCNEikehq3QwpBOzF2NYkhpee1C66kA&bvm=bv.41934586,d.dmQ

AsylumLaw.Org. (2010). Gay life in modern Guatemala 2010. Retrieved from www.asylumlaw.org/docs/sexualminorities/Guatemal043010.pdf

Australian Human Rights Commission (AHRC). (2009). *The sex and gender diversity project.* Retrieved from https://www.humanrights.gov.au/sites/default/files/document/publication/SFR_2009_Web.pdf

Balsam, K. F., Huang, B., Fieland, K. C., Simoni, J. M., & Walters, K. L. (2004). Culture, trauma, and wellness: A comparison of heterosexual and lesbian, gay, bisexual, and two-spirit Native Americans. *Cultural Diversity and Ethnic Minority Psychology, 10*, 287–301.

BBC. (2016). The sudden intensity of Indonesia's anti-gay onslaught. Retrieved from http://www.bbc.com/news/world-asia-35657114

Benkov, E. J. (2000). Middle ages, European. In G. Haggerty & B. Zimmerman (Eds.), *Encyclopedia of lesbian and gay histories and cultures* (Vol. 1, pp. 497–500). New York: Taylor and Francis.

Ben-Natan, M., & Adir, O. (2009). Screening for cervical cancer among Israeli lesbian women. *International Nursing Review, 56*(4), 433–441.

Boehmer, U., & Bowen, D. J. (2007). Health promotion and disease prevention. In H. Makadon, K. Mayer, J. Potter, & H. Goldhammer (Eds.), *The Fenway guide to lesbian, gay, bisexual, and transgender health* (pp. 159–186). Philadelphia: American College of Physicians.

Bottassi, M., & Fernandes, M. (2000). Brazil. In B. Zimmerman (Ed.), *Lesbian histories and cultures: An encyclopedia* (pp. 129–130). New York: Garland Publishing

Bronski, M. (2011). *A queer history of the U.S.A.* Boston: Beacon Press.

Butler, A. H., & Astbury, G. (2005). South Africa: LGBT issues. In J. T. Sears (Ed.), *Youth, education, and sexualities: An international encyclopedia* (pp. 810–814). Westport, CT: Greenwood.

Canadian Rainbow Health Coalition. (2004). *Health and wellness in the gay, lesbian, bisexual, transgendered and two-spirit communities*. Retrieved from http://www.rainbowhealth.ca

Carrara, S. (2012). Discrimination, policies, and sexual rights in Brazil. *Cadernos de Saúde Pública, 28*(1), 184–189.

Cartabia, M. (2008). *Legal study on homophobia and discrimination on grounds of sexual orientation—Italy*. Vienna: European Union Agency for Fundamental Rights.

Carter, B. J. (2011). Removing the offending member: Iran and the sex-change or die option as the alternative to the death sentencing of homosexuals. *The Journal of Gender, Race, and Justice, 14*, 797–832.

Center of Development of People, Center for Human Rights, & International Gay and Lesbian Human Rights Commission. (2011). *Shadow report on the implementation of the ICCPR in Malawi*. Retrieved from http://www.iglhrc.org/cgi-bin/iowa/article/publications/reportsandpublications/1445.html

Chamberland, L., Blais, M., Corriveau, P., Lévy, J. J., Richard, G., & Ryan, B. (2010). Canada. In C. Stewart (Ed.), *The greenwood encyclopedia of LGBT issues worldwide* (Vol. 1, pp. 49–72). Santa Barbara, CA: ABC-CLIO.

Chen, G., Li, Y., Zhang, B., Yu, Z., Li, X., Wang, L., & Yu, Z. (2012). Psychological characteristics in high-risk MSM in China. *BMC Public Health, 12*(1), 58.

Cho, J., & Chan, C. (2011). *Hong Kong government advocates conversion therapy for gays*. Retrieved from http://www.iglhrc.org/cgi-bin/iowa/article/takeaction/partners/1418.html

Clements-Nolle, K., Marx, R., & Katz, M. (2006). Attempted suicide among transgender persons: The influence of gender-based discrimination and victimization. *Journal of Homosexuality, 51*(3), 53–69.

Committee on Lesbian, Gay, Bisexual, Transgender Health Issues, Research Gaps, Opportunities, Board on the Health of Select Populations, & Institute of Medicine. (2011). *The health of lesbian, gay, bisexual, and transgender people: Building a foundation for better understanding.* Washington DC: National Academy Press.

Corleto, C., & Sullivan, G. (2010). Australia. In C. Stewart (Ed.), *The Greenwood encyclopedia of LGBT issues worldwide* (Vol. 1, pp. 317–332). Santa Barbara, CA: ABC-CLIO.

The Court. (2012). *Pride in Ontario: Amending the Ontario human rights code.* Retrieved from http://www.thecourt.ca/2012/06/23/amici-curiae-tobys -act-u-s-s-battle-against-solitary-confinement-and-canadas-new-copyright -reforms/

Cviklová, L. (2012). Advancement of human rights standards for LGBT people through the perspective of international human rights law. *Journal of Comparative Research in Anthropology and Sociology, 3*(2), 45–60.

Dworkin, S. H., & Yi, H. (2003). LGBT identity, violence, and social justice: The psychological is political. *International Journal for the Advancement of Counseling, 25*(4), 269–279.

Fish, J. (2009). Cervical screening in lesbian and bisexual women: A review of the worldwide literature using systematic methods. *NHS Cervical Screening Programme.* Retrieved from http://www.glhv.org.au/files/screening-lesbians -bisexual-women.pdf

Freedom and Roam Uganda & International Gay and Lesbian Human Rights Commission. (2010). *Uganda: Violation of the human rights of lesbian, bisexual, transgender (LBT) and kuchu people in Uganda.* Retrieved from http://www.iglhrc.org/cgi-bin/iowa/article/publications/reportsandpub lications/1241.html

Fried, S. T., & Teixeira, A. (n.d.). International gay and lesbian human rights com- mission input memo to the UN secretary general's study on violence against women. Retrieved from http://www.un.org/womenwatch/daw /vaw/ngocontribute/International%20Gay%20and%20Lesbian%20Human %20Rights%20Commission.pdf

Galgani, J. (2010). Chile. In C. Stewart (Ed.), *The Greenwood encyclopedia of LGBT issues worldwide* (Vol. 1, pp. 73–88). Santa Barbara, CA: ABC-CLIO.

Gay and Lesbian Rights Lobby. (2009). *Overview of the same-sex law reforms.* Retrieved from http://glrl.org.au/index.php/Rights/Relationships/Overview -of-the-Same-Sex-Reforms

Global Rights & International Gay and Lesbian Human Rights Commission. (2007). *Chile: Shadow report on the status of lesbian, gay, bisexual and transgender individuals.* Retrieved from http://www.iglhrc.org/cgi-bin /iowa/article/publications/reportsandpublications/413.html

Global Rights, International Gay and Lesbian Human Rights Commission, & International Human Rights Clinic. (2010). *Mexico: Shadow report, the violations of the rights of lesbian, gay, bisexual and transgender persons.* Retrieved from http://www.iglhrc.org/cgi-bin/iowa/article/publications /reportsandpublications/1485.html

Global Rights & International Human Rights Clinic. (2006a). *Bosnia and Herzegovina: Shadow report on the status of lesbian, gay, bisexual and transgender (LGBT) individuals.* Retrieved from http://www.iglhrc.org/cgi-bin/iowa/article/publications/reportsandpublications/309.html

Global Rights & International Human Rights Clinic. (2006b). *Honduras: Shadow report on the status of lesbian, gay, bisexual and transgender (LGBT) individuals.* Retrieved from http://www.iglhrc.org/cgi-bin/iowa/article/publications/reportsandpublications/308.html

Government to conduct first study of HIV among gays, prostitutes. (2013). *The Moscow Times.* Retrieved from http://www.themoscowtimes.com/news/article/government-to-conduct-first-study-of-hiv-among-gays-prostitutes/484007.html

Greenberg, D. F. (1990). *Construction of homosexuality.* Chicago: The University of Chicago Press.

Grungras, N., Levitan, R., & Slotek, A. (2009). Unsafe haven: Security challenges facing LGBT asylum seekers and refugees in Turkey. *Praxis: The Fletcher Journal of Human Security, 14,* 41–62.

Gueboguo, C. (2010). Cameroon. In C. Stewart (Ed.), *The Greenwood encyclopedia of LGBT issues worldwide* (Vol. 3, pp. 23–28). Santa Barbara, CA: ABC-CLIO.

Home Office. (2011). Advancing transgender equality—a plan for action. Retrieved from http://www.homeoffice.gov.uk/publications/equalities/lgbt-equality-publications/transgender-action-plan?view=Binary

Human Rights Campaign. (2013). Resources: DOMA: Get the facts. Retrieved from http://www.hrc.org/resources/entry/doma-get-the-facts

ILGA. (2012). Lesbian and gay rights in the world. Retrieved from http://old.ilga.org/Statehomophobia/ILGA_map_2012_A4.pdf

ILGA-Europe. (2011a). IGLA-Europe annual review 2011 on Italy. Retrieved from http://ilga-europe.org/home/guide/country_by_country/italy/ilga_europe_annual_review_2011_on_italy

ILGA-Europe. (2011b). IGLA-Europe annual review 2011 on United Kingdom. Retrieved from http://ilga-europe.org/home/guide/country_by_country/united_kingdom/review_2011

ILGA-Europe. (2012). "Homosexual Propaganda" bans in Russia. Retrieved from http://lib.ohchr.org/HRBodies/UPR/Documents/Session16/RU/ILGA_UPR_RUS_S16_2013_ILGAEurope_E.pdf

ILGA-Europe. (2013). ILGA-Europe's briefing note on the human rights situation of LGBTI people and other minority groups in Russia. Retrieved from http://www.ilga-europe.org/home/guide_europe/country_by_country/russia/russia_what_s_on/keep_hope_alive

IGLA-Europe. (2016). Russian Ministry of Health proposes sexologist offices in mental hospitals to address sexual orientation and gender identity. Retrieved from http://www.ilga-europe.org/resources/news/latest-news/russian-ministry-health-proposes-sexologist-offices-mental-hospitals

International Gay and Lesbian Human Rights Commission. (1995). Russia: Gay, lesbian & bisexual group denied legal registration. Retrieved from http://

www.iglhrc.org/content/russia-gay-lesbian-bisexual-group-denied-legal
-registration

International Gay and Lesbian Human Rights Commission. (2003). India. Retrieved from http://www.iglhrc.org/binary-data/ATTACHMENT/file/000 /000/45-1.pdf

International Gay and Lesbian Human Rights Commission (IGLHRC) & Iranian Queer Organization (IRQO). (2011). *Human rights violations on the basis of sexual orientation, gender identity, and homosexuality in the Islamic Republic of Iran.* Retrieved from http://www.iglhrc.org/cgi-bin/iowa/article /publications/reportsandpublications/1437.html

Irwin, L. (2007). Homophobia and heterosexism: Implications for nursing and nursing practice. *Australian Journal of Advanced Nursing, 25*(1), 70–76.

Itaborahy, L. P. (2012). State-sponsored homophobia: A world survey of laws criminalizing same-sex sexual acts between consenting adults. Retrieved from http://old.ilga.org/Statehomophobia/ILGA_State_Sponsored_Homo phobia_2012.pdf

It's time for Thailand to end state homophobia. (2010). *The Nation.* Retrieved from http://www.nationmultimedia.com/2010/11/20/opinion/Its-time-for -Thailand-to-end-state-homophobia-30142726.html

Kapila, K. (2012). HIV and MSM abroad: The Fenway Institute's work in Malawi. Retrieved from http://fenwayfocus.org/2012/02/hiv-and-msm-abroad-the -fenway-institutes-work-in-malawi/

Katz, A. (2011). Gay and lesbian patients with cancer. In J. Mulhall, L. Incrocci, I. Goldstein, & R. Rosen (Eds.), *Cancer and sexual health* (pp. 397–406). New York: Springer.

Kaufman, R. (2007). Introduction to transgender identity and health. In H. Makadon, K. Mayer, J. Potter, & H. Goldhammer (Eds.), *The Fenway guide to lesbian, gay, bisexual, and transgender health* (pp. 331–363). Philadelphia: American College of Physicians.

King, M., Semlyen, J., Tai, S. S., Killaspy, H., Osborn, D., Popelyuk, D., & Nazareth, I. (2008). A systematic review of mental disorder, suicide, and deliberate self harm in lesbian, gay and bisexual people. *BMC Psychiatry, 8*, 70.

Likhitpreechakul, P. (2009). *Thailand: Without equality, tolerance is just a myth.* Retrieved from http://www.iglhrc.org/cgi-bin/iowa/article/takeaction /resourcecenter/883.html

Marcus, E. (2002). *Making gay history: The half-century fight for lesbian and gay equal rights.* New York: Harper Collins.

Marsiaj, J. (2011). Brazil: From AIDS to human rights. In M. Tremlay, D. Paternotte, & C. Johnson (Eds.), *The lesbian and gay movement and the state: Comparative insights into transformed relationship* (pp. 57–71). Burlington, VT: Ashgate.

McNair, R., Anderson, S., & Mitchell, A. (2001). Addressing health inequalities in Victorian lesbian, gay, bisexual and transgender communities. *Health Promotion Journal of Australia: Official Journal of Australian Association of Health Promotion Professionals, 11*(1), 32.

Meem, D. T., Gibson, M. A., & Alexander, J. (2010). *Finding out: An introduction to LGBT studies.* Thousand Oaks, CA: Sage.

Mertus, J. (2007). The rejection of human rights framings: The case of LGBT advocacy in the U. S. *Human Rights Quarterly, 29, 1036-1064.*

Meyer, I. H. (2003). Prejudice, social stress, and mental health in lesbian, gay, and bisexual populations: Conceptual issues and research evidence. *Psychological Bulletin 129,* 674–697.

Meyer, I. H., Dietrich, J., & Schwartz, S. (2008). Lifetime prevalence of mental disorders and suicide attempts in diverse lesbian, gay, and bisexual populations. *American Journal of Public Health, 98*(6), 1004–1006.

Mieses, A. (2009). Gender inequality and corrective rape of women who have sex with women. *Gay Men's Health Crises Treatment Issues,* 1–3. Retrieved from http://www.gmhc.org/files/editor/file/ti-1209.pdf

Minton, H. L. (2002). *Departing from deviance: A history of homosexual rights and emancipatory science in America.* Chicago: The University of Chicago Press.

Misra, G. (2009). Decriminalising homosexuality in India. *Reproductive Health Matters, 17*(34), 20–28.

Mountford, T. (2009). China: The legal position and status of lesbian, gay, bisexual, and transgender people in the People's Republic of China. Retrieved from http://www.iglhrc.org/cgi-bin/iowa/article/takeaction/resourcecenter /1107.html

Mulé, N., Ross, L. E., Deeprose, B., Jackson, B. E., Daley, A., & Travers, A. (2009). Promoting LGBT health and wellbeing through inclusive policy development. *International Journal for Equity in Health, 8,* 18.

Najmabadi, A. (2008). Transing and transpassing across sex-gender walls in Iran. *Women's Studies Quarterly, 36*(3), 23–42.

Najmabadi, A. (2011). Verdicts of science, rulings of faith: Transgender/sexuality in contemporary Iran. *Social Research: An International Quarterly, 78*(2), 533–556.

O'Donnell, S., Meyer, I. H., & Schwartz, S. (2011). Increased risk of suicide attempts among Black and Latino lesbians, gay men, and bisexuals. *American Journal of Public Health, 101*(6), 1055–1059.

Office of the High Commissioner for Human Rights. (2011). *UN report on discriminatory laws and practices and acts of violence against individuals based on their sexual orientation and gender identity.* Retrieved from http://www.ohchr.org/EN/HRBodies/HRC/RegularSessions/Session19 /Pages/ListReports.aspx

Office of the High Commissioner for Human Rights. (2013). Human rights bodies. Retrieved from http://www.ohchr.org/EN/HRBodies/Pages/HumanRights Bodies.aspx

Organización Trans Reinas de la Noche, Red Latinoámericana y del Caribe de Personas Trans, International Gay and Lesbian Human Rights Commission, Heartland Alliance for Human Needs and Human Right, & International Human Rights Clinic. (2012). *Human rights violations of lesbian, gay, bisexual, and transgender (LGBT) people in Guatemala: A shadow report.* Retrieved from http://www.iglhrc.org/cgi-bin/iowa/article/publications /reportsandpublications/1511.html

Ortiz-Hernández, L., Gómez Tello, B. L., & Valdés, J. (2009). The association of sexual orientation with self-rated health, and cigarette and alcohol use in Mexican adolescents and youths. *Social Science & Medicine, 69*(1), 85–93.

Peters, R. (2005). *Crime and punishment in Islamic law: Theory and practice from the sixteenth to the twenty-first century.* New York: Cambridge University Press.

Pillay, N. (2011). No place for homophobia here. Retrieved from http://www.iglhrc .org/cgi-bin/iowa/article/publications/reportsandpublications/1416.html

Pitts, M. K., Fox, C., Willis, J., & Anderson, J. (2007). What do gay men know about human papillomavirus? Australian gay men's knowledge and experience of anal cancer screening and human papillomavirus. *Sexually Transmitted Diseases, 34*(3), 170–173.

Polders, L. A., Nel, J. A., Kruger, P., & Wells, H. L. (2008). Factors affecting vulnerability to depression among gay men and lesbian women in Gauteng, South Africa. *South African Journal of Psychology, 38*(4), 673–687.

Quinn, S. (2006). Accessing health: The context and the challenges for LGBT people in Central and Eastern Europe. Retrieved from http://www.ilga-europe .org/home/publications/reports_and_other_materials/%28offset%29/30

Safren, S. A., & Heimberg, R. G. (1999). Depression, hopelessness, suicidality, and related factors in sexual minority and heterosexual adolescents. *Journal of Consulting and Clinical Psychology, 67*(6), 859–866.

Sambria, J. (2012). Making waves: Malawi revives debate on gay rights. Retrieved from http://www.un.org/africarenewal/web-features/making-waves-malawi -revives-debate-gay-rights

Sandfort, T. G., de Graaf, R., Bijl, R. V., & Schnabel, P. (2001). Same-sex sexual behavior and psychiatric disorders: findings from the Netherlands Mental Health Survey and Incidence Study (NEMESIS). *Archives of General Psychiatry, 58*(1), 85.

Sexual Health and Rights Project. (2007). Access to Health Care for LGBT People in Kyrgyzstan. Retrieved from http://www.opensocietyfoundations.org /sites/default/files/kyrgyzstan_20071030.pdf

Simon, R. J., & Brooks, A. (2009). *Gay and lesbian communities the world over.* Lanham, MD: Lexington Books.

Social Policies Gender Identity and Sexual Orientation Studies Association (SPoD), Kaso GL Association, & International Gay and Lesbian Human Rights Commission (IGLHRC). (2012). *Human rights violations of lesbian, gay, bisexual and transgender (LGBT) people in Turkey: A shadow report.* Retrieved from https://www2.ohchr.org/english/bodies/hrc/docs/ngos /IGLHRC_Turkey_HRC106.pdf

Stewart, C. (2010). Introduction. In C. Stewart (Ed.), *The Greenwood encyclopedia of LGBT issues worldwide* (Vol. 1, pp. 3–12). Santa Barbara, CA: ABC-CLIO.

Tafoya, T. (1997). Native gay and lesbian issues: The Two-Spirited. In B. Greene (Ed.), *Psychological perspectives on lesbian and gay issues: Vol. 3. Ethnic and cultural diversity among lesbians and gay men* (pp. 216–239). Thousand Oaks, CA: Sage.

Ugwu, D. (2012). Malawi suspends sodomy laws. Retrieved from http://www.iglhrc .org/cgi-bin/iowa/article/pressroom/pressrelease/1610.html

UNAIDS. (2008). Policy brief: HIV and international labour migration. Retrieved from   http://www.unaids.org/en/media/unaids/contentassets/dataimport /pub/manual/2008/jc1513a_policybrief_en.pdf

UN Free & Equal. (2013). UN Free & Equal. Retrieved from https://www.unfe.org /en/actions/freedom-of-expression

United Nations. (2013). *The universal declaration of human rights.* Retrieved from http://www.un.org/en/documents/udhr/index.shtml

UN News Center. (2013). UN unveils "Free & Equal" campaign to promote lesbian, gay, bisexual, transgender rights. Retrieved from http://www.un.org /apps/news/story.asp?NewsID=45503&Cr=lesbian&Cr1#.UkC8GD8pczA

U.S.A. Citizen and Immigration Services. (2010). Human immunodeficiency virus (HIV) infection removed from CDC list of communicable diseases of public health significance. Retrieved from http://www.uscis.gov/portal/site /uscis/menuitem.5af9bb95919f35e66f614176543f6d1a/?vgnextoid=1a05cc 5222ff5210VgnVCM100000082ca60aRCRD&vgnextchannel=68439c7755 cb9010VgnVCM10000045f3d6a1RCRD

Wells, H. (2006). *Levels of empowerment among lesbian, gay, bisexual, and transgender (LGBT) people in Kwa-Zulu Natal, South Africa.* Retrieved from http://www.out.org.za/index.php/library/reports

Wilets, J. D. (2010). Honduras. In C. Stewart (Ed.), *The Greenwood encyclopedia of LGBT issues worldwide* (Vol. 1, pp. 141–150). Santa Barbara, CA: ABC-CLIO.

Williams, W. L. (2010). Thailand. In C. Stewart (Ed.), *The Greenwood encyclopedia of LGBT issues worldwide* (Vol. 1, pp. 505–522). Santa Barbara, CA: ABC-CLIO.

Wolfe, M. (2000). Bars. In G. Haggerty & B. Zimmerman (Eds.), *Encyclopedia of lesbian and gay histories and cultures* (Vol. 1, pp. 95–96). New York: Taylor and Francis.

Wu, H. (2016). LGBT Indians dare to hope as supreme court rules on anti-gay law. Retrieved from http://www.cnn.com/2016/02/02/asia/india-gay-law-court -challenge/

Yogyakarta Principles: The application of international human rights law in relation to sexual orientation and gender identity (2007). Retrieved from: http://www.yogyakartaprinciples.org/

About the Editors and Contributors

EDITORS

JASON S. SCHNEIDER, MD, is an associate professor of medicine in the Division of General Medicine and Geriatrics at the Emory University School of Medicine. He works as a clinician educator at Grady Memorial Hospital in Atlanta, Georgia, where he provides direct care to general adult and transgender patients. Dr. Schneider has clinical interests in sexual health and sexuality; the interaction of psychiatry and general medicine; and primary care for lesbian, gay, bisexual, and transgender patients. He served on the board of directors of GLMA: Health Professionals Advancing LGBT Equality for over 13 years, serving two years as president.

LAURA ERICKSON-SCHROTH, MD, MA, is an assistant professor of psychiatry at Columbia University Medical Center and a consulting psychiatrist at Hetrick-Martin Institute, a nonprofit dedicated to empowerment, education, and advocacy for LGBTQ youth. She is the editor of *Trans Bodies, Trans Selves*, a resource guide written by and for transgender people, and coauthor of *"You're in the Wrong Bathroom!" and 20 Other Myths and Misconceptions about Transgender and Gender Nonconforming People.*

VINCENT M. B. SILENZIO, MD, MPH, is an associate professor of psychiatry, Public Health Sciences and Family Medicine, and director of the Laboratory of Informatics and Network Computational Studies (LINCS)/ Network Science Lab at the University of Rochester. He was a founding faculty member of the Columbia University Program in LGBT Health and served as coeditor of the *Journal of the Gay and Lesbian Medical Association.* His current research focuses on applications of machine learning and network analysis in suicide prevention research with LGBT adolescents and young adults and in studies of behavioral health and HIV prevention with gender and sexual minority communities in North America and around the globe.

CONTRIBUTORS

REBECCA ALLISON, MD, is a cardiologist with the Heart and Vascular Center of Arizona. She served on the board of directors of the World Professional Association for Transgender Health and was president of the board of directors of GLMA.

ELIE G. AOUN, MD, is an addiction psychiatrist, currently a forensic psychiatry fellow at Columbia University, and sits on the American Psychiatric Association's Council on Addiction Psychiatry. He performs forensic evaluations on individuals involved with the criminal justice system and works on program development and implementation in reentry models for individuals with substance use disorders, examining interventions that reduce crime recidivism in this population.

DEBORAH (DEB) BOWEN, PhD, is a professor in the Department of Bioethics and Humanities at the University of Washington. She was previously a professor and chair in the Department of Community Health Sciences of the School of Public Health at Boston University. She has been the principal investigator of several grants and projects involving cancer risk feedback and communication, health behavior change, and community-based intervention.

DIANE BRUESSOW, PA-C, DFAAPA, divides her time between clinical practice, organizational governance, health policy, and academic pursuits. She practices medicine in New York and New Jersey at Healthy Transitions LLC and specializes in transgender health across the life span.

FAYE CHAO, MD, is an assistant professor of Psychiatry at Icahn School of Medicine at Mount Sinai and site director of the Mount Sinai Addiction Psychiatry Fellowship at the James J. Peters VA Medical Center. She is board certified in both general psychiatry and addiction psychiatry, and her interests include LGBT issues, Internet addiction, and the management of pain in the addicted population.

JUSTIN A. CHEN, MD, MPH, is a psychiatrist at the Massachusetts General Hospital Depression Clinical and Research Program and associate director of Medical Student Education in Psychiatry at Harvard Medical School, where he also holds an appointment as assistant professor. He is interested in cross-cultural psychiatry, stigma, racial/ethnic disparities in mental health service utilization, and medical education.

JOHN A. DAVIS, PhD, MD, is an associate professor in the Division of Infectious Diseases and the associate dean for curriculum at the University of California, San Francisco. His clinical interests center on infections in the immunocompromised host, including those living with HIV, and his academic interests are in medical education, including curriculum development, related to sexual and gender minority populations.

BRIAN HURLEY, MD, MBA, DFASAM, is an addiction psychiatrist, works for the Los Angeles County Department of Mental Health, and is an assistant professor of addiction medicine at the David Geffen School of Medicine of UCLA. Brian previously served on the board of directors for GLMA: Health Professionals Advancing LGBT Equality, was Chair of the AMA's Advisory Committee on LGBT Issues, and served on the Association of American Medical College's Advisory Committee on Gender, Sexuality, and Difference of Sex Development.

JENNIFER JABSON, PhD, is an assistant professor at the University of Tennessee in the Department of Public Health. She has contributed to the scientific field of LGBT health and health disparities with her research, including: behavioral interventions with lesbian, bisexual men and women, and gay men; physician and nurse attitudes about LGBT people in the health care setting; health, behavioral risks, and psychosocial experiences of LGBT cancer survivors; biological indicators of stress as mediators of health outcomes among LGBT people; and elevated behavioral health disparities among LGBT people in rural regions.

DAVID M. LATINI, PhD, MSW, is a clinical health psychologist and oncology social worker who has worked in genitourinary cancer survivorship since 2000. He has a particular focus on access to care for underserved groups with cancer—the LGBT community, persons with low health literacy, and communities of color. He has published more than 80 peer-reviewed articles and a dozen chapters describing his work. He is currently an associate professor of urology and psychiatry at Baylor College of Medicine, where he is course codirector for two medical student electives annually—Human Sexuality and LGBT Health.

MEGAN C. LYTLE, PhD, is an assistant professor of psychiatry at the University of Rochester Medical Center. Dr. Lytle's clinical and research expertise is in multiculturalism, with a particular focus on the health and suicide disparities among lesbian, gay, bisexual, transgender, queer, and questioning (LGBTQQ) individuals. Her current research integrates computational methods with traditional approaches to investigate the unique experiences among diverse trans communities.

DARRYL MITTELDORF, LCSW, is the founder and executive director of Malecare, the world's first nonprofit organization to develop psychosocial support for gay and bisexual men diagnosed with prostate cancer. Mr. Mitteldorf is also the founder of the United States–based National LGBT Cancer Project and is an oncology social worker and researcher focused on clinical care and psychosocial support in the LGBT cancer survivor community since 1997.

HENRY NG, MD, MPH, is an academic internist-pediatrician and past president of GLMA: Health Professionals Advancing LGBT Equality. He is the cofounder of the Pride Clinic, Ohio's first Medical home for LGBTQ patients.

LOUIS OSTROWSKY, MD, is a child and adolescent psychiatrist at the Cambridge Health Alliance, in Cambridge, Massachusetts, where he works in their school-based clinics and as a consultant to local schools. He is also a staff psychiatrist in the Mental Health and Counseling Service at the Massachusetts Institute of Technology (MIT Medical). Ostrowsky is an instructor of psychiatry part time at Harvard Medical School.

GERALD PERLMAN, PhD, is in private practice in New York City, where he specializes in psychodynamic and bioenergetic psychotherapy. For almost a decade, he facilitated a group for gay men with prostate cancer under the auspices of Malecare Inc. From his experience with this group came *A Gay Man's Guide to Prostate Cancer*, which he coedited with Dr. Jack Drescher.

NFN SCOUT, MA, MPH, PhD, is the vice president at social justice for an international think tank, The Torvus Group. He trains extensively on LGBT cultural competence as well as tobacco and cancer disparities. He is a member of the National Institutes of Health's Council of Councils and for over a decade ran the CDC-funded LGBT tobacco and cancer disparity network.

TRAVIS P. SHERER, PA-C, MBA, AAHIVS, is a physician's assistant at Golden Gate Urgent Care in San Francisco, California. Travis is actively involved in LGBT health and HIV/AIDS prevention and treatment. He is a founder of the Health Equity Project, a nonprofit that provided medical care to marginalized populations in sub-Saharan Africa and recently served on New York governor Cuomo's Ending AIDS Task Force.

CARL G. STREED JR., MD MPH, is an assistant professor in the Section of General Internal Medicine at Boston University and primary care provider in Boston Medical Center, where his research focuses on the health and well-being of sexual and gender minorities, particularly transgender individuals. He has served nationally on the board of GLMA and has chaired the American Medical Association Advisory Committee on LGBTQ Issues.

JOHN B. TAYLOR, MD, MBA, is a psychiatrist at Massachusetts General Hospital, where he serves as medical director of the Urgent Care Psychiatry Clinic, director of outcomes assessment for population health management for the Department of Psychiatry, associate director of the Psychosomatic Medicine Fellowship, and assistant director of the MGH/McLean Adult Psychiatry Residency Training Program. He is an instructor in psychiatry at Harvard Medical School.

HECTOR VARGAS, JD, is executive director of GLMA: Health Professionals Advancing LGBT Equality, a multidisciplinary membership organization of LGBT health professionals and their allies whose mission is to ensure equality in health care for lesbian, gay, bisexual, and transgender (LGBT) individuals and health care professionals. GLMA (formerly known as the Gay and Lesbian Medical Association) is a leading voice on LGBT health and employs the expertise of its health professional members in policy, advocacy, and education to advance the health and well-being of the LGBT community.

CATHY E. WELCH, MSc, is a feminist counselor who has worked in community antiviolence agencies and the mental health system since the mid-1980s. She has been instrumental in bringing attention to and advocating for services to address issues of violence in same-sex/same-gender relationships throughout most of her career. She currently works as a therapist in private practice and is part of an advisory committee to the Safe Choices Program in British Columbia, Canada, providing support and education on violence in queer relationships.

AMY WILSON-STRONKS is a lifetime advocate for health care improvement. Her professional experience includes research conducted at the Joint Commission to inform the development of quality standards to guide the provision of LGBT culturally competent care. As an independent consultant, she worked directly with health care organizations to create more culturally competent systems of care. Her past board appointments include GLMA: Health Professionals Advancing LGBT Equality, where she served as the vice president of education. She is now retired.

LAZARO ZAYAS, MD, is a staff child, adolescent, and adult psychiatrist at the Massachusetts General Hospital Eating Disorders Clinical and Research Program and is an instructor in psychiatry at Harvard Medical School. He also has a private practice in Newton Centre, Massachusetts, where he works largely with children and adolescents in long-term psychotherapy and psychoanalysis, primarily focusing on issues of sexual and gender identity.

Index

Page numbers followed by *t* indicate tables and *f* indicate figures.